MELVIN LEWIS, MBBS, FRCPsych, DCH
CONSULTING EDITOR

CHILD AND ADOLESCENT PSYCHIATRIC CLINICS
OF NORTH AMERICA

Mood Disorders

GABRIELLE A. CARLSON, MD, AND
JAVAD H. KASHANI, MD, GUEST EDITORS

VOLUME 11 • NUMBER 3 • JULY 2002

W.B. SAUNDERS COMPANY
A Division of Elsevier Science
PHILADELPHIA LONDON TORONTO MONTREAL SYDNEY TOKYO

W.B. SAUNDERS COMPANY
A Division of Elsevier Science

The Curtis Center • Independence Square West • Philadelphia, Pennsylvania 19106

http://www.wbsaunders.com

CHILD AND ADOLESCENT PSYCHIATRIC CLINICS
OF NORTH AMERICA   Volume 11, Number 3
July 2002   ISSN 1056-4993
Editor: Sarah E. Barth

The ideas and opinions expressed in *Child and Adolescent Psychiatric Clinics of North America* do not necessarily reflect those of the Publisher. The Publisher does not assume any responsibility for any injury and/or damage to persons or property arising out of or related to any use of the material contained in this periodical. The reader is advised to check the appropriate medical literature and the product information currently provided by the manufacturer of each drug to be administered to verify the dosage, the method and duration of administration, or contraindications. It is the responsibility of the treating physician or other health care professional, relying on independent experience and knowledge of the patient, to determine drug dosages and the best treatment for the patient. Mention of any product in this issue should not be construed as endorsement by the contributors, editors, or the Publisher of the product or manufacturers' claims.

Child and Adolescent Psychiatric Clinics of North America (ISSN 1056-4993) is published quarterly by W.B. Saunders Company. Corporate and editorial offices: The Curtis Center, Independence Square West, Philadelphia, PA 19106-3399. Accounting and circulation offices: 6277 Sea Harbor Drive, Orlando, FL 32887-4800. Periodicals postage paid at Orlando, FL 32862, and additional mailing offices. Subscription prices are $155.00 per year (US individuals), $207.00 per year (US institutions), $179.00 per year (Canadian individuals), $246.00 per year (Canadian institutions), $198.00 per year (foreign individuals), and $246.00 per year (foreign institutions). Foreign air speed delivery is included in all *Clinics* subscription prices. All prices are subject to change without notice. POSTMASTER: Send address changes to *Child and Adolescent Psychiatric Clinics of North America*, W.B. Saunders Company, Periodicals Fulfillment, Orlando, FL 32887-4800. **Customer Service: 1-800-654-2452 (US). From outside the US, call 1-407-345-4000. E-mail:** hhspcs@harcourt.com.

Child and Adolescent Psychiatric Clinics of North America is covered in *Index Medicus, ISI, SSCI, Research Alert, Social Search, Current Contents,* and *EMBASE/Excerpta Medica.*

Printed in the United States of America.

CONSULTING EDITOR

MELVIN LEWIS, MBBS, FRCPsych, DCH, Professor of Child Psychiatry and Pediatrics, Yale Child Study Center, Yale University School of Medicine, New Haven, Connecticut

GUEST EDITORS

GABRIELLE A. CARLSON, MD, Professor of Psychiatry and Pediatrics; Director, Child and Adolescent Psychiatry, Stony Brook University, Stony Brook, New York

JAVAD H. KASHANI, MD, Department of Child and Adolescent Psychiatry, University Hospitals Health System, Laurelwood Hospital, Willoughby, Ohio

CONTRIBUTORS

MARTIN ANDERSON, University of California at Los Angeles, School of Medicine, Los Angeles, California

CLARA ARBALAEZ, MD, Visiting Psychiatrist, Colombian School of Medicine, Bogotá, Colombia

JOAN ROSENBAUM ASARNOW, University of California at Los Angeles, School of Medicine, Los Angeles, California

ROBINDER K. BHANGOO, MD, Senior Staff Fellow, Pediatrics and Developmental Neuropsychiatry Branch, National Institute of Mental Health, National Institutes of Health, Bethesda, Maryland

BORIS BIRMAHER, MD, Professor of Psychiatry, University of Pittsburgh School of Medicine, Western Psychiatric Institute and Clinic, Pittsburgh, Pennsylvania

KELLY N. BOTTERTON, MD, Assistant Professor of Psychiatry and Radiology, Division of Child and Adolescent Psychiatry, Washington University School of Medicine, St. Louis, Missouri

DAVID BRENT, MD, Professor of Psychiatry, Pediatrics and Epidemiology, University of Pittsburgh School of Medicine, Western Psychiatric Institute and Clinic, Pittsburgh, Pennsylvania

MAUREEN E. BUCKLEY, MA, Department of Psychology, State University of New York at Stony Brook, Stony Brook, New York

ARMAN K. DANIELYAN, MD, Department of Psychiatry, University of Pennsylvania, Philadelphia, Pennsylvania

DENISE DELPORTO-BEDOYA, MA, Department of Psychiatry, University Hospitals of Cleveland, Case Western Reserve University, Cleveland, Ohio

CHRISTINE DEMETER, BA, Department of Psychiatry, University Hospitals of Cleveland, Case Western Reserve University, Cleveland, Ohio

MARK ELLENBOGEN, PhD, Department of Psychology, Université de Montréal, Montréal, Québec, Canada

ALAN B. ETTINGER, MD, Long Island Jewish Comprehensive Epilepsy Center, Department of Neurology, Albert Einstein College of Medicine, New Hyde Park, New York

BRIGITTE FAUCHER, MSc, Department of Psychology, Université de Montréal, Montréal, Québec, Canada

NORAH C. FEENY, PhD, Department of Psychiatry, University Hospitals of Cleveland, Case Western Reserve University, Cleveland, Ohio

ROBERT L. FINDLING, MD, Director, Child and Adolescent Psychiatry, Department of Psychiatry, University Hospitals of Cleveland, Case Western Reserve University, Cleveland, Ohio

IRA GLOVINSKY, PhD, Private Practice Psychologist, West Bloomfield, Michigan

SHEILAGH HODGINS, PhD, Department of Psychology, Université de Montréal, Montréal, Québec, Canada

LISA H. JAYCOX, RAND, Arlington, Virginia

DANIEL N. KLEIN, PhD, Department of Psychology, State University of New York at Stony Brook, Stony Brook, New York

MARIA KOVACS, PhD, University of Pittsburgh School of Medicine, Pittsburgh, Pennsylvania

ELLEN LEIBENLUFT, MD, Chief, Unit on Mood Disorders, Pediatrics and Developmental Neuropsychiatry Branch, National Institute of Mental Health, National Institutes of Health, Bethesda, Maryland

PETER M. LEWINSOHN, PhD, Oregon Research Institute, Eugene, Oregon

CYNTHIA R. PFEFFER, MD, Professor of Psychiatry, Weill Medical College of Cornell University, New York Presbyterian Hospital, White Plains, New York

JOHN R. SEELEY, PhD, Oregon Research Institute, Eugene, Oregon

JOEL T. SHERRILL, PhD, University of Pittsburgh School of Medicine, Pittsburgh, Pennsylvania

ROBERT J. STANSBREY, MD, Department of Psychiatry, University Hospitals of Cleveland, Case Western Reserve University, Cleveland, Ohio

RICHARD D. TODD, PhD, MD, Blanche F. Ittleson Professor of Psychiatry; Professor of Genetics; and Director, Division of Child and Adolescent Psychiatry, Washington University School of Medicine, St. Louis, Missouri

DEBORAH M. WEISBROT, MD, Division of Child and Adolescent Psychiatry, Department of Psychiatry and Behavioral Sciences, State University of New York at Stony Brook, Stony Brook, New York

ELIZABETH B. WELLER, MD, Department of Child and Adolescent Psychiatry, Children's Hospital of Philadelphia, Philadelphia, Pennsylvania

RONALD A. WELLER, MD, Department of Psychiatry, University of Pennsylvania, Philadelphia, Pennsylvania

ANICA ZARAC, Department of Psychology, Université de Montréal, Montréal, Québec, Canada

CONTENTS

> The concept of bipolar disorder in children has its roots in
> ancient medicine. This article reviews the history of bipolar dis-
> order, beginning from its early history in ancient Greece
> through 1980, when diagnostic criteria for children were being
> considered. The acceptance of bipolar disorder in children was
> highly controversial after the first criteria were developed by
> Anthony and Scott in 1960. The concept was rejuvenated when
> Robert DeLong investigated the use of lithium in children with
> symptoms of mania. In the late 1970s and early 1980s, diagnostic
> criteria began to define the major criteria for bipolar disorder
> in children.

> The purpose of this article is to present findings from the Oregon
> Adolescent Depression Project regarding full-syndrome and
> subthreshold bipolar disorder (BD) in adolescence and young
> adulthood. BD first incidence peaked around age 14 years.
> Adolescent BD showed significant continuity across developmental

periods and was associated with adverse outcomes during young adulthood. Subthreshold BD results provide partial support for a bipolar spectrum.

This article emphasizes the promise of efforts to improve care for depression within the primary care setting. These efforts, however, face a number of potential obstacles. After reviewing the literature on the detection and treatment of depression among youth in primary care settings, the authors argue that primary care offers underutilized potential for reaching out to youth and improving access to high-quality care for depression. Much work remains to be done before this potential can be realized.

This article reviews what is currently known regarding the etiology and familial and genetic nature of early-onset mood disorders and the relationship of early-onset illness to adult illness. The primary focus is on epidemiology and genetic and imaging studies. This article updates and expands two recent reviews of early-onset mood disorders. In this article, the term early-onset refers to an index episode occurring in childhood or early adolescence.

This article introduces the basic concepts of affective neuroscience and demonstrates how they can be applied to research on the normal development of the regulation of emotion. The discussion focuses on the biologic mechanisms mediating emotional processes and the regulation of emotion. The development of such mechanisms is influenced by endogenous and environmental factors. The most important environmental influences are the relationships with caregivers. This article describes techniques that can be used to identify the neural circuitry underlying the regulation of emotions and to study how such circuitry functions differently in patients with bipolar and other mood disorders than in control subjects. In particular, this article highlights research techniques of relevance to the study of childhood bipolar disorder.

involve parents directly. Parents may be critical to the success of interventions with depressed children and should be regarded as potentially important agents of change.

Although many classes of psychotropic medications, including mood stabilizers, antidepressants, anticonvulsants, antipsychotics, and psychostimulants, have been used to treat bipolar disorder in recent years, mood stabilizers seem to be the most efficacious agents for bipolar patients, regardless of age. Although the biopsychosocial approach to treatment is recommended for all patients, this article focuses only on the somatic treatment of bipolar disorder in children and adolescents.

Major depressive disorder (MDD) is a familial recurrent illness that significantly interferes with the child's normal development and is associated with increased risk for suicidal behaviors and psychiatric and psychosocial morbidity. Although most children and adolescents recover from their first depressive episode, 30-70%, in particular those with familial history of MDD, comorbid psychiatric disorders, dysthymia, subsyndromal symptoms of depression, anxiety, negative cognitive style, and exposure to negative life events (eg, family conflicts and abuse) will experience one or more depressive recurrences during their childhood, adolescence, and adulthood. Depressed youth who present with psychosis, psychomotor retardation, pharmacological induced hypomania/mania, and/or family history of bipolar disorder are at high risk to develop bipolar disorder.

This article reviews the risk factors for fatal and nonfatal suicidal behavior in children and adolescents. Numerous empirical studies suggest that mood disorders are among the most important risk factors for youth suicidal behavior. In addition, other psychosocial factors increase risk for youth suicidal behavior independent of mood disorders. Prevention strategies for suicidal behavior should incorporate methods to identify children and adolescents who suffer from major depressive, dysthymic, and bipolar disorders. Such strategies should identify children and adolescents who have a history of suicidal ideation and/or suicide attempts.

FORTHCOMING ISSUES

RECENT ISSUES

VISIT THESE RELATED WEB SITES

MD Consult—A comprehensive online clinical resource:
http://www.mdconsult.com

For more information about Clinics:
http://www.wbsaunders.com

Child Adolesc Psychiatric Clin N Am
11 (2002) xiii–xiv

CHILD AND
ADOLESCENT
PSYCHIATRIC
CLINICS

Foreword

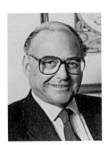

Melvin Lewis, MBBS, FRCPsych, DCH
Consulting Editor

This volume offers a timely and comprehensive account of bipolar disorder in children, from the earliest descriptions found in the era of ancient Greece to our contemporary views of the condition using the DSM-IV criteria for diagnosis.

The causes, genetics, and developmental neuropathology of early-onset mood disorders are thouroughly discussed, as are high risk factors for major affective disorders.

The use of somatic and nonsomatic interventions for depressive illnesses in children and adolescents are reviewed. The review ranges from the earlier use of tricyclic antidepressants through to contemporary use of serotonin-selective reuptake inhibitors. Light theraphy for seasonal affective disorders also is discussed. Electroconvulsive therapy is briefly considered for youth who are not responsive to any other form of therapy. Many other possible medications, including the use of lithium, are extensively discussed, and important side effects of such medications are judiciously noted.

Potential treatment in the context of the primary care setting also is considered.

The course and outcome for children and adolescents with major depressive disorder are thoroughly discussed.

The relationship between suicide and mood-disordered children and adolescents is described, and the importance of the clinical of aggression and mood also is described, particularly in relation to violent behavior.

This volume is a reliable, thoughtful, and highly informed account of virtually everything that a child psychiatrist would want to know about mood disorders in children and adolescents.

I am truly grateful to Grabrielle A. Carson and Javad H. Kashani for bringing together such an outstanding group of authors for this masterly account of an important topic.

Melvin Lewis, MB BS, FRCPsych, DCH
Yale Child Study Center
Yale University School of Medicine
230 South Frontpage Road
New Haven, CT 06510-8009, USA

CHILD AND
ADOLESCENT
PSYCHIATRIC
CLINICS

Child Adolesc Psychiatric Clin N Am
11 (2002) xv–xxii

Preface

What is new in bipolar disorder and major depressive disorder in children and adolescents

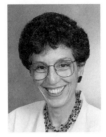 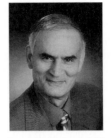

Gabrielle A. Carlson, MD   Javad H. Kashani, MD
Guest Editors

When we initially were asked to edit this series of articles on mood disorders, we questioned the necessity of yet another series on the topic; however, since the publication of the Mood Disorders issue compiled by Dr. Dennis Cantwell in July 1992, which actually initiated the *Child and Adolescent Phychiatric Clinics of North America*, considerable progress has been made in the field of childhood mood disorders. In fact, after reviewing the articles submitted by the distinguished authors for this issue, we became convinced that not only was another series needed, but also that periodic review is essential to keeping abreast of new and emerging knowledge in the field of mood disorders in children.

Efforts to classify mental illness are as old as mental illness itself, and these classifications seem to vary, over time, from broader and more liberal to narrower and more conservative conceptualizations. Although the controversy surrounding the diagnosis of depression in children has largely subsided, and the handling of comorbidity is not a major issue, it is useful to recognize that cycles in the understanding of the disorder have occurred and continue to occur. Even the names given to the disorder reflect an evolution from a narrow emphasis on psychosis (eg, folie circulaire and manic-depressive insanity) to a broader emphasis on illness (eg, manic depressive illness and bipolar disorder) [1–5]. Glovinsky discusses the evolution of the understanding of bipolar manic depression and the early descriptions of the condition in children. As Glovinsky points out, the willingness to consider bipolar manic depression as a condition afflicting children and adolescents has waxed and waned. Glovinsky uses the term *manic depression* to refer to the narrower, episodic condition.

Astute clinicians interested in mental illness and youth have probably always recognized the existence of manic depression in young people. The major issues continue to be (1) the age limits that define childhood (many accounts describe young adolescents, and there is less controversy about manic depression's increasing in frequency at puberty) and (2) how broadly one defines manic depression or bipolar disorder. Despite attempts to categorize illnesses, most conditions seem to have at least some measure of dimensionality. With manic depression, the spectrum seems to merge with temperament and development at one end and with schizophrenia at the other. Within the spectrum of bipolar disorder (which includes bipolar disorder I, bipolar disorder II, bipolar not otherwise specified, cyclothymia, and possibly recurrent depression with a positive family history of bipolar disorder), there are subclassifications based on cyclicity, polarity, psychosis, mood severity, and sensitivity to environmental stress. Environmental stress can arise from physical illness, medication, or the use of alcohol or illicit drugs.

In 1968, the term *manic-depressive psychosis* still included both recurrent depression and circular manic depression and was considered endogenous [2]. The circular subclassification of manic-depressive psychosis involved concurrent euphoria and irritability, with depression occurring as a separate episode. Psychosis could occur in either state but only within the context of mood congruence, and the definition required that phases be manifest.

During the next 30 years, the definition of manic depression changed in several ways. The recognition of hypomanic (brief) bipolar disorder II episodes and rapid cycling has led to changes in the definition of a bipolar or manic-depressive episode. It was observed that extreme disorganization during an acutely psychotic state, although often seen in schizophrenia, is not exclusive to it [6]. This observation led to changes in handling the content of psychosis and in the degree of mood congruence required to meet the diagnostic criteria. According to Goodwin and Jamison [7], the significant change in *The Diagnostic and Statistical Manual of Mental Disorders*, 3rd edition (DSM–III) [3] was to redefine mood disorders as unipolar or bipolar disorders. All non–bipolar depressions were subsumed in the unipolar (major depression) type; the category of bipolar disorder included conditions involving mania or hypomania, with or without depression. Complicating this neat division, however, were the symptoms that occur in both unipolar depression and mania, namely irritability and agitation, difficulty in concentrating, and reduced sleep (although in the case of mania, sleep is unwanted). Because of the recognition of these overlaps, mixed states became increasingly described.

Finally, there have been changes in understanding secondary mania, in treating pathologic central nervous system conditions, and in use of medications and other substances. *The Diagnostic and Statistic Manual of Mental Disorders*, 4th edition, (DSM–IV) [5] largely abandoned the previous classification of disorders as functional or organic. The DSM–IV also abandoned a condition designated "organic affective personality." The descriptors of this condition would include many children now diagnosed as bipolar. An organic affective personality was described as a persistent personality disturbance marked by affective instability (eg, marked shifts from normal mood to depression, irritability, or anxiety; recurrent outbursts of aggression or rage that are grossly out of proportion to any precipitating psychosocial stressors; marked impairment of social judgment, sometimes manifested by sexual indiscretions; marked apathy and indifference; and suspiciousness or paranoid ideation) [3,4].

The diagnosis of bipolar disorder now includes what was earlier defined as manic-depressive psychosis but is a much broader concept. To meet the diagnostic criteria, psychosis no longer need be mood congruent, so the term bipolar disorder covers a spectrum ranging from eccentricity to mood-congruent symptoms to paranoia to bizarre delusions or hallucinations. Irritability, a highly disturbing symptom of mania that sometimes leads to volatile and aggressive behavior resulting in hospitalization or imprisonment, can occur without euphoria, in depression, and in conditions comorbid with mania. The diagnostic criteria no longer require separate phases of mania and depression, as they did when Anthony and Scott wrote their seminal paper [8]. These phases may occur simultaneously with gradients of either mania or depression (ie, mixed episodes). The criteria also consider the degree of mood instability and the ease with which the patient moves from euphoria to dysphoria; this dimension of episodicity ranges from momentary fluctuations to discrete phases. Finally, whereas the DSM–I [1] and the DSM–II [2] combined bipolar and non–bipolar depressions in a single (and confusing) designation, the DSM–III [3] and the DSM–IV [5] equate mania with bipolar disorder, making it difficult to determine whether a case report describes a patient's lifetime course of illness or a current episode.

These changes are especially significant for child psychiatry. Narrowly defined manic-depressive psychosis is rare in children, becoming more common after puberty. As more broadly defined, bipolar disorder seems to be considerably more common at all ages and especially in prepubertal children. Prominent symptoms of early-onset bipolar disorder include poor regulation of emotion with rapid mood shifts, very low tolerance of frustration with high levels of irritability, hyperarousal with poor sleep and generalized anxiety, intense energy, poor attention, and often a multiplicity of other developmental difficulties. These difficulties are described as comorbidity, but they translate to children who have a vast array of serious symptoms that affect their families, peers, and education. This condition seems to start early, to be chronic, to merge frequently with severe behavior disorders, and to be highly resistant to monotherapy with lithium, as Weller describes.

Epidemiology

Lewinsohn, Seeley, Buckley, and colleagues are conducting the first large-scale study of bipolar disorder in teenagers as part of the Oregon Adolescent Depression Project. Their article highlights some of the measures available to ascertain the presence of bipolar disorder and the spectrum of related symptoms. Some of the participants in their study have been followed though ages 24 or

30 years, providing cross-sectional and longitudinal perspectives. Their findings provide several insights. First, based on Schedule for Affective Disorders and Schizophrenia for School-Age Children (K-SADS) interviews with the participants, they report weighted first-incidence rates of mania, hypomania, and cyclothymia of 1.4%, roughly equal to rates found in other studies (although studies in adults are usually only of acute mania). Emotional lability (called subthreshold bipolar disorder by the authors), as defined by at least 1 week of "elated, expansive or irritable mood," occurred at a rate of 4.5%. Teenagers who reported these symptoms had higher rates of nonaffective comorbidity (anxiety, disruptive behavior disorders, and substance abuse), suicidal behavior, and impairment than seen in the sample of teenagers who had never been mentally ill. The rates of major depressive disorder and bipolar disorder were higher among the family members of these adolescents than in the families of the never-mentally-ill comparators. The teenagers with subthreshold bipolar symptoms, however, never evidenced emergence of mania and, if anything, indicated higher rates of new-onset depression as they grew older. Emotional lability itself declined with age. Finally, of the new cases of bipolar depression occurring between ages 19 and 23 years, only three had had a prior history of major depression, a switch rate much lower than has been reported in adolescents diagnosed as clinically depressed or hospitalized for depression. The hazard rate of bipolar depression peaked at age 14 years and declined through young adulthood, a trend opposite that described in clinical samples (eg, by Loranger and Levine [9]). These data suggest that certain aspects of manic symptoms may be developmental in nature, reminiscent of the previous diagnosis of "emotionally unstable character disorder," a condition that responded to lithium but became less severe with age [10]. The level of impairment and family history suggest that the condition is not trivial and may be related to bipolar disorder. The data also suggest, however, that not every young person who reports an elated, expansive, and irritable mood is destined to develop manic depression.

Etiology

Although the causes of bipolar disorder are unknown, its familiality has long been recognized. Todd and Botteron note heritability estimates between 40% and 70%, although no data address whether the heritability of early-onset bipolar disorder is different from that derived in studies of adults. The possibility of genetic transmission is being addressed by studying the impact on brain morphology. Although data are still preliminary, it is hoped that ultimately genetic vulnerabilities will be detectable with brain-imaging studies. Specific prefrontal and cortico-limbic structures seem to be involved in regulating emotion. Data from imaging studies of adults with affective disorder suggest abnormalities in the ventral medial prefrontal cortex, orbital frontal cortex, cingulate, amygdala, and in highly interconnected limbic portions of the striatum and mediodorsal thalamus.

Bhanghoo and Leibenluft review the developmental aspects of the regulation of emotion. They point out that newborns, whose inhibitory structures have not yet myelinated, cannot manage their emotions or regulate the intensity of their responses. They depend on adult caretakers to modulate their emotions by changing the conditions causing the emotions. Throughout the preschool years, children achieve management of negative emotion (expressed as tantrums and crying) as frontal lobes mature and executive functions develop. Among the repertoire of executive functions are focusing attention, shifting sets (transitioning from one task to another), and effortful control. Finally, development of language allows young children to communicate their needs to caregivers and to increase their tolerance of frustration. Although perinatal distress and birth difficulties are part of the neurodevelopmental risk traditionally associated with schizophrenia [11], some data suggest that these risk factors may also be found in some children with bipolar disorder [12,13]. One might hypothesize, then, that some children with prepubertal bipolar disorder have a developmental delay or arrest in these neural structures. The delay could be genetically determined or result from in utero or perinatal stressors, from subsequent traumatic experiences, or from illness. In this last context, a secondary mania might be a more appropriate designation.

Examination of persons at high risk, namely offspring of bipolar adults, is informative but sobering. At a practical level, according to a meta-analysis done by Hodgins and colleagues [14], as many as half the offspring of bipolar parents meet criteria for a psychiatric disorder. Mood and behavior disorders are most common in this population. Adults being treated for bipolar depression, however, are rarely asked about their child's mental health or to determine whether or not the child needs an assessment.

In trying to understand the ontogeny of bipolar disorder, this Canadian research team examined both the genetic and interfamilial impacts of bipolar disorder. Their early data have led them to hypothesize that emotional lability and susceptibility to negative affect as a response to stress (called neuroticism) is a core feature of bipolar disorder and is inherited. This trait in the parent is associated with poor parenting practices (eg, with high-risk behaviors during pregnancy) and with emotional overreactions that create a chaotic environment and model poor coping techniques for the child. It is a short step from the parent's early difficulty in providing adequate external management of the infant's hyperarousal (which may have been inherited) to meeting Patterson's model [15] for the development of behavior disorders with a coercive parenting style. This model, however, assumes that the trait of neuroticism underpins an episodic disorder or reflects a condition that may not be adequately treated. Another Canadian team has found that offspring of lithium-responding bipolar parents have far fewer psychologic and behavior problems than those whose parents are less well controlled [16].

Treatment

Treatment of major depression is reviewed from two points of view. Findling and colleagues review the somatic treatment and discuss pharmacotherapy, light therapy, and electroconvulsive therapy. Sherrill and Kovacs examine the knowledge base for psychologic therapies. They describe the view of the Task Force on Promotion and Dissemination of the Psychological Procedure and examine the roles of cognitive behavior therapy, interpersonal psychotherapy, and family therapy.

Treatment of manic-depressive illness, classic variety, consists of lysing the mania, stopping the depression, or preventing future episodes of disorder. Older studies disagreed whether intermorbid abnormalities occur in classic manic depression, but the consensus was that the patients would function well if they were rid of the disease that disrupted their lives. The broadened concept of bipolar disorder includes many people, particularly children and many adolescents, who require considerably more treatment than the use of a single mood stabilizer [17]. The deplorable state of child mental health services means that many children cannot be seen intensively enough to have a complete assessment, let alone receive treatment. These children must be treated within family and educational settings that are not prepared to manage them as comprehensively as needed. In treating them, combinations of medications are used for which there is little to no evidence-based support other than reports of success in open trials of some adults with bipolar disorder. Weller describes the current state of somatic treatment of bipolar disorder in children and adolescents.

Outcome

Among the vexing diagnostic questions involved in child and adolescent depression is whether the patient will continue to have relapses and recurrences, will develop a bipolar disorder, or will attempt or succeed in suicide. The articles by Todd and Botteron and by Birmaher, Arbelaez, and Brent conclude that in both clinical and community settings early-onset mood disorders have a high likelihood of continuing into adulthood. Suicide, as Pfeffer discusses, is the third-leading cause of death among young people. She suggests that, as in adults, there is a relationship in young people between hopelessness and suicide. Several empiric studies suggest that mood disorders (along with other psychosocial factors) are among the most important risk factors for suicidal behavior in youth. Finally, the percentage of depressed youth who will develop a bipolar course varies but is not quite as high as the percentage of youth who remain depressed or dysthymic.

Although this issue does not specifically address the outcome of bipolar disorders, some data indicate that a child or adolescent whose symptoms of mania are severe enough to cause hospitalization probably has an even more serious condition than one who has symptoms in childhood or adolescence but is not hospitalized until adulthood. Two studies by Carlson and colleagues illustrate this point. The first, involving a sample of adults hospitalized at the National Institute of Mental Health about 30 years ago, compared manic depressive patients who had onset of symptom before age 19 years with those whose symptoms appeared after age 45 years. About 60% of those with early-onset symptoms functioned well (even with an episodic course), 20% had poor outcomes, and the rest were in between [18]. A sample of patients with bipolar disorder and psychosis hospitalized in Suffolk County, New York, between 1989 and 1995 revealed that those hospitalized before the age of 20 years were more likely to have incomplete remissions (odds ratio [OR], 6.23; confidence interval [CI], 2.30–16.9) and were more likely to have a poor psychosocial outcome 2 years after admission (OR, 2.83; CI, 1.17–6.86) than those first hospitalized after the age of 20 years [19]. Further inspection of the latter data, however, revealed that the comorbidity of childhood psychopathology with the bipolar disorder, not only the age of onset, accounted for the poorer outcomes.

When aggressive behavior is a chronic concomitant with bipolar disorder, all the negative outcomes attributed to aggression might be thought to add a further dimension to the bipolar condition. As Weisbrot and Ettinger explain, the relationship between aggression and mood is far from simple. Nevertheless, outcome studies of young children who are seriously aggressive suggest such aggression is an enduring trait and is likely to lead to continued behavioral problems in adulthood [20]. If childhood neurocognitive problems, temperament, and behavioral problems are associated with continued delinquency in adulthood [21], and parental psychopathology adds further to risk factors, the outcome of children is likely to be grim indeed unless effective interventions are found. Whether rages are considered as "rapid cycles," severe temper tantrums, affective dysregulation, or affective aggression, there is abundant evidence that problems are complex, enduring, do not develop into classic manic depressive illness, and require better treatment strategies than are currently available.

Although this issue covers a wide variety of topics, many others are not included. Among topics not discussed are the definite differences in the symptom expression of mood disorders in different age groups (ie, preschool, school-age, adolescent, young adult) and the increasing knowledge about strategies other than medication for treatment of bipolar disorder in youth. During the next decade the understanding of the biology, genetics, and treatment of mood disorders in youth will increase further.

References

[1] Diagnostic and statistical manual for psychiatric disorders. Washington, DC: American Psychiatric Association; 1952.

[2] Diagnostic and statistical manual for psychiatric disorders. 2nd edition. Washington, DC: American Psychiatric Association; 1968.

[3] Diagnostic and statistical manual for psychiatric disorders. 3rd edition. Washington, DC: American Psychiatric Association; 1980.

[4] Diagnostic and statistical manual for psychiatric disorders. 3rd edition, revised. Washington, DC: American Psychiatric Association; 1987.

[5] Diagnostic and statistical manual for psychiatric disorders. 4th edition. Washington, DC: American Psychiatric Association; 1994.

[6] Carlson GA, Goodwin FK. The stages of mania—a longitudinal analysis of the manic episode. Arch Gen Psychiatry 1973;23:221–8.

[7] Goodwin FK, Jamison KR. Manic depressive illness. New York: Oxford University Press; 1990. p. 56–69.
[8] Anthony EJ, Scott P. Manic depressive psychosis in childhood. J Child Psychol Psychiatry 1960; 1:53–72.
[9] Loranger AW, Levine PM. Age at onset of bipolar affective illness. Arch Gen Psychiatry. 1978;35(11):1345–8.
[10] Rifkin A, Levitan SJ, Galewski J, et al. Emotionally unstable character disorder–a follow-up study. I. description of patients and outcome. Biol Psychiatry. 1972;4(1):65–79.
[11] Geddes JR, Verdoux H, Takei N, et al. Schizophrenia and complications of pregnancy and labor: an individual patient data meta-analysis. Schizophr Bull 1999;25(3):413–23.
[12] Marcelis M, van Os J, Sham P, et al. Obstetric complications and familial morbid risk of psychiatric disorders. Am J Med Genet 1998;81:29–36.
[13] Kinney DK, Yurgelun-Todd DA, Levy DL, Medoff D, Lajonchere CM, Radford-Paregol M. Obstetrical complications in patients with bipolar disorder and their siblings. Psychiatry Res 1993;48:47–56.
[14] Lapalme M. Hodgins S. LaRoche C. Children of parents with bipolar disorder: a metaanalysis of risk for mental disorders. Can J Psychiatry–Revue Canadienne de Psychiatrie 1997;42:623–31.
[15] Patterson GR, DeBaryshe BD, Ramsey E. A developmental perspective on antisocial behavior. Am Psychol 1989;44:329–35.
[16] Duffy A, Alda M, Kutcher S, et al. Psychiatric symptoms and syndromes among adolescent children of parents with lithium-responsive or lithium-nonresponsive bipolar disorder. Am J Psychiatry 1998;155:431–3.
[17] Post RM, Frye MA, Leverich GS, et al. The role of complex combination therapy in the treatment of refractory bipolar illness. CNS Spectrums 1998;3:66–86.
[18] Carlson GA, Davenport YB, Jamison KR. A comparison of outcome in adolescent and late onset bipolar manic depressive illness. Am J Psychiatry 1977;134:919–22.
[19] Carlson GA, Bromet EJ, Driessens C. Age of onset, childhood psychopathology, and 2-year outcome in psychotic bipolar disorder. Am J Psychiatry 2002;159:307–9.
[20] Offord DR, Bennett KJ. Conduct disorder. In: Hechtman L, editor. Do they grow out of it? Long-term outcomes of childhood disorders. Washington, DC: American Psychiatric Association; 1996. p. 77–99.
[21] Moffitt TE, Caspi A. Childhood predictors differentiate life-course persistent and adolescence-limited antisocial pathways among males and females. Dev Psychopathol 2001;13(2):355–75.

Gabrielle A. Carlson, MD
Professor of Psychiatry and Pediatrics
Director
Child and Adolescent Psychiatry
Stony Brook University
Stony Brook, NY 11794-8790, USA

Javad H. Kashani, MD
Professor of Psychiatry
Case Western Reserve University
Director
Child and Adolescent Services
University Health System
Laurelwood Hospital
Willoughby, OH 44094, USA

CHILD AND
ADOLESCENT
PSYCHIATRIC
CLINICS

Child Adolesc Psychiatric Clin N Am
11 (2002) 443–460

A brief history of childhood-onset bipolar disorder through 1980

Ira Glovinsky, PhD

Private Practice, 2001 Pauline Court, Ann Arbor, MI 48103, USA

Bipolar disorder in children has only recently received the attention it deserves in the psychiatric literature. In June 1995, the American Academy of Child and Adolescent Psychiatry devoted a section of its journal to the disorder [1]. In the same month, the *Harvard Review of Psychiatry* published an article on pediatric-onset bipolar disorder by Faedda et al [2] describing it as "a neglected clinical and public health problem." More recently, Geller and Luby [3] reviewed the literature on the last 10 years' research in pediatric bipolar disorder.

This article traces the history of the concept of childhood-onset bipolar disorder from its roots in the descriptions of bipolar adults in ancient texts, through more recent scientific literature on bipolar adults, and its emergence in the pediatric literature. By 1980, specific criteria for childhood-onset bipolar disorder had begun to be developed.

Early roots of the concept of bipolar disorder

Today's concept of bipolar disorder can be traced to ancient Greece. Depression, or melancholia, and mania were two of the three forms of madness described by Alcmaeon of Crotona and other Greek physicians, who described melancholia as resulting from an interaction between bile, one of the four bodily fluids, and the brain. Melancholia and mania were described as chronic diseases, without fever; phrenitis was an acute disease characterized by fever and delirium [4].

Melancholia and mania, as described in the earliest medical writings, encompassed a wider range of disorders than the twentieth-century definitions of the same terms. Melancholic symptoms included dejected states, delusions, subdued behavior, insomnia, discouragement, and fear. Symptoms of mania included

E-mail address: cindyglovin@cs.com (I. Glovinsky).

excited states, delusions, wild behavior, grandiosity, and related affects. It was also noted that behaviors generally associated with one state were often found in the other: dejection was often seen in mania, and grandiosity sometimes predominated in melancholia [4]. In the second century CE the link between melancholia and mania was described by Aretaeus of Cappadocia [5], who wrote, "It appears to me that melancholy is the commencement and a part of mania." In interpreting Aretaeus' work in his *History of Ancient Psychiatry,* Roccataliata [6] used the term "cyclothymia" for a form of mental disease in which phases of depression alternate with mania. He credited Aretaeus with identifying bipolar cyclothymia, monopolar cyclothymia consisting of only a manic phase, and paranoid psychosis that he considered akin to schizophrenic mania. Roccataliata stated that the classic form of mania is bipolar:

> The patient who previously was gay, euphoric and hyperactive suddenly has a tendency towards melancholy; he becomes at the end of the attack languid, sad, taciturn, he complains that he is worried over the future, feels ashamed, when the depressive phase is over, such patients go back to feeling gay.

From antiquity to the present, controversies have centered on the terms *melancholia* and *mania,* the relationship between them, and the differences between their presentations in childhood and in adulthood. The ancients viewed melancholia and mania as disorders of reason rather than primarily as affective disorders. Their focus was much more cognitive than affective. They described these disorders as occurring only in adults. The ancients observed melancholia most frequently in middle-aged men and rarely in women and in younger or older men. Similarly, they encountered mania most often in young and middle-aged men, rarely in old men, and most infrequently in women and children [7].

Jackson [4] summarized the important points in the understanding of the relationship between melancholia and mania from antiquity through medieval times:

1. They continue to appear together among the diseases of the head;
2. To be grouped together as chronic diseases or forms of madness;
3. To be described as being without fever;
4. To be presented in adjacent chapters or sections, if not in the same chapter;
5. Mania continued to refer to excited psychotic states;
6. The clinical description changed little.

Connecting melancholia and mania

The first documented connection between melancholia and mania can be found in Théophile Bonet's *Sepelchretum sine Anatomia Practica ex Cadaveribus Morbo Donatis* [4,8]. Bonet first used the term "melancholicus mania" in 1679, and it appeared again in 1700 in an edition of Bonet's work revised by Johannes and Jacob Mangetus [9].

The connection between melancholia and mania was also discussed in the seventeenth century by Thomas Willis (1621–1675) [4,10]. In *Two Discourses Concerning the Soul of Brutes* ..., Willis described melancholia and mania as two "distempers of raving." Melancholia was "raving without feavour or fury," associated with sadness and fear. Mania was "without feavour but it entailed a fury...add boldness, strength."

Willis saw melancholia and mania as two distinct but closely related diseases. "Melancholy," he wrote, "being a long time protracted 'may' pass into other diseases, including madness (mania)." Concerning madness [mania] he wrote,

> ...both which are so much akin that these distempers often change, and pass from one into the other, for the Melancholik disposition growing worse brings on fury; and fury or madness growing less hot, often times ends in a Melancholick disposition. These two, like smoke and flame, mutually receive and give place to one another.

Other key figures in the seventeenth century also contributed to the evolution of the concept of manic depression. In his *Aphorisms* [4,11] Herman Boerhaave (1668–1738) stated,

> If melancholy increases so far, that from the great Motion of the Liquid of the Brain, the patient be thrown into a wild fury, it is call'd Madness. Which differs only in degree from the sorrowful kind of melancholy, is its Offspring, produced from the same causes, and cured by the same Remedies.

Robert James (1705–1776) [4,12] stated that "violent anger" was the likely cause of melancholia becoming mania and that the two disorders are really a single entity. Richard Mead (1673–1754) [13] wrote that the two disorders replaced one another and combined in various ways. Melancholia frequently changed into mania, and when insanity decreased, the sadness returned.

Jackson [4] summarizes the understanding during this period:

> In the 17th century it was usual to conceive of melancholia as partial insanity, that is, the derangement limited to a single idea or small number of related ideas, and mania as universal insanity, that is the derangement extended through the person's thinking. Thus, a continuum of increasingly disordered intellectual functioning became a representation of the ideas of melancholia degenerating into mania or worsening to become mania.

The birth of the modern concept of bipolar disorder

The major shift in considering manic depression as a distinct entity did not occur until the nineteenth century. In 1850 and 1851, Jules Pierre Falret, a resident under Esquirol at La Salpêtrière, in France, began a series of weekly lectures on the "general symptomatology of mental illness" [14]. In his tenth lecture he briefly described a form of insanity that he named "folie circulaire." In a book published in 1854 [15] Falret wrote,

The transformation of mania into melancholia, and visa versa, has always been mentioned as an accidental fact, but it has not until now been realized that there is a category of insanity in which succession of mania and melancholia manifests itself in nearly a regular manner. We have considered this fact to be of sufficient importance to become the basis for a special form of mental illness we call circular madness (la folie circulaire) because the course of this type of insanity runs in a repetitive circle of pathological states...separated only by rational intervals of fairly short duration.

Just after the publication of Falret's book in 1854, Baillarger, another resident at La Salpetriere, presented a lecture entitled, "A note on a type of madness whose attacks are characterized by regular periods of depression and excitement." He proposed the term "folie à double forme" to describe a disorder that had two phases, one of depression followed by an immediate, either sudden or gradual, switch to mania. In this disturbance there was no interval of rationality as described in Falret's folie circulaire. The manic period was seen as a "reaction" to the preceding depressed phase and as proportional to it [14]. The controversy over who had first described the disorder was not resolved until both Falret and Baillarger received joint credit for their work by the Académie de Médecine at a ceremony at La Salpêtière in 1894.

Following their acceptance in France, the concepts of folie circulaire and folie à double forme were accepted in other European countries, particularly in Germany. Griesinger [16], in his *Pathologie und Therapie der psychischen Krankheiten*, described the transition from melancholia to mania and the alternations of these forms as being common. Kahlbaum [17] supported Falret's concept of folie circulaire—continuous cycles of depression, mania, and intervals free of the disorder, varying in length.

Emil Kraepelin [18–21] was the next major figure in psychiatry to concern himself with bipolarity. He dichotomized the "endogeneous psychoses" into dementia praecox and manic-depressive insanity and eliminated the distinctions between unipolar forms of the disorder. All types of affective disorders were brought together in a unified concept of manic-depressive illness. The primary features distinguishing manic depression from dementia praecox are that manic depressive insanity has a periodic or episodic course, is a more benign psychosis, and includes a family history of manic-depressive illness [22]. By the sixth edition of Kraepelin's textbook, *Psychiatrie,* in 1899, the unification was complete.

Although there was some opposition to Kraepelin's work; Kraepelin's influence remained powerful for almost 70 years, until the distinction between unipolar and bipolar disorders became generally accepted. The opposition in Germany came from Karl Wernicke [23], who differentiated affective syndromes into smaller categories and supported the earlier views of Falret and Baillarger. Karl Leonhard [24] classified the phasic psychoses into pure phasic psychoses and polymorphous phasic disorders and included manic depression within this second category.

In Europe, the medical model of illness remained dominant. In this model, the symptoms of an individual's disorder were understood in terms of a specific disease, with a specific history and pathophysiology [22]. By identifying the underlying pathophysiology, one could understand and treat the disorder. This model, however, made understanding manic depression problematic because the underlying pathophysiology could not be identified.

In the United States the medical model was generally regarded as having little use for understanding the functional psychoses, including manic depression [22]. The field of psychiatry in the United States was heavily influenced by psycho-analytic theory and by the theories of Adolf Meyer during the first half of the twentieth century.

Meyer [25] emphasized the interaction between an individual's biologic and genetic characteristics and the social environment. Biologic and genetic factors created a vulnerability that could be affected by specific social or psychologic factors. Goodwin and Jamison [22] stated that this perspective influenced the first diagnostic manual that was published by the American Psychiatric Association in 1952 that included a diagnosis of "manic-depressive reaction."

Psychoanalytic theory placed a heavy emphasis on psychodynamic factors contributing to the origins of psychopathology. The theory posited stages of vulnerability for the later development of manic depression. Because children lack higher-level cognitive structures, it was thought that manic depression could not be a viable diagnosis in childhood.

For example, Karl Abraham [26,27] discussed early psychosexual stages of child development as being influential in the evolution of manic depression. He proposed that the oral, anal, and phallic stages of development were divided into early and late components. Abraham related mania to the cannibalistic (later) oral stage of libidinal development and suggested a number of etiologic factors, both constitutional and psychodynamic, that were involved in the "circular" insanities.

Glover [28] stated that the manic-depressive sequence corresponded to the alternation of reactions of infants who were traumatically frustrated at an oral level and then subsequently satisfied: "alternating states are also exploited as a defensive maneuver to *prevent* the development or reactivation of primary ambivalence, a state of mind which must be at first completely baffling as well as psychically painful to the infant."

Melanie Klein [29], conducting psychoanalytic work with children, described two normal psychologic "positions" during the first year of life. These were the "paranoid-schizoid" position during the first 6 months and the "depressive" position during the second 6 months of life. During the depressive position, the infant no longer split the "good mother" and "bad mother": the infant's heightened sense of reality increased its awareness that the "good" and "bad" external object (mother) were identical and that the mother was a "whole object" with good and bad parts.

Hypomania or mania reflected the overuse of these defense mechanisms. Other manic defenses included omnipotence, identification with the superego, introjec-tion, manic triumph, and extreme idealization. Klein maintained that manic-depressive patients had been unable to establish securely a good inner object in infancy and had not been able to work through the infantile depressive position.

Psychoanalytic theory and psychoanalytic developmental theory continued to influence the psychiatric literature on manic depression through the 1970s. Pao [30], citing the work of Lewin [31], stated that in mania the ego is overwhelmed by the experience of loss and by destructive impulses. Consequently, it regresses, and many ego functions are impaired.

Finally, Mahler [32], working with children, suggested that the "practicing phase" of the separation-individuation process is a period of vulnerability for the development of manic depression. During the practicing phase, elation is the predominant mood because the child is increasingly mobile and exploratory. The child's world is expanding through exploration. Both mania and hypomania occur as a result of defenses against object loss. In hypomania, denial is the predominant defense; in mania, additional defenses operate relating to the intensification of aggressive impulses.

Psychoanalytic theory posited stages of vulnerability for the later development of manic depression. Because children lack higher-level cognitive structures, however, manic depression was not considered a viable diagnosis in childhood.

In Europe, psychoanalysis and psychosocial theories were not widely accepted psychiatric traditions: the medical or disease model continued to exercise primary influence on psychiatric thought. Thus, manic depression was still understood in terms of the medical model, although there were disputes regarding the distinction between unipolar and bipolar disorder. In addition to the work of Wernicke [23,33], Kliest [34], and Leonhard [24], who described subtle distinctions among affective illnesses, Eugen Bleuler [35] departed from the Kraepelian tradition and described the relationship between manic depression and dementia praecox as a continuum without specific boundaries. Patients were placed on a "spectrum," which had a fluid quality: they could move from one position to another along the continuum, depending on the number of manifested symptoms of each disorder. Bleuler's use of subcategories and his use of the term *affective illness* influenced both the eighth and ninth editions of the *International Classification of Diseases* [36,37] and the earliest versions of the American Psychiatric Association's *The Diagnostic and Statistical Manual of Mental Disorders* (DSM-I and DSM-II) [38,39].

Bleuler's broader concepts of schizophrenia were widely used in the United States and contributed to the tendency to label all psychoses as "schizophrenia," even when there were prominent mood symptoms. Also contributing to this broad definition of schizophrenia, to the exclusion of diagnoses of bipolar disorder, were some of the ideas of Kurt Schneider, a contemporary of Kraepelin. Schneider had defined "first rank" symptoms that were thought by many to occur only in schizophrenia. They included the delusion that others could hear one's thoughts because they were being broadcast, delusions that one's thoughts and feelings are controlled by outside forces; and hallucinations that outside voices are constantly commenting on every detail of one's behavior. These symptoms are now seen as occurring in mania as well as in schizophrenia.

That many patients who would be diagnosed as schizophrenic in the United States were likely to be diagnosed as having mood disorder in Europe was demonstrated in the 1970s. Anglo-American researchers compared diagnoses of patients hospitalized in England and patients hospitalized in America. Hospital diagnoses varied widely, but when standard criteria were applied to the same patients, the diagnoses were similar in the two countries [40].

In more recent editions of the DSM, manic-depressive disorders are differentiated into unipolar (major depressive) and bipolar disorders. Kurt Leonhard had observed in the mid-twentieth century that some patients had histories of both mania and depression as well as a higher incidence of mania in their families, whereas other patients had histories of depression only and few manic relatives. A decade later, Angst and Perris in separate studies provided systematic data from family histories to support Leonhard's unipolar/bipolar distinction. The first American researchers to emphasize this distinction were Winokur, Clayton, and Reich [41–43].

Historic roots of the childhood bipolar disorder concept: mania in children

Before the nineteenth century no scientific studies of pediatric psychopathology existed. The prevailing belief before that time was that children were essentially miniature adults, to be introduced to economic responsibilities as soon as they were ready [44]. Scientific interest in children began in the mid-nineteenth century with the emergence of pediatrics as a specialty. No specialty at that time was called "child psychiatry." Even before the nineteenth century, however, isolated descriptions of childhood mental illness, including mania, appeared in European literature. Crichton translated Greding's *Medical Aphorisms on Melancholy* [40,45], in which a case of mania in an infant was reported. The case has a strikingly organic quality:

> On the 20th, January, 1763, was brought to bed without any assistance, a male child, who was raving mad. When he was brought to our workhouse, which was on the 24th, he possessed so much strength in his legs and arms, that four women could, at times, with difficulty restrain him. These paroxysms either ended in indescribable laughter for which no evident reason could be observed, or else he tore in anger everything near him, cloaths, linen, bed, furniture, even thread when he could get hold of it. We durst not allow him to be alone, otherwise he would get on the benches and table, and even attempt to climb the walls. Afterwards, however, when he began to have teeth, he fell into a general wasting or decline, and died.

Haslam [46] described a 10-year-old boy who was referred for treatment because of mischievous and uncontrollable behavior that had grown worse since the child was 2 years old. The child was described as violent, cruel, destructive — "an unrelenting foe to all china, glass, and crockery."

In the American literature there were isolated descriptions of mania in children before the twentieth century [47]. Crichton-Browne [48] described melancholia and mania in "the early life of the child":

> This disease appears incompatible with early life, but it is so only in appearance, for the buoyancy and gladness of childhood may give place to despondency and

despair, and faith and confidence be superceded by doubt and misery ...
Melancholia may be sudden or insidious in its attack; it may be a primary
disorder, or it may be a sequel to some other form of insanity. Those suffering
from it are gloomy and taciturn, and indifferent. And with respect to mania,
Mania is a more general disorder ... in all its various forms, may occur in
infancy and childhood. In mania the mental faculties, as a whole are deranged.
And the mind is in a state of confusion and excitement. The ideas are incoherent
and disconnected. The language is loose, voluble, and wild. The mental affection
consists of a supremacy exercised by the lower over the higher faculties of the
mind, and is often accompanied by bodily disease. During its continuance, the
incoherence of language is due to electric rapidity with which the mind acts, to
the impossibility of giving utterance to all 'fast coming fancies,' and not to any
loss of the knowledge of meanings of words and phrases. Delusions are more
frequent in this form of insanity, than positive hallucinations.

Beach [49] described a 13-year-old boy who evidenced "folie circulaire":

> He was a dull child, and had been so often punished at school, on account of his
> slow progress, that he became deeply melancholy and tried to kill himself. The
> melancholy alternated with mania, in which he whistled and sang all day and
> night, tore his clothes and was filthy at his habits.

Kraepelin [18–21] referred to the possibility of manic depression occurring in
early childhood, although he saw this disorder in childhood as extremely rare.
During the same period of time, in Germany, Theodor Ziehen [50] described
occurrences of the disorder in younger children. He categorized the disorder
under "composite or periodic psychoses." Ziehen's eloquent description of the
disorder can be compared with present day descriptions:

> A simple, non-recurring mania occurs only exceptionally during childhood. In
> most cases a mania is characterized by periodic recurrences or regular alternation
> with melancholy, that means either by so-called periodic mania or circular
> insanity. The two mental diseases are clinically distinctive and therefore shall be
> treated separately under the heading *Composite Psychoses.* ...
>
> Among the symptoms, pathological mirth is the most striking. It is reflected in
> the entire features of the child: the eyes gleam; the facial expression is smiling;
> sometimes children cannot stop laughing for hours. Even during pain symptoms,
> reproaches, and invectives the mirthful psychosis continues to exist. Not rarely is
> it joined by anger. In severe cases, fierce outbursts of rage may follow.
>
> The accelerated association of ideas, the so-called flight of ideas, manifests itself
> in an incessant, quick speech, the so-called logorrhea. Frequently, the child does
> not let his parents or teachers get a word in, butts in during class time and rambles
> from one subject to another. In slighter attacks the coherence of this flighty chit-
> chat remains. Severe cases entail the so-called *secondary incoherence*: the child
> constantly loses his thread, strings together sentences and words that either have
> no or a purely superficial context based on sound patterns (rhyme).
>
> Pathological distraction of attention, the so called *hypervigilance*, is closely
> related to the accelerated association of ideas. Each noise, each change in the
> environment, creates ideas and triggers off flighty remarks. ... It is also very

noticeable that children with mania may suffer exceptionally from paroxysms even though they never occurred before the outbreak nor recurred after the cure of mania. The symptoms of the paroxysms resemble those of real epilepsy. Almost never absent in childhood mania, troubled sleep (agrypnia) stands in direct relation with the accelerated movement compulsion and accelerated association of ideas. In more severe cases a nearly total sleeplessness persists. Sensory derangement, i.e., hallucinations and illusions, is an inconstant symptom of mania.

In describing the development of the disorder, Ziehen stated that the onset is often sudden and that the apex of the disorder is reached quickly. The disorder rarely lasts only a few days and most often lasts for several weeks or months. A period of depression following the mania is common. According to Ziehen, "almost all cases can be cured."

Early research studies of mania in children

In the early 1920s, group studies of mania in children began to appear. Strecker [51] reported 10 cases of manic depression in children under age 15 years in 5000 consecutive hospital admissions. Nine of the 10 children were in the pubertal age range, and 7 evidenced depression primarily.

In 1931, Barrett [52] reviewed 100 cases of manic depression and found that 5% had had a first attack before age 12 years. Barrett suggested a constitutional component to the disorder, stating that children evidencing the disorder appear to have a "nervous endowment." He believed that early episodes of the disorder are precursors for later periodic psychoses. In reviewing the cases of childhood manic depression, Barrett concluded that (1) the first attack was one of depression; (2) depression or "excitement" is less severe than in cases where the symptomatology emerged in later years; (3) depression is characterized by emotional sadness, psychomotor retardation, and limited thought productivity, with no prominent delusions and with subsequent attacks being uniformly more intense and more severe than first attacks; (4) there is a conspicuous "hereditary tainting."

During the same period, Kasanin [53] studied affective psychoses in children. Describing the clinical picture of mania, he noted mild elation, overactivity, irritability, and pressured speech. The picture of depression, on the other hand, included withdrawal, under-talkativeness, general retardation, and occasional refusal of food.

Leo Kanner [54] described different presentations of manic depression in young children. Using the terminology of Adolf Meyer, he depicted two "reaction patterns." Hyperthymergasia consisted of exaggerated happiness, hilariousness, acceleration of thinking, flight of ideas, and increased psychomotor activity. In contrast, hypothymergasia consisted of profound sadness and downheartedness, slowing of thought processes, and depressed psychomotor activity. These presented in five different patterns: (1) manic phase—depressive phase—interval; (2) depressive phase—manic phase—interval; (3) manic phase—interval—depressive phase; (4) depressive phase—interval—manic phase; (5) depressive phase—interval—depressive phase.

The duration of intervals, according to Kanner, could vary from very short periods to periods that might last years or even decades. Kanner's 1935 edition of *Child Psychiatry* was the last to describe the disorder. This subsequent silence probably reflected general resistance to the diagnosis of manic depression in early childhood and the influence of psychoanalytic theory in understanding childhood psychopathology.

Bradley [55] illustrated the resistance to the diagnosis of manic depression in children:

> In children, sustained elevation of mood and exhilaration are not encountered except in response to reasonably appropriate stimuli. Hyperactivity is a frequent symptom of conflict in children but is not observed in attacks that are reminiscent of adult mania. Hyperactivity resulting from emotional conflict is usually accompanied by irritability and negativism in children, and to observe it as a pathological symptom in conjunction with exhilarated emotional responses would be a most unusual experience worth reporting.
>
> It is likely that in the rare reported cases of manic psychoses in children there may well have been confusion either in observation or interpretation of motor activity, impulsiveness, or other similar childhood symptoms, and attempts to fit the patient into an adult psychiatric classification which *does not apply to children* [italics supplied] seems unwarranted. . . . For the present it is best to avoid the diagnosis of manic-depressive psychosis or affective psychosis in children.

Barton-Hall [56] found support for the prevailing belief that manic depression did not occur before adolescence. Of 1000 children between the ages of 5 and 16 years who were examined in a psychiatric practice between 1944 and 1949, a diagnosis of affective disorder was made in only six patients, all of whom were age 13 years or older. Furthermore, in a group of 1200 patients observed over an 8-year period in biweekly visits to male and female observation wards, no cases of mania or melancholia were reported in children younger than 15 years of age. Barton-Hall concluded "these facts endorse the general belief that manic-depressive states are illnesses of maturing or the matured personality."

Whereas Barton-Hall and other investigators [57–60] rejected the diagnosis of manic depression in young children, others believed that manic depression was a valid pediatric diagnosis. Harms [61] suggested that symptoms of manic depression in children existed but went unnoticed by family members. Sadler [43] described adult cases that he had followed from childhood:

> Many children who puzzled me twenty-five years ago, and whose condition I diagnosed merely as nervous irritability, high tension, and overactivity, I have since observed, as they have grown up, to have developed into definite cycloid personalities–manic-depressives, . . . I am inclined to think that, in more typical cases, it would be possible to recognize this cycloid tendency even in the nursery. . . . Many cycloid temperaments early disclose the tendency by indulging in a glorified type of "mood swing." These youngsters are often emotionally unstable throughout childhood, and the majority of these cycloid deviates belong to the extrovert or ambivalent type of personality. . . . Early in childhood they tend to develop this 'roller coaster' type of disposition.

Campbell [62] expressed his disagreement with Bradley's [55] conclusions as a result of his work with manic-depressive patients. Campbell suggested that observations of the disorder in children were accurate and that perhaps these cases were being misdiagnosed:

> There was a noted proclivity among psychiatrists to classify milder cyclothymic reactions in the psychoneurotic category and the more severe manic and depressive reactions with schizophrenic classification disregarding the possibility of manic-depressive psychosis in the younger age group.

From his research with manic-depressive children and adolescence Campbell concluded that

1. A study of 18 children . . . emphasizes the frequency and importance of this psychosis among children, the strong familial tendency of the disease . . . and over-emphasis that has been placed on conventional and dynamic factors in the psychiatric illness of children.
2. Cyclothymic personality and manic-depressive psychosis among children are too often diagnosed as psychoneurosis or schizophrenia or the patients are classified as "problem children."
3. As a general rule, the earlier in life the cyclothymic process reaches a clinical degree, the more pronounced will the manic depression be found in the patient's stock.
4. Generally, it appears that when cyclothymic disease manifests itself early in life the individual is strongly burdened with manic-depressive disposition and may expect either a chronic course or many recurrent episodes.

The first attempt to systematize the literature on manic-depressive psychosis in childhood was made by Anthony and Scott [42] in 1960. After reviewing 28 papers published between 1884 and 1954, they developed 10 criteria for manic depression in children:

1. Evidence of an abnormal psychiatric state at some time of the illness approximating the *classical clinical descriptions* as given by Kraepelin, Bleuler, Meyer, and others.
2. Evidence of a "positive" family history suggesting manic-depressive "diathesis."
3. Evidence of an *early* tendency to a manic-depressive type of reaction as manifested in:
   A. A cyclothymic tendency with gradually increasing amplitude and length of "oscillations."
   B. Delirious manic or depressive outbursts occuring during pyrexial illnesses.
4. Evidence of a *recurrent* or *periodic* illness. This evidence entails the observation of at least two episodes, separated by a period of time (gauged in months or years), and regarded as clinically similar. There should be diagnostic agreement by different clinical judges on the nature of any one

episode, and diagnostic agreement by different clinical judges on the identity of different episodes.

5. Evidence of a *diphasic* illness showing swings of pathological dimension from states of elation to states of depression and vice-versa.
6. Evidence of an *endogenous* illness indicating that the phases of the illness alternate with minimal reference to environmental events.
7. Evidence of *severe* illness as indicated by a need for in-patient treatment, heavy sedation, and electroconvulsive therapy (ECT).
8. Evidence of an *abnormal underlying personality* of an extroverted type as demonstrated by objective test procedures.
9. An *absence* of features that might indicate other abnormal conditions such as schizophrenia, organic states (alcohol, delerium, GPI, hysteria, etc).
10. The evidence of *current*, not retrospective, assessments.

After reviewing these cases, Anthony and Scott concluded that manic depression is a rare disorder in childhood. They found only 3 of 60 cases that could meet their criteria for manic depression. Although this was a pioneer effort at systemization, the inclusion of Kraepelin's symptoms and of criteria inconsistent with DSM-IIIR [63] criteria for adult mania resulted in cases being excluded and made underdiagnosis more probable. By setting up their own criteria, Anthony and Scott essentially swept away the concept of manic depression in children.

Revival of the concept of manic depression in children

In the 1970s, some clinicians presented cases of manic behavior in young children. Feinstein and Wolpert [65], for example, described the behavior of a 5-year-old girl who had first been seen at the age of 3 years presenting with hyperactive behavior, low frustration tolerance, impulsivity, destructiveness, and inability to concentrate. The child slept only in short spurts and ate poorly. She began to walk at 14 months, and her behavior was impulsive, hyperactive, and, uncontrollable. She was subject to rapid mood shifts. After playing calmly, she would suddenly shift into a state in which she would hit, bite, scratch, and become very destructive. Her family history was marked by affective disorders.

Thompson and Shindler [66] described a pattern of "embryonic mania" in a 5-year-old boy The term *embryonic mania* was used by Anthony and Scott [42] to indicate an *embryonic stage* of mania in which there were internal fantasies with manic-depressive qualities, including heightened self-esteem and thoughts of omnipotence that were not of psychotic proportions. When this fantasy life was externalized, behavior patterns included "manic utterances," overactive behavior, flight of ideas, distractibility, emotional lability, and omnipotent fantasies to defend against feelings of low self-esteem. The patient had a short attention span, "a mind that seemed to be wandering," and behaved disruptively in the kindergarten classroom. His elevated mood, shifting attention, and language problems affected his school performance.

LaGrone [67] described a child of 11.5 months whose behavior pattern was suggestive of early-onset bipolar disorder. Christopher was referred for hyperactivity, sleeplessness, and extreme irritability. He had been described as overactive from birth and subject to variable mood swings, shifting from irritability and crying to "days of brightness and increased activity." The shifts did not correlate with external events in his life. Christopher had a short attention span and was easily frustrated. His sleep period was unpredictable. In the nursery he responded to limit-setting with increased irritability. The constants in Christopher's overall behavior pattern were his high activity level and irritability. Christopher's mother expressed concern about his periods of "sadness." She herself had had periods of depression in the past, and his father was described as a man of "boundless energy" and aggressive behavior. The family history was strong for affective disturbances.

DeLong's [68,69] pioneer work led to the revival of the concept of bipolar disorder in children. DeLong successfully used lithium in some children and adolescents with hyperaggressive behaviors who were also manifesting symptoms of manic depression but who had not been diagnosed as such. His successes rekindled interest in bipolar disorder in children.

During the 1970s a number of clinicians and researchers began to report using lithium with children. Youngerman and Canino [70], reviewing the literature on the use of lithium with children, concluded:

> In children and adolescents the published literature seems to suggest that aggressivity per se and hyperactivity per se are sufficient indications for the use of lithium carbonate. However, aggressive or hyperactive patients with major affective components to their behavior may well warrant a trial of lithium carbonate.

The next major attempt to establish diagnostic criteria for mania in children was carried out by Weinberg and Brumback [71]. Adapting the criteria from the classification system developed by Feighner et al [64], which was being used to diagnose adult mania, Weinberg and Brumback included the following behaviors:

1. Euphoric or irritable mood, and
2. Three or more of the following, which should reflect a change from the child's normal behavior:
   a. hyperactive, intrusive behavior
   b. push of speech
   c. flight of ideas
   d. grandiosity
   e. decreased amount of sleep or unusual pattern of sleep
   f. distractibility
   g. symptom duration of 1 month

The 1970s closed with an important paper published by Davis [72], in which he described a "manic-depressive variant syndrome of childhood." Davis proposed that an identifiable syndrome exhibited by children and adolescents below the age of 16 years was characterized by five primary features and one or more secondary features. The primary features included:

1. affective storms, defined as a loss of control that is highly intense, disruptive, and transient
2. significant family histories of affective disturbances
3. mental, verbal, and physical hyperactivity
4. high level of distractibility
5. rapid talk or a "rapid progression of interest"

Davis pointed out that hyperactivity and emotional upheaval in children differ from the grandiosity of manic adults and that there were no delusions or hallucinations. Manic-depressive children also had highly troubled interpersonal relationships because of their erratic behavior. Davis included one exclusion characteristic in his description, the absence of psychotic thought disorder. Although their behavior might appear psychotic-like, the manic-depressive children's thoughts were not bizarre. Secondary characteristics included sleep disturbances, possible minimal brain dysfunction, occasionally abnormal EEG patterns, possible enuresis, and associated neurologic problems.

Investigators were now beginning to find more support for the reports of some adult patients with manic depression, that some of the symptoms of manic depression had been experienced in childhood. Loranger and Levine [41] found that 5% of patients with well-established diagnoses of manic depression reported their age at the onset of their illnesses as between 5 and 9 years.

While Davis was studying manic depression in children in the United States, Coll and Bland [73] were studying it in Canada. They proposed that manic depression did occur in childhood but was underdiagnosed because it was not expressed the same way in children as in adults. The presentation of bipolar disorder—as manic depression was now being called—included either or both of symptoms 1 and 2 and three or more of symptoms 3–8:

1. Euphoria
   a. Denial of problems or illness
   b. Inappropriate feelings of well-being, inappropriate cheerfulness, giddiness, and silliness
2. Irritability and/or agitation (particularly belligerence, destructiveness, and anti- social behavior)
3. Hyperactivity, "motor drive," intrusiveness
4. Push of speech (may become unintelligible), garrulousness
5. Flight of ideas
6. Grandiosity (may be delusional)
7. Sleep disturbance (decreased sleep and unusual sleep pattern)
8. Distractibility (short attention span).

By the beginning of the 1980s it was increasingly accepted that young children could present bipolar symptomatology. Carlson [74,75] concluded that certain children aged 15 months to 8 years presented a bipolar pattern marked by hyperactivity, an absence of discrete episodes, greater irritability and emotional lability as opposed to euphoria, and a relative absence of grandiosity and paranoia. In contrast, slightly older children—but still of prepubertal age—and older children seemed to present a more classic pattern marked by discrete episodes, euphoria, irritability, and grandiosity. In the depressive phase of the disorder younger children again did not evidence specific episodes. There was a relative absence of depressed appearance, guilt, paranoia, morbid preoccupation, or psychomotor retardation. More typically, they were agitated and irritable, a pattern also seen in unipolar depressed children.

Thus, although by the 1980s many clinicians agreed on the diagnosis of childhood-onset bipolar disorder, the diagnosis was still controversial. The continued use of adult criteria contributed to the controversy. In the early 1980s, developmental research that suggested that childhood-onset bipolar disorder might present differently from adult-onset bipolar disorder. Developmental factors contribute to certain characteristics consistent with the disorder, but these characteristics look different in children than in adults because the children are at a different point in their development. From the 1980s through the turn of the twenty-first century bipolar disorder has been studied within a developmental framework.

The concept of bipolar disorder in children, which has its roots in ancient medicine, has always been highly controversial, paralleling controversies in the adult literature. Not until the mid-nineteenth century were mania and depression first seen as two phases of a single disorder. Although Anthony and Scott were the first to delineate criteria for bipolar disorder in children in 1960, these criteria essentially abolished the diagnosis of the disorder because they excluded almost all children. Psychopharmacologic studies in the 1970s restored the concept of childhood-onset bipolar disorder, and research and clinical work with young children beginning in 1970 significantly altered the criteria defining the disorder. These changes resulted in more widespread treatment of children suffering from bipolar disorder and in help to families overwhelmed by this devastating illness.

Acknowledgments

The author thanks Cindy Glovinsky, MSW, for her help in editing this manuscript. He also thanks Nancy Austin, PsyD, Ross Baldessarini, MD, Gaye Carlson, MD, Georgia DeGangi, PhD, Robert DeLong, MD, Gianni Faedda, MD, and Stanley Greenspan, MD, for reviewing and commenting on earlier drafts.

References

[1] Nottelmann EDC, editor. Bipolar affective disorders in children and adolescents. J Am Acad Child Adolesc Psychiatry 1995;34:705–61.
[2] Faedda GL, Baldessarini R, Suppes T, et al. Pediatric-onset bipolar disorder: a neglected clinical and public health problem. Harv Rev Psychiatry 1995;34:171–95.

[3] Geller G, Luby J. Child and adolescent bipolar disorder: a review of the past ten years. J Am Acad Child Adolesc Psychiatry 1997;36:1168–76.

[4] Jackson SW. Melancholia and depression. New Haven: Yale University Press, 1986.

[5] Aretaeus. The extant works of Aretaeus, the Cappadocian. [Adams F, editor and trans.] London: Sydenham Society; 1856.

[6] Roccataliata G. History of ancient psychiatry. New York: Greenwood Press; 1986.

[7] Drabkin IE. Remarks on ancient psychopathology. Isis 1995;46:223–34.

[8] Boneti T. Sepelchretum sine anatomia practica ex cadaveribus morbo donatis. Geneva: Leonardi Chouët; 1679.

[9] Altschule M. The development of traditional psychotherapy: a sourcebook. New York (NY): Hemisphere Publishing; 1986.

[10] Willis T. Two discourses concerning the soul of brutes which is that of the vital and sensitive of man. [Perdage S, Trans.] London: Thomas Dring, Ch. Harper, and John Leigh; 1683.

[11] Boerhaave H. Boerhaave's aphorisms: concerning the knowledge and cure of diseases. London: W. and J. Innys; 1735.

[12] James R. A medicinal dictionary, vol 2. London: T. Osborne; 1743–5.

[13] Mead R. The medical works of Richard Mead, M.D. London: T. Osborne; 1743–5.

[14] Pichot P. The birth of the bipolar disorder concept. Eur Psychiatry 1995;10:1–10.

[15] Falret JP. Leçons cliniques de médecine mentale. Paris: J.-B. Baillière. 1854.

[16] Griesinger W. Pathologie und therapie der psychischen krankheiten. Stuttgart: Adolf Krabbe Verlag, 1845.

[17] Kahlbaum K. Die gruppirung der psychischen krankheiten und die eintheilung der seelenstörungen. Danzig: Kafemann; 1863.

[18] Krapelin E. Manic-depressive insanity and paranoia. [Barkely M, Trans.] Edinburgh: Livingstone; 1921.

[19] Krapelin E. Psychiatrie 4. Auflage. Leipzig: Barth; 1893.

[20] Krapelin E. Psychiatrie. 5. Auflage. Leipzig: Barth; 1896.

[21] Krapelin E. Psychiatrie.6. Auflage. Leipzig: Barth; 1899.

[22] Goodwin FK, Jamison K. Manic-depressive illness. New York: Oxford University Press; 1990.

[23] Wernicke C. Grundriss der psychiatrie. Leipzig: Thieme; 1900.

[24] Leonhard K. Aufteilung der endogener psychosen. Berlin: Akademie Verlag; 1957.

[25] Meyer A. Collected papers of Adolph Meyer. Winters EE, editor. Baltimore (MD): Johns Hopkins Press; 1950–2.

[26] Abraham K. Notes on the psychoanalytic investigation of manic-depressive insanity and allied conditions. In: Jones E, editor. Selected papers on psychoanalysis. London: Hogarth Press; 1949. p. 137–56.

[27] Abraham K. A short study of the development of the libido, viewed in the light of mental disorders. In: Jones E, editor. Selected papers on psychoanalysis. London: Hogarth Press; 1949. p. 418–501.

[28] Glover E. Psychoanalysis: a handbook for medical practitioners and students of comparative psychology. London: Staples Press; 1949.

[29] Klein M. Mourning and its relation to manic-depressive states. In: Klein P, editor. Contributions to psychoanalysis, 1921–1945. London, Hogarth Press; 1952. p. 311–338.

[30] Pao P. Elation, hypomania, and mania. J Am Psychoanal Assoc 1971;19:787–98.

[31] Lewin SD. Some psychoanalytic ideas applied to elation and depression. Am J Psychiatry 1959;116:38–43.

[32] Mahler MS, Pine F, Bergman A. The psychological birth of the human infant. New York: Basic Books; 1975.

[33] Wernicke C. Grundrisse der psychiatrie in klinischen vorlesungen. Leipzig: Thieme; 1906.

[34] Kliest K. Die gliederung der neuropsychischen erkrankungen. Mon Psychiatrie Neurol 1953; 125:526–54.

[35] Bleuler E. Textbook of psychiatry. [Brill AA, editor, English language edition.] New York: The Macmillan Co; 1924.

[36] International classification of diseases. 8th edition. Geneva: World Health Organization; 1967.
[37] International classification of diseases. 9th edition. Washington, DC: US Department of Health and Human Services; 1989.
[38] Diagnostic and statistical manual of mental disorders I. Washington, DC: American Psychiatric Association; 1952.
[39] Diagnostic and statistical manual of mental disorders II. Washington, DC: American Psychiatric Association, 1968.
[40] Crichton A. An inquiry into the nature and origin of mental derangement: comprehending a concise system of physiology and pathology of the human mind and a history of passions and their effect. London: T. Cadell, Jr and W. Davies, 1798.
[41] Loranger AW, Levine PM. Age at onset of bipolar affective illness. Arch Gen Psychiatry 1978;35:1345–8.
[42] Anthony EJ, Scott P. Manic-depressive psychosis in childhood. J Child Psychol Psychiatry 1960;1:53–72.
[43] Sadler WS. Juvenile manic activity. Nervous Child 1952;9:363–8.
[44] Parry-Jones W. The history of child and adolescent psychiatry: its present day relevance. J Child Adolesc Psychiatry 1989;30:3–11.
[45] Greding JE. Medical aphorisms on melancholy, etc. In: Crichton A, editor. An inquiry into mental derangement II. London: T. Cadell, Jr and W. Davies; 1798. p. 349–435.
[46] Haslam J. Observations on madness and melancholy: including practical remarks on those diseases; together with cases; and an account of the morbid appearances on dissection. London: J Callow; 1809.
[47] Marneros A, Angst J. Bipolar disorders: 100 years after manic-depressive insanity. Dordrecht: Kluwer Academic Publishers; 2000.
[48] Crichton-Browne J. Psychical disease in early life. Journal of Mental Science 1860;6:284–320.
[49] Beach F. Insanity of children. Journal of Mental Science 1898;44:459–74.
[50] Ziehen TG. Die geiteskrankheiten des kindersalters. [Federhofer K, Trans.] Berlin: Van Reuther & Reichard; 1917. Ann Arbor: University of Michigan; 1999.
[51] Strecker EA. The prognosis in manic-deppressive psychosis. NY Med J 1921;114:209–11.
[52] Barrett AM. Manic depressive psychosis in childhood. International Clinics 1931;3:205–17.
[53] Kasanin J. The affective psychoses in children. Am J Psychiatry 1931;10:897–903.
[54] Kanner L. Child psychiatry. Springfield (IL): CC Thomas; 1935.
[55] Bradley C. Psychoses in children. In: Lewis N, Pacella B, editors. Modern trends in child psychiatry. New York: International Universities Press, 1945. p 135–54.
[56] Barton-Hall M. Our present knowledge about manic-depressive states in childhood. Nervous Child 1952;9:319–25.
[57] Lurie LA, Tietz EB, Hertzman J. Functional psychoses in children. Am J Psychiatry 1936; 92:1169–84.
[58] Lurie LA, Luriem ML. Psychoses in children: a review. J Pediatr 1950;36:801–9.
[59] Ituarte RD, Olaizola J. Report on the First International Congress of Psychiatry. Paris: Section VII 1950.
[60] Sole-Sagarra J. Endogenous childhood psychoses. Arch Psychiatry 1951;187:131–8.
[61] Harms E. Differential patterns of manic-depressive disease in childhood. Nervous Child 1952;9:326–56.
[62] Campbell JD. Manic-depressive psychoses in children: report of 18 cases. J Nerv Ment Dis 1952;116:424–39.
[63] Diagnostic and statistical manual of mental disorders III-R. Washington, DC: American Psychiatric Association; 1980.
[64] Feighner JP, Robins E, Guze SD, et al. Diagnostic criteria for psychiatric research. Arch Gen Psychiatry 1972;116:702–6.
[65] Feinstein SC, Wolpert EA. Juvenile manic-depressive illness: clinical and therapeutic considerations. J Am Acad Child Adolesc Psychiatry 1975;12:123–36.
[66] Thompson J, Shindler FH. Embyonic mania. Child Psychiatry Hum Dev 1976;6(3):149–54.

[67] LaGrone D. Manic-depressive illness in early childhood: the case of Christopher. South Med J 1981;74(4):479–81.
[68] DeLong GR. Lithium treatment and bipolar disorders in childhood. N C Med J 1990;51:152–4.
[69] DeLong GR, Nieman GW. Lithium-induced behavior changes in children with symptoms suggesting manic-depressive illness. J Pediatr 1983;93:689–94.
[70] Youngerman J, Canino IA. Lithium carbonate use in children and adolescents: a survey of the literature. Arch Gen Psychiatry 1978;35(2):216–24.
[71] Weinberg WA, Brumback RA. Mania in childhood: case studies and literature review. American Journal of Disorders in Children 1976;130:380–5.
[72] Davis RE. Manic-depressive variant syndrome of childhood. Am J Psychiatry 1979;136:702–6.
[73] Coll PG, Bland MB. Manic-depressive illness in adolescence and childhood: review and case report. Can J Psychiatry 1979;24:255–62.
[74] Carlson G. Bipolar affective disorder in childhood and adolescence. In: Cantwell D, Carlson G, editors. Affective disorders in childhood and adolescence. New York: Spectrum Publications; 1983. p 61–83.
[75] Carlson G. Annotation: child and adolescent mania – diagnostic considerations. J Child Psychol Psychiatry 1990;31:331–41.

CHILD AND
ADOLESCENT
PSYCHIATRIC
CLINICS

Child Adolesc Psychiatric Clin N Am
11 (2002) 461–475

Bipolar disorder in adolescence and young adulthood

Peter M. Lewinsohn, PhD [a],[*], John R. Seeley, PhD[a],
Maureen E. Buckley, MA [b], Daniel N. Klein, PhD[b]

[a]Oregon Research Institute, 1715 Franklin Boulevard, Eugene, OR 97403-1983, USA
[b]Department of Psychology, State University of New York at Stony Brook,
Stony Brook, NY 11794, USA

It is currently accepted that the classic (ie, Kraepelinian) form of bipolar disorder can be manifested in children and adolescents [1]. There is also consensus that, with relatively minor modifications, the *Diagnostic and Statistical Manual of Mental Disorders,* 3rd edition, revised (DSM–III-R) [2] and the *Diagnostic and Statistical Manual of Mental Disorders*, 4th edition (DSM–IV) [3] criteria for bipolar disorder can be used with children and adolescents. The DSM–IV criteria for manic and hypomanic episodes are presented in the box.

DSM-IV definition of a manic or hypomanic episode

Criterion A: A distinct period of elevated, expansive, or irritable mood (manic ≥ 1 week; hypomanic 4–6 days)
Criterion B: During the mood disturbance, three or more of the following (four if criterion A is met only by irritable mood):
1. Inflated self-esteem
2. Decreased need for sleep
3. More talkative than usual
4. Flight of ideas
5. Distractibility
6. Increase in goal-directed activity
7. Excessive involvement in pleasurable activities

This work was supported by Grant Nos. R01 DA12951 from the National Institute on Drug Abuse, R01 MH50522 and R01 MH40501 from the National Institute of Mental Health.
* Corresponding author.
E-mail address: pete@ori.org (P.M. Lewinsohn).

Recent studies in the epidemiology of bipolar disorder in adults have indicated that the lifetime prevalence of bipolar I and bipolar II disorder ranges from 3% to 6% across a variety of countries and cultures [4]. Although data on the prevalence of bipolar disorders in community samples of older adolescents are limited, the Oregon Adolescent Depression Project (OADP) [5] suggests that the lifetime prevalence of bipolar spectrum disorders (primarily bipolar II and cyclothymia) is approximately 1%. Lifetime prevalence of subthreshold bipolar disorder, defined as manifesting the manic core symptom (DSM–IV criterion A) plus one or more other manic symptoms (DSM–IV criterion B), but never meeting criteria for bipolar disorder, was approximately 5%. Although there are no community data on the prevalence of what has been called prepubertal, juvenile, or pediatric bipolar disorder, several recent investigators have argued that the disorder is more common in clinically referred children than previously thought [6].

The manifestations of childhood and adolescent mania and hypomania differ. For example, the symptoms of grandiosity and excessive involvement in pleasurable activities can vary as a function of age and developmental level [7,8]. Juvenile-onset bipolar disorder is typically characterized by high rates of comorbidity with attention deficit-hyperactivity disorder (ADHD) [9,10] and conduct disorder [11]. Some investigators have reported high levels of rapid cycling (eg, >365 cycles per year) in children with bipolar disorder [10,12]. Childhood-onset bipolar disorder may also differ from adolescent bipolar disorder in such nonclassic presentations as mixed or dysphoric mania, irritability, aggressiveness, and the absence of clear-cut episodes that follow good premorbid adjustment. Juvenile bipolar disorder seems to be a much more chronic condition that has a very early age of onset [13]. These patients are severely impaired, showing a great deal of emotional lability, impulsivity, aggressiveness, and destructiveness. According to Geller et al [14], the more prevalent pattern for juvenile bipolar disorder is a period of illness lasting more than 3 years, during which time multiple episodes occur on a daily basis. Young children with the clinical manifestations described by Geller and colleagues and by Biederman et al are encountered in clinical practice. What is controversial is whether juvenile bipolar disorder and the classic form of manic disorder [15] are manifestations of the same disorder [1,9,13,16]. Further research is needed to determine whether juvenile bipolar disorder is an early manifestation of the classic form of bipolar disorder and a precursor for fully syndromal bipolar disorder and whether developmental taxa exist similar to those postulated for other disorders [1].

This article presents some selected findings from the OADP. Following a brief overview of the OADP, assessment measures appropriate for identifying adolescent and young-adult patients with bipolar disorder are briefly summarized. The OADP findings are then presented regarding

1. Epidemiology and clinical characteristics of fully syndromal and subthreshold bipolar disorder
2. Family history of psychopathology in probands with bipolar disorders

3. Course of bipolar disorder in young adults \course and outcome of adolescent bipolar disorder
4. Associations between suicidal behavior and bipolar disorder

Finally, the authors discuss the clinical implications of these findings and point to future directions for research in this area.

The Oregon Adolescent Depression Project

The OADP is an epidemiologic, family-history, and follow-up study of a large cohort of community adolescents [17]. The initial (T_1) sample consisted of a randomly selected cohort of 1709 high school students who were administered semistructured diagnostic interviews and completed a comprehensive battery of inventories. Approximately 1 year later (T_2), 1507 of the adolescents were re-evaluated with the same measures. At age 24 years (T_3), participants with a history of major depressive disorder or non–mood disorders and a randomly selected subset of adolescents with no psychiatric diagnosis through T_2 were evaluated for a third time using semistructured diagnostic interviews [18,19]. The authors are currently collecting a fourth wave (T_4) of assessments from the participants at age 30 years. They have attempted also to interview all the first-degree relatives of the probands selected to participate at T_3 about their own history of psychopathology. Direct interviews with relatives were supplemented with family history information about all relatives from the probands. A second family member was asked for information concerning relatives who could not be interviewed [20]. Some of the results concerning bipolar disorder and subthreshold bipolar disorder have been reported in greater detail in previous papers [5,21,22].

As to the distinction between prepubertal and adolescent bipolar disorder, a review of the write-ups for all of the cases of bipolar disorder by OADP diagnostic interviewers did not reveal a single case of rapid cycling as defined by Geller [23], and there were only three cases with an age of onset below 10 years. The low number of cases with prepubertal bipolar disorder may result from sample selection (ie, juvenile bipolar disorder may be so impairing as to preclude enrollment in public high schools), from the failure of the OADP version of the Schedule for Affective Disorders and Schizophrenia for School-Age Children (K-SADS) [24] diagnostic interview to probe for the rapid cycling, which is purported to be a key feature of juvenile bipolar disorder, or from the investigators' reliance on interviews with the adolescents rather than collecting data from parents.

Assessment instruments

To identify adolescents with bipolar disorder, it is necessary to determine which assessment instruments are most effective in identifying the presence of bipolar-spectrum disorders and subthreshold manifestations of bipolar disorder and in differentiating the features of bipolar disorder from those of frequently encountered comorbid conditions such as ADHD. Currently available assessment instruments may be categorized as interviewer-based and questionnaire measures.

Diagnostic interviews

Several interviewer measures have proved useful in identifying bipolar-spectrum disorders. The K-SADS and the Diagnostic Interview Schedule for Children-Version 4 (DISC-IV) [25] contain standardized stems that assess the presence of core manic or hypomanic features (eg, "Has there been a time when you were feeling so good or hyper that other people around you thought you were not your normal self or so hyper that you got into trouble?" or "How about times when you feel super angry, grouchy, cranky [or irritable] all the time?") and the additional symptoms associated with manic and hypomanic episodes (eg, "Did you talk more or faster than usual?" "Were you more restless or fidgety than usual?"). If positive responses are obtained from the core item stems, both the K-SADS and DISC-IV include detailed follow-up questions, including the assessment of the onset and resolution of episodes, the specific symptoms exhibited during an episode, and the severity of symptoms. The K-SADS and the DISC-IV also include sections assessing the level of functional impairment in the domains of school, peer interactions, and family interactions. It should also be noted that Geller et al [26] have recently expanded the K-SADS to assess prepubertal mania and rapid cycling. This assessment tool is the Washington University in St. Louis Kiddie Schedule for Affective Disorders and Schizophrenia (WASH-U-K-SADS).

The Child and Adolescent Psychiatric Assessment (CAPA) [27] is a relatively recent interviewer-based measure that is available in different developmentally appropriate versions from preschool through young adulthood. Parent- and teacher-report interview measures that correspond to the CAPA are also available to compare information across sources. These measures also contain standardized stems to evaluate a wide range of internalizing and externalizing psychologic difficulties, and responses are compared with a detailed "glossary" of symptom descriptions to determine the duration and intensity of symptoms as well as levels of psychosocial impairment.

Questionnaires

Several informant-report questionnaire measures have also been suggested as means to identify bipolar disorder in prepubertal and adolescent samples. For example, Biederman et al [28] found the Child Behavior Checklist (CBCL) [29] useful to distinguish a structured-interview diagnosis of ADHD and mania in children younger than age 12 years. Specifically, they found excellent correspondence between the Delinquent Behavior, Aggressive Behavior, Somatic Complaints, Anxious/Depressed, and Thought Problems scales of the CBCL and a prepubertal diagnosis of mania. The investigators suggest that although these results still require cross-validation, the CBCL may provide a quick and useful way to screen for mania in children. Geller et al [30] also found that the CBCL significantly distinguished juvenile bipolar disorder from ADHD.

Other instruments that specifically assess manic symptoms in children and adolescents include the Child Symptom Inventory [31] which has been used in studies of both inpatient and outpatient children and adolescents to assess the presence of manic and hypomanic symptoms using parent- and teacher-report questionnaires, and the Young Mania Rating Scale which has been used to assess manic and hypomanic symptoms by adolescent self-reporting. The General Behavior Inventory (GBI) [32] and the Hypomanic Personality Scale [33], originally developed for assessing full-spectrum symptoms of bipolar disorder in adults, may also be appropriate for use with adolescents. In the OADP, the Hypomanic Personality Scale predicted significant increases in social and academic dysfunction and depressive symptomatology between T_1 and T_2 [21]. An abbreviated eight-item version of the GBI was also examined in the OADP [34]. At T_1, adolescents scoring in the upper quartile of the abbreviated GBI were significantly more likely to have had a history of bipolar disorder or subthreshold bipolar disorder and were also more likely to develop bipolar disorder or subthreshold bipolar disorder by T_3 than were adolescents scoring in the lower three quartiles. These data suggest that the GBI may provide an economical means of screening for and identifying adolescents and young adults in the community who are at significantly increased risk of developing full- or subthreshold manifestations of bipolar disorder.

Incidence and prevalence

Based on the K-SADS interview in the OAPD, the weighted first incidence of bipolar disorder was 1.4% through age 18 years and 0.7% from ages 19 through 23 years. Of the 18 cases of bipolar disorder identified in the T_1 and T_2 evaluations, 2 met criteria for bipolar I disorder, 11 met criteria for bipolar II disorder, and 5 met criteria for cyclothymic disorder. The hazard functions of the first incidence of bipolar disorder are presented separately for male and female participants in Fig. 1. The incidence rates peak at age 14 years and decline sharply by early adulthood. Based on the subsample who have participated in the T_4 assessment to date ($n = 256$), no new cases were detected between 24 and 30 years of age. These rates are comparable to those reported in Carlson and Kashani's study of adolescents [35] and more recent community studies of bipolar disorder in adults [4,36]. These rates of bipolar spectrum disorders are also consistent with those found in a register-based investigation of manic-depressive psychosis in Denmark (1.2%) [37].

The OADP also examined rates of subthreshold bipolar disorder. The weighted lifetime prevalence of subthreshold bipolar disorder through age 18 years was found to be 4.5%, roughly comparable to the rate reported in Angst's community sample [38]. The rate of new cases of subthreshold bipolar

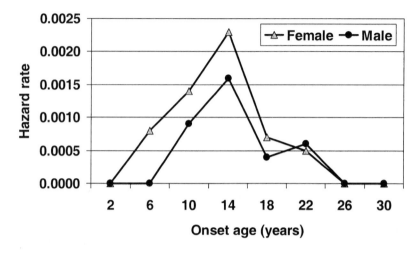

Fig. 1. Hazard functions of the first incidence of bipolar disorder in male and female participants of the Oregon Adolescent Depression Project.

disorder in the OAPD sample decreased after age 18 years: the weighted first incidence from ages 19 through 23 years was only 0.9%. The point prevalence of bipolar disorder was 0.6%, 0.5%, and 0.7% at T_1, T_2, and T_3, respectively. The point prevalence of subthreshold bipolar disorder was 1.2%, 0.3%, and 0.0% at T_1, T_2, and T_3, respectively, again indicating that the rate of subthreshold bipolar disorder diminishes as participants approach and enter young adulthood.

There were six new cases of bipolar disorder in OADP participants between the ages of 19 through 23 years. Three of these cases had a history of major depressive disorder before age 19. These cases, however, comprised only 1% of the adolescents with major depressive disorder in the OADP sample. This switch rate is lower than those reported in most previous studies of major depressive disorder, which have all used clinical samples. For example, Geller et al reported a switch rate of 32% [12], and Strober et al reported a switch rate of 20% [39]. Given the disparity between rates of switching in clinical and community samples, the question arises whether switching from major depressive disorder to mania in children and adolescents may be associated with antidepressant medications

Demographic correlates, clinical characteristics, and comorbidity

Adolescents with a lifetime history of bipolar disorder and subthreshold bipolar disorder did not differ from adolescents with no history of mental illness in sex, age, race, or parental education. Adolescents with bipolar disorder, however, were significantly more likely to come from disrupted homes than adolescents with no history of mental illness.

The mean age of onset of the first affective episode for the 18 bipolar cases through T_2 was 11.8 years (range, 7–15 years). In most cases, the first episode was depressed rather than manic. The mean duration of the most recent episode was 10.8 months.

A substantial portion of the adolescents with bipolar disorder exhibited impairment in social (67%), family (56%), and especially school (83%) functioning. Although to a lesser degree, adolescents with subthreshold bipolar disorder also exhibited impairment in social (49%), family (54%), and school (53%) functioning. Current functioning, as assessed by the DSM-III-R Global Assessment of Functioning (GAF) scale, was significantly poorer among adolescents with bipolar disorder than among those with subthreshold bipolar disorder. Both groups of adolescents with bipolar conditions exhibited significantly lower functioning on the GAF than adolescents with no history of mental illness and those with a history of major depressive disorder. Because these differences may have resulted from comorbid conditions, the authors identified a subgroup of adolescents with subthreshold bipolar disorder but no history of any mental disorder. This subgroup's functioning as measured by the GAF did not differ from that of adolescents with no history of mental illness.

Although adolescents with subthreshold bipolar disorder had fewer manic symptoms (mean [M] = 2.9, SD = 2.0) than adolescents with bipolar disorder (M = 4.5, SD = 1.4), the relative frequency of symptoms was similar in both groups, with a Spearman correlation of 0.74. In addition, the majority of adolescents with subthreshold bipolar disorder had a history of major depressive disorder (48.5%) or dysthymia (12.4%).

Adolescents with bipolar disorder and subthreshold bipolar disorder had high rates of nonaffective comorbidity. Both groups had high lifetime rates of anxiety (32.0% and 33.3%, respectively, versus 7.7% of the never mentally ill controls) and disruptive behavior disorders (18.6% and 22.2%, respectively, versus 6.9% for the controls). Adolescents with bipolar disorder and subthreshold bipolar disorder also had significantly elevated rates of substance abuse or dependence (22.2% and 23.7%, respectively, versus 10.4% for the controls). It is important to note that although comorbidities with ADHD (8.2% and 11.1%, respectively, versus 2.7% for controls) and conduct disorder (8.2% and 3.0%, respectively, versus 3.0% for controls) were significantly elevated, they were substantially below those reported by Biederman et al [11] and by Geller et al [10] for prepubertal bipolar disorder.

Family history of psychopathology

Family studies provide an important means of testing the validity of diagnostic constructs and exploring the links between disorders. Therefore, the OADP used the data from family studies to explore the validity of a diagnosis of bipolar disorder in adolescents and the relationship between full-symptom and subthreshold bipolar disorder.

The first-degree relatives of adolescents with bipolar disorder exhibited significantly higher rates of major depressive disorder and subthreshold bipolar disorder than did the first-degree relatives of adolescents with no history of mental disorder through age 18 years (Table 1). In addition, the first-degree relatives of adolescents with subthreshold bipolar disorder had significantly higher rates of bipolar I and bipolar II disorder and major depressive disorder than did relatives of the adolescents who had never been mentally ill. Eighty-one percent of the relatives with bipolar disorder exhibited the classic picture of elated or euphoric mood, as opposed to being diagnosed solely on the basis of irritable mood.

Interestingly, there were also significantly higher rates of anxiety disorders in the relatives of adolescents with bipolar disorder and subthreshold bipolar disorder than in the relatives of adolescents with no history of psychopathology. The groups of relatives did not differ, however, in rates of alcohol or drug use disorders.

These data support the validity of the diagnosis of bipolar disorder in adolescents, in that adolescent bipolar disorder is associated with elevated rates of major depressive disorder in relatives. They also indicate that subthreshold bipolar disorder may lie on a continuum with fully syndromal bipolar disorder, because there was an elevated rate of subthreshold bipolar disorder in the

Table 1
Kaplan-Meier age-corrected (to age 60 years) morbid risk estimates of psychiatric disorders among first-degree relatives by adolescent diagnostic group (age 0–18 years)

	Diagnostic group 0–18 years					Planned contrasts[a]	
Disorder	BD (N = 52)	SUB (N = 136)	MDD (N = 774)	DBD (N = 145)	ND (N = 885)	BD	SUB
MDD % (SE)	43.3 (7.6)	40.3 (5.9)	47.4 (3.4)	48.6 (6.3)	26.9 (2.0)	ND[c]	ND[c]
BD % (SE)	3.9 (2.7)	4.8 (2.2)	1.3 (0.5)	2.1 (1.2)	1.4 (0.5)		ND[c]
SUB % (SE)[b]	9.6 (4.5)	2.9 (1.4)	3.8 (0.7)	4.8 (1.9)	1.7 (0.5)	ND[c]	
Anxiety % (SE)	24.1 (7.5)	23.1 (4.0)	15.2 (1.4)	12.6 (3.3)	10.8 (1.2)	ND[c]	DBD[c]NND[d]
Alcohol abuse % (SE)	34.9 (7.2)	38.3 (4.7)	39.2 (2.1)	35.1 (4.4)	29.0 (2.1)		
Drug abuse % (SE)	27.9 (6.8)	24.2 (3.9)	20.7 (1.6)	30.1 (4.1)	13.8 (1.2)		
Antisocial PD % (SE)[b]	11.5 (5.3)	4.4 (1.7)	5.0 (0.8)	4.8 (1.7)	3.1 (0.6)		
Borderline PD % (SE)[b]	7.7 (3.5)	3.7 (1.5)	3.1 (0.6)	3.5 (1.5)	1.8 (0.4)	ND[c]	

Diagnostic groups listed in the BD and SUB planned contrasts columns indicate a significant difference at $P < 0.05$; differences between BD and SUB appear only in the BD column.

Data from Lewinshon PM, Klein DN, Seeley JR. Bipolar disorder during adolescence and young adulthood in a community sample. Bipolar Disorders 2000;2:281–93; with permission.

SE, standard error; BD, bipolar disorder; SUB, subthreshold bipolar disorder; MDD, major depressive disorder; DBD, disruptive behavior disorder; ND, no disorder; PD, personality disorder.

[a] Contrasts were based on Taylor series variance estimation and adjusted for gender of proband, gender of relative, relationship to proband, education of relative, direct interview participation, and number of informant interviews.

[b] Uncorrected rates are presented because of indeterminate age of onset.

[c] $P < 0.05$

[d] $P < 0.001$

relatives of adolescents with bipolar disorder, and there were elevated rates of bipolar disorder and major depressive disorder in the relatives of adolescents with subthreshold bipolar disorder.

Outcome of bipolar disorder in young adults

Some of the adolescents who developed bipolar disorder before age 19 years experienced a chronic or recurrent course; 35% had not remitted by age 19; and 12% had not remitted by age 24. Of those who were in remission at age 18 years, 27% had another episode between the ages of 19 and 24 years.

To examine the diagnostic stability of adolescent bipolar disorder in young adulthood, the authors compared rates of disorders from ages 19 through 23 years in adolescents with bipolar disorder, subthreshold bipolar disorder, major depressive disorder, disruptive behavior disorder, or no mental disorder [5]. Adolescents with bipolar disorder had a significantly higher rate of manic or hypomanic episodes in young adulthood (27.3%) than adolescents with subthreshold bipolar disorder (2.1%), major depressive disorder (0.7%), disruptive behavior disorder (0.0%), and no history of psychopathology (0.3%). The rates of major depressive disorder episodes (40.9%) and anxiety disorders (13.3%) were significantly higher in adolescents with subthreshold bipolar disorder than in adolescents with no history of mental illness (18.9% and 2.3%, respectively). The groups did not differ significantly in rates of alcohol or drug use disorders in young adulthood. The subgroup of adolescents with subthreshold bipolar disorder and no lifetime history of major depressive disorder through age 18 years had a significantly higher first incidence of major depressive disorder during young adulthood (39.3%) than did adolescents with no history of psychopathology (18.9%). Thus, subthreshold bipolar symptomatology in adolescence was found to be a significant risk factor for the subsequent development of a major mood disorder.

Bipolar disorder and subthreshold bipolar disorder in adolescence also presaged significant functional impairment in young adulthood (Table 2). Compared with adolescents with no history of mental illness before age 19 years, adolescents with bipolar disorder had significantly higher scores on a composite measure of psychosocial impairment, exhibited significantly poorer functioning on the DSM-IV GAF scale, and had significantly greater use of mental health services in young adulthood. Adolescents with subthreshold bipolar disorder also exhibited significantly greater psychosocial impairment, poorer functioning on the GAF scale, greater use of mental health services, and were significantly less likely to graduate from college than were adolescents with no history of mental illness.

Suicidal behavior

Although it is firmly established that adults with bipolar disorder are at extremely high risk for suicidal behaviors (studies report a suicide completion

Table 2
Young adulthood functioning (age 24 years) by adolescent diagnostic group (age 0–18 years)

	Diagnostic group 0–18 years					Planned contrasts	
Functioning measure	BD (N = 17)	SUB (N = 48)	MDD (N = 275)	DBD (N = 49)	ND (N = 307)	BD	SUB
Psychosocial	0.27	0.20	0.25	0.05	-0.32	ND[a]	ND[c]
impairment (M, SD)	(0.90)	(0.96)	(1.04)	(0.99)	(0.91)		
GAF (M, SD)	75.6	78.5	76.1	77.6	81.9	ND[b]	ND[a]
	(9.59)	(9.0)	(10.1)	(7.9)	(7.6)		
Mental health treatment utilization (%)	41.2	27.1	28.0	20.4	9.1	ND[c]	ND[c]
Suicide attempt	5.9	6.3	5.5	4.1	1.6		
Years of education	13.8	13.9	13.7	13.0	14.5	DBD[a]	ND[a]
(M, SD)	(2.2)	(1.8)	(1.8)	(1.8)	(1.8)		
Bachelor's degree (%)	29.4	22.9	19.6	12.2	41.7		ND[a]
Income (per 10,000;	2.1	2.3	2.1	2.4	2.4		
M, SD)	(1.5)	(1.7)	(1.4)	(1.5)	(1.5)		
Unemployed (%)	5.9	4.2	7.6	2.0	6.5		
Ever married (%)	35.3	37.5	43.6	30.6	37.5		
Parent (%)	23.5	29.2	32.6	22.4	20.7		

Diagnostic groups listed in the BD and SUB planned contrasts columns indicate a significant difference at $P < 0.05$; differences between BD and SUB only appear in the BD column.
Data from Lewinshon PM, Klein DN, Seeley JR. Bipolar disorder during adolescence and young adulthood in community sample. Bipolar Disorders 2000;2:281–93; with permission.
Note SD, standard deviation; M, mean; BD, bipolar disorder; SUB, subthreshold bipolar disorder; MDD, major depressive disorder; DBD, disruptive behavior disorder; ND, no disorder.
[a] $P < 0.05$,
[b] $P < 0.01$,
[c] $P < 0.001$

rate ranging from 12% to 50% and an attempt rate from 25% to 50%), information about the suicide attempt and completion rates among adolescent patients with bipolar disorder is relatively sparse [40–42].

To examine the association between bipolar disorder and suicidal behavior, the OADP defined four groups based on lifetime history of psychopathology through 18 years: (1) bipolar disorder ($n = 18$), (2) subthreshold bipolar disorder ($n = 51$), (3) major depressive disorder without bipolar disorder or subthreshold bipolar disorder ($n = 294$), and (4) no mental disorder ($n = 233$). The lifetime history of suicidal behavior through age 18 years was assessed with the T_1 through T_3 K-SADS interviews. For those who attempted suicide, the groups were compared regarding age at first attempt, percentage with multiple attempts, suicidal intent, and medical lethality. Suicidal intent was rated by the diagnostic interviewer on a six-point scale ranging from no intent to extreme intent. Medical lethality was rated on an 11-point scale ranging from death as an improbable outcome to death as a highly probable outcome.

The rate of suicide attempts in the group with bipolar disorder was significantly higher (44.4%) than in the other three groups. The rate of suicide attempts in the group with subthreshold bipolar disorder was significantly higher (17.6%)

than in the group with no mental disorders (1.2%) but did not differ from that of the group with major depressive disorder (21.8%). Suicidal ideation was also higher in the group with bipolar disorder than in the groups with subthreshold bipolar disorder or with no mental disorder but did not differ significantly from the group with major depressive disorder. The group with bipolar disorder had a younger age of first suicide attempt and a higher percentage of multiple suicide attempts than either the group with major depressive disorder or that with subthreshold bipolar disorder. Based on medical lethality ratings, the suicide attempts in the group with bipolar disorder were more serious than those in the other groups.

In sum, the group with bipolar disorder exhibited a greater degree of suicidal behavior than their counterparts with major depressive disorder, subthreshold bipolar disorder, or no mental disorder. Lifetime suicide attempts and suicidal ideation were higher in the group with subthreshold bipolar disorder than in the group with no mental disorder. In the group with subthreshold bipolar disorder, however, the higher rate of suicide attempts and suicidal ideation may have been confounded by the high degree of psychopathologic comorbidity. Even after the participants with comorbid psychopathology were removed from comparison, however, the rate of suicide attempts remained significantly higher in the group with subthreshold bipolar disorder than in the group with no mental disorder (12.5% versus 1.2%). The difference in the rate of suicidal ideation was not as significant (12.5% versus 5.9%).

Clinical implications and future directions

The classic form of bipolar disorder (conforming to the criteria in the DSM-IV) clearly exists in adolescence. Consistent with the findings of earlier and more recent investigators, the OADP data provide partial support for the existence of a bipolar spectrum (ie, a continuum extending from subthreshold symptoms and elevated levels of hypomanic personality traits through fully symptomatic bipolar disorder). Although in prospective analyses the authors did not find a significant escalation from subthreshold bipolar disorder to fully syndromal bipolar disorder, subthreshold bipolar disorder was a risk factor for subsequent major depressive disorder. Furthermore, the family histories of persons with subthreshold bipolar disorder showed increased rates of bipolar disorder and significant psychosocial dysfunction during young adulthood. Clinicians need to be sensitive to the presence of the full-blown bipolar disorder syndrome and also to the milder and less easily perceived manifestations of this disorder. Bipolar disorder, even at the subthreshold level, has serious negative consequences for adolescents and affects their ability to cope with psychosocial demands during young adulthood. Detecting, mediating, and, better still, preventing bipolar disorder disorders in children and adolescents should be a high public-health priority. Cost-effective screening tools that can detect potential cases in a timely, nonstigmatizing, and inexpensive way are essential.

Consistent with findings on adult bipolar disorder, suicidal behavior is highly prevalent in the OADP participants with a history of bipolar disorder. Seventy-two percent have had suicidal ideation, and 44% have attempted suicide. The severity of the attempts was more serious among those with bipolar disorder than in their counterparts with major depressive disorder. The rates of suicidal behavior in the OADP participants with bipolar disorder are commensurate with the rates reported for referred cases. Clinicians need to be sensitive to the potential for suicidal acts among youth with both full-blown and subthreshold bipolar disorder.

Suicidal ideation and suicide attempts among youth almost always occur in the context of psychopathology [43]. Given the greater prevalence and seriousness of suicidal behavior among youth with bipolar disorder, the potential mechanisms by which bipolar disorder potentiates suicidal behavior must be investigated from a theoretical perspective. As Shaffer [44] points out, to determine the diagnostic specificity of suicidal behavior, it is necessary to compare the clinical characteristics of those with suicidal behavior and those without. Thus, future comparative studies should be conducted to identify the factors that differentiate adolescents with bipolar disorder who have a history of suicide attempt from those without such a history.

To facilitate the development and evaluation of preventative and therapeutic interventions, the psychosocial antecedents and consequences of prepubertal and adolescent bipolar disorder need to be identified through future research. Research to delineate the psychosocial concomitants of bipolar disorder in children and adolescents is also important. Discussions of the spheres of functioning that may evidence impairment can be found in the work of Alloy [45], Hammen et al [46], and Miklowitz and Goldstein [47]. An understanding of the early manifestations of bipolar disorder would be especially important in devising interventions at the youngest possible age to prevent at-risk youth from developing bipolar disorder. Indeed, the incidence functions presented in Fig. 1 suggest that the risk for bipolar disorder escalates during pre-adolescence and peaks during early adolescence. Longitudinal follow-up and family history studies of the prepubertal and juvenile-onset cases of bipolar disorder identified, studied, and treated by Geller, Biederman, and their colleagues must be conducted to establish whether bipolar disorder in very young children and bipolar disorder in adolescents are different manifestations of the same disorder.

The authors would like to end on a positive note by suggesting that the characteristics that predispose children and adolescents to bipolar disorder may bestow some advantages. These advantages, of course, would result from bipolar characteristics that remain within normal range of variation, not those at pathologic levels of intensity. As has been shown by Andreasen [48], Ludwig [49], Jamison [50], and Richards et al [51], highly creative individuals experience bipolar disorder more often than do other groups in the general population. An area for investigation is which characteristics of the bipolar spectrum contribute to creative achievement. In her review of this literature, Jamison [50] suggests features that should be considered: sharpened and unusually original thinking;

high activity and energy levels; optimism perhaps verging on grandiosity; verbal fluency; and enhanced motivation to work on ambitious goals. To these traits, one might add the enjoyment of being with people, social competence, and the ability to persuade and to inspire others. The challenge is to allow youngsters to take advantage of these traits without escalating to destructive and pathologic levels.

The OADP data provide some support for the existence of a bipolar spectrum early in the lifespan. With early detection and remediation, the many adverse consequences associated with bipolar disorder, such as suicidal behavior, may be prevented. Because of the pernicious course of prepubertal and adolescent bipolar disorder, such efforts should be a high public health priority.

References

[1] Nottelmann E, Biederman J, Birmaher B, et al. National Institute of Mental Health research roundtable on prepubertal bipolar disorder. J Am Acad Child Adolesc Psychiatry 2001;40: 871–8.

[2] American Psychiatric Association. Diagnostic and statistical manual of mental disorders, III-R. Washington, DC: American Psychiatric Association; 1987.

[3] American Psychiatric Association. Diagnostic and statistical manual of mental disorders. 4th edition. Washington, DC: American Psychiatric Association; 1994.

[4] Weissman MM, Bland RC, Canino GJ, et al. Cross-national epidemiology of major depression and bipolar disorder. JAMA 1996;276:293–9.

[5] Lewinsohn PM, Klein DN, Seeley JR. Bipolar disorder during adolescence and young adulthood in a community sample. Bipolar disorders 2000;2:281–93.

[6] Wozniak J, Biederman J, Kiely K, et al. Mania-like symptoms suggestive of childhood-onset bipolar disorder in clinically referred children. J Am Acad Child Adolesc Psychiatry 1995;34: 867–76.

[7] Bowring MA, Kovacs M. Difficulties in diagnosing manic disorders among children and adolescents. J Am Acad Child Adolesc Psychiatry 1992;31:611–4.

[8] Geller B, Luby J. Child and adolescent bipolar disorder: a review of the past 10 years. J Am Acad Child Adolesc Psychiatry 1997;36:1168–76.

[9] Biederman J. Resolved: Mania is mistaken for ADHD in prepubertal children. J Am Acad Child Adolesc Psychiatry 1998;37:1091–9.

[10] Geller B, Zimerman B, Williams M, et al. Diagnostic characteristics of 93 cases of a prepubertal and early adolescent bipolar disorder phenotype by gender, puberty and comorbid attention deficit hyperactivity disorder. J Child Adolesc Psychopharmacol 2000;10:157–64.

[11] Biederman J, Faraone SV, Hatch M, et al. Conduct disorder with and without mania in a referred sample of ADHD children. J Affect Disord 1997;44:177–88.

[12] Geller B, Fox LW, Clark KA. Rate and predictors of prepubertal bipolarity during follow-up of 6- to 12-year old depressed children. J Am Acad Child Adolesc Psychiatry 1994;33:461–8.

[13] Carlson GA. Identifying prepubertal mania. J Am Acad Child Adolesc Psychiatry 1995;34: 750–3.

[14] Geller B, Craney JL, Bolhofner K, et al. One year recovery and relapse rates of children with a prepubertal and early adolescent bipolar disorder phenotype. Am J Psychiatry 2001;158:303–5.

[15] Kraepelin E. Manic-depressive insanity and paranoia. Edinburgh: E & S Livingstone; 1921.

[16] Carlson GA. Mania and ADHD: comorbidity or confusion. J Affect Disord 1998;51:177–87.

[17] Lewinsohn PM, Hops H, Roberts RE, et al. Adolescent psychopathology: I. prevalence and incidence of depression and other DSM-III-R disorders in high school students. J Abnorm Psychol 1993;102:133–44.

[18] Lewinsohn PM, Rohde P, Klein DN, et al. Natural course of adolescent major depressive

disorder: I. continuity into young adulthood. J Am Acad Child Adolesc Psychiatry 1999;38: 56–63.

[19] Lewinsohn PM, Rohde P, Seeley JR, et al. Natural course of adolescent major depressive disorder in a community sample: predictors of recurrence in young adults. Am J Psychiatry 2000;157:1584–91.

[20] Klein DN, Lewinsohn PM, Seeley JR, et al. A family study of major depressive disorder in a community sample of adolescents. Arch Gen Psychiatry 2001;58:13–20.

[21] Klein DN, Lewinsohn PM, Seeley JR. Hypomanic personality traits in a community sample of adolescents. J Affect Disord 1996;38:135–43.

[22] Lewinsohn PM, Klein DN, Seeley JR. Bipolar disorders in a community sample of older adolescents: prevalence, phenomenology, comorbidity, and course. J Am Acad Child Adolesc Psychiatry 1995;34:454–63.

[23] Geller B, Cook Jr EH. Ultraradian rapid cycling in prepubertal and early adolescent bipolarity is not in transmission disequilibrium with Val/Met COMT Alleles. Society of Biological Psychiatry 2000;47:605–9.

[24] Orvaschel H, Puig-Antich J, Chambers WJ, et al. Retrospective assessment of prepubertal major depression with the Kiddie-SADS-E. J Am Acad Child Psychiatry 1982;21:392–7.

[25] Shaffer D, Schwab-Stone M, Fisher P, et al. The Diagnostic Interview Schedule for Children-Revised Version (DISC-R): I. preparation, field testing, interrater reliability, and acceptability. J Am Acad Child Adolesc Psychiatry 1993;32:643–50.

[26] Geller B, Zimerman B, Williams M, et al. Reliability of the Washington University in St. Louis Kiddie Schedule for Affective Disorders and Schizophrenia (WASH-U-KSADS) mania and rapid cycling sections. J Am Acad Child Adolesc Psychiatry 2001;40:450–5.

[27] Angold A, Costello EJ. The Child and Adolescent Psychiatric Assessment (CAPA). J Am Acad Child Adolesc Psychiatry 2000;39:39–48.

[28] Biederman J, Wozniak J, Kiely K, et al. CBCL clinical scales discriminate prepubertal children with structured interview-derived diagnosis of mania from those with ADHD. J Am Acad Child Adolesc Psychiatry 1995;34:464–71.

[29] Achenbach TM. Child behavior checklist/4–18 years (CBCL/4–18). Burlington (VT): University of Vermont Department of Psychiatry; 1991.

[30] Geller B, Warner K, Williams M, et al. Prepubertal and young adolescent bipolarity versus ADHD: assessment and validity using the WASH-U-KSADS, CBCL, and TRF. J Affect Disord 1998;51:93–100.

[31] Gadow K, Sprafkin J. Child symptom inventories manual. Stony Brook (NY): Checkmate Plus; 1994.

[32] Depue RA, Slater JF, Wolfsetter-Kausch H, et al. A behavioral paradigm for identifying persons at risk for bipolar depressive disorder: a conceptual framework and five validation studies. J Abnorm Psychol 1981;90:381–437.

[33] Eckblad M, Chapman LJ. Development and validation of a scale for hypomanic personality. J Abnorm Psychol 1986;95:214–22.

[34] Lewinsohn PM, Seeley JR, Klein DN. Bipolar disorder in a community sample of adolescents: epidemiology and suicidal behavior. In: Geller B, DelBello M, editors. (Child and early adolescent bipolar disorder. New York (NY): Guilford; in press.

[35] Carlson GA, Kashani JH. Manic symptoms in a non-referred adolescent population. J Affect Disord 1988;15:219–26.

[36] Kessler RC, Rubinow DR, Holmes C, et al. The epidemiology of DSM-III-R bipolar I disorder in a general population survey. Psychol Med 1997;27:1079–89.

[37] Thomsen PH, Moller LL, Dehlholm B, et al. Manic-depressive psychosis in children younger than 15 years: A register-based investigation of 39 cases in Denmark. Acta Psychiatr Scand 1992;85:401–6.

[38] Angst J. The emerging epidemiology of hypomania and bipolar II disorder. J Affect Disord 1998;50:143–51.

[39] Strober M, Lampert C, Schmidt S, et al. The course of major depressive disorder in adolescents:

I. recovery and risk of manic switching in a follow-up of psychotic and nonpsychotic subtypes. J Am Acad Child Adolesc Psychiatry 1993;32:34–42.

[40] Guze S, Robins E. Suicide and primary affective disorders. Br J Psychiatry 1970;117:437–8.

[41] Jamison KR. Suicide and bipolar disorders. In: Mann JJ, Stanley M, editors. Psychobiology of suicidal behavior. New York (NY): New York Academy of Sciences; 1986. p. 301–15.

[42] Robins E, Murphy GE, Wilkinson Jr. RH, et al. Some clinical considerations in the prevention of suicide based on a study of 134 successful suicides. Am J Public Health 1959;49:888–99.

[43] Lewinsohn PM, Rohde P, Seeley JR. Adolescent suicidal ideation and attempts: prevalence, risk factors and clinical implications. Clinical Psychology: Science and Practice 1996;3:25–46.

[44] Shaffer D. Depression, mania, and suicidal acts. In: Rutter M, Hersov L, editors. Child and adolescent psychiatry: modern approaches. 2nd edition. Oxfor (UK): Blackwell; 1985, p. 698–719.

[45] Alloy LB, Just N, Panzarella C. Attributional style, daily life events, and hopelessness depression: subtype validation by prospective variability and specificity of symptoms. Cognitive Therapy and Research 1997;21:321–44.

[46] Hammen C, Burge D, Burney E, et al. Longitudinal study of diagnoses in children of women with unipolar and bipolar affective disorder. Arch Gen Psychiatry 1990;47:1112–7.

[47] Miklowitz DJ, Goldstein MJ. Bipolar disorder: a family-focused treatment approach. New York (NY): Guilford; 1997.

[48] Andreasen NC. Creativity and mental illness: prevalence rates in writers and their first-degree relatives. Am J Psychiatry 1987;144:1288–92.

[49] Ludwig LD. Elation-depression and skill as determinants of desire for excitement. J Pers 1975;43:1–22.

[50] Jamison KR. Manic-depressive illness and creativity. Sci Am 1995;272:62–7.

[51] Richards R, Kinney DK, Lunde I, et al. Creativity in manic-depressives, cyclothymes, their normal relatives, and control subjects. J Abnorm Psychol 1988;97:281–8.

CHILD AND
ADOLESCENT
PSYCHIATRIC
CLINICS

Child Adolesc Psychiatric Clin N Am
11 (2002) 477–497

Depression among youth in primary care
Models for delivering mental health services

Joan Rosenbaum Asarnow, PhD[a],*, Lisa H. Jaycox, PhD[b],
Martin Anderson, MD, MPH[a]

[a]*School of Medicine, University of California at Los Angeles, Los Angeles, CA 90024-1759, USA*
[b]*RAND, 1200 South Hayes Street, Arlington, VA 22202, USA*

The high costs of health care and the need to extend service capacity have resulted in primary care providers serving as gatekeepers to specialty care, including specialty mental health care. Consistent with the priority placed on promoting mental health in *Healthy People 2010*, recommendations from the United States Public Health Service call for a review of children's mental health in routine pediatric examinations [1–3]. This increased emphasis on the role of the primary care provider has stimulated efforts to develop and test models for delivering mental health services through primary care; however, are primary care providers ready to meet this challenge?

This article focuses specifically on the knowledge and tools available to the primary care provider to treat depression in youth. Depressive disorders are common: it is estimated that roughly 20% of the youth in the United States experience a depressive episode by the age of 18 years [4]. Moreover, depression is associated with significant current and future disability. The Global Burden of Disease Study predicts that major depression will become the second leading cause of disability in the world by the year 2010 [5]. Although depressive disorders are associated with significant risk of dysfunction, there are psychosocial and pharmacologic treatments with demonstrated efficacy [6–9]. Current treatments can be improved, and additional data are needed on treatment efficacy and effectiveness in real-world practice settings. There is also a critical need to improve access to efficacious treatments. Because most youth in the United States have contact with primary care providers, efforts within the primary care setting have great potential for improving access to high quality care for depression in youth.

To guide this review and discussion, we first present a heuristic model to guide the delivery of effective care for depression in youth seen in primary care

---

* Corresponding author.
E-mail address: jasarnow@mednet.ucla.edu (J.R. Asarnow).

settings. We then review extant research and literature on (1) patterns of primary care use, (2) detection of depression among youths seen in the primary care setting, (3) the presentation of depression in primary care populations, (4) current practice patterns for treating depression through primary care, (5) settings in which youth receive mental health care, and (6) intervention and treatment strategies for depression among youth in primary care. To illustrate one approach to improving care for depression through primary care, we emphasize our ongoing study of adolescent depression funded by the Agency for Health Care Research and Quality. The article concludes with recommendations regarding directions for further clinical and research initiatives.

A heuristic model

Efforts to develop models for delivering mental health services through primary care confront several potential barriers. Fig. 1, which illustrates the paths a youth must follow to receive care for depression through primary care, highlights some of these potential access problems. First, the youth must present for a primary care visit. As reviewed later in this article, most youth have some contact with a primary care provider each year. Universal access to primary care is not guaranteed in the United States, however, and some youth, particularly the uninsured or disadvantaged, never reach primary care. Additional barriers to optimal use of primary care during adolescence include the tendencies of adolescents to seek care in settings with fewer resources for detecting and treating mental health problems (eg, obstetric-gynecologic services, urgent care, or the emergency department) and their lower levels of well-child primary care visits. These impediments underscore the need to improve the use of primary care in this age group.

Second, depression must be detected in the youth who require care. Screening and identification of youth who need mental health services occurs within the context of a health care visit and in a patient-provider relationship that emphasizes physical health care. Further, primary care visits tend to be brief in comparison to the lengthier visits typically scheduled in specialty mental health care, and the evaluation of mental health needs and psychosocial risk factors competes with a wide range of health issues, including inoculations, medical conditions, and the diverse array of health risk behaviors (eg, diet, exercise, substance use, sexual behavior and safe practices, sexually transmitted diseases, seat belt use, safe driving practices). Indeed, mental health clinicians working with primary care physicians are frequently confronted with questions about the wisdom of focusing on screening for depression when there is already too little time to evaluate and treat other health conditions.

Third, once youth who need mental health services have been identified, those youth and their family members must be receptive to services. Treatment will not occur unless the youth and family members are motivated to adhere to treatment recommendations. This hurdle can be particularly complicated in primary care settings, because patients and family members have not sought mental health

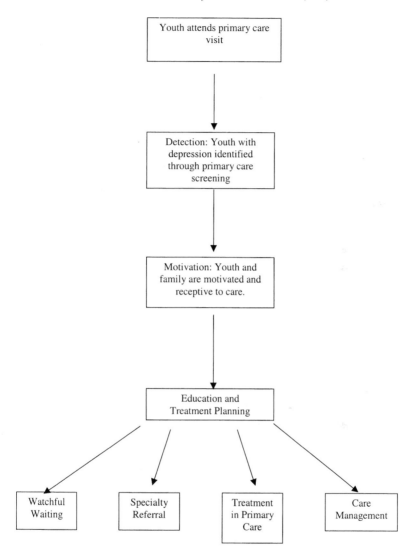

Fig. 1. Pathways to care for depression through primary care.

services. Indeed, youth and family members may not perceive a need for mental health services, may view mental health treatment as stigmatizing, and may be reluctant to accept mental health services. Furthermore, unlike mental health settings, in which youth or parents are aware of the mental health problem and have sought treatment, parents of youth whose depression is detected through primary care may be unaware of the youth's distress; the youth may have concerns about revealing difficulties to parents; and these complexities may create further barriers to mental health treatment.

Fourth, the youth and family need to be educated about treatment options, and an appropriate treatment plan needs to be developed. Primary care providers must therefore be able to offer viable treatment options. There has been increasing interest in integrating mental health care within primary care settings, and a variety of service-delivery strategies have been used and evaluated [10]. To date, this work has primarily focused on adults, but recent attention has turned to child and adolescent populations. A number of potential barriers remain to be addressed. For instance, many primary care practices lack easily accessible mental health services. Moreover, despite emerging evidence for the efficacy of structured psychothera-pies such as cognitive behavior therapy and interpersonal psychotherapy for the treatment of depression in youth [6–8], these treatments are frequently unavailable in primary care settings. Frequently, the only feasible treatment option through primary care is antidepressant medication, which may not be an appropriate treatment choice for all youth. Indeed, there is some consensus that psychosocial intervention should be tried first, and antidepressant medication trials should be initiated after there is evidence that the youth is not likely to respond to psychosocial intervention alone [9]. Current data, however, do support the short-term safety and efficacy of selective serotonin reuptake inhibitors (SSRIs) for the treatment of depression in youth [9,11,12].

Fifth, the youth and family must use the services and follow through with the treatment plan. Inadequate mental health care resources and a variety of other obstacles—transportation problems, limited time, conflicting demands, resistance to mental health services, and discomfort with available services—may interfere with adherence to the treatment plan. Additionally, attitudes towards mental health issues are influenced by culture. All these factors need to be addressed to ensure that minority populations do not experience disparities in access, avail-ability, and appropriateness of mental health care [13].

Finally, treatments that have demonstrated efficacy in other settings may not be as effective when delivered through primary care. Research on treatment efficacy for youth in primary care is scarce, and information is lacking on the general-izability of the efficacy data to primary care populations. Given the differences between primary care and specialty care populations, as discussed later, it is likely that current treatments may need to be adapted to meet the needs of typical primary care patients. Even assuming that treatments are equally effective with primary care populations, quality-of-care problems may lead to treatment that is ineffective.

Patterns of primary care use by youth

Current literature suggests that most children and adolescents have some contact with a primary care provider each year for well-child visits, school- or sports-mandated physical examinations, or acute care [14]. National data indicate that 70% of youth between the ages of 10 and 18 years visit a physician during a year, averaging 3 visits [15,16]. Primary care visits seem to be less frequent for adolescents between the ages of 13 and 16 years. Analyses of computer records for a general practice in London indicated that 53.5% of adolescents registered for that practice visited the practice during a 1-year period [14]. This rate is significantly lower than the national rate of 78% for all age groups in the United Kingdom. A reason for this low rate of visits for this middle adolescent age group may be that the settings in which youth receive primary care tend to shift during adolescence. Whereas children tend to visit pediatric practices, adolescents begin to seek medical care in a wider variety of settings, including pediatric, family practice, adolescent medicine, urgent and emergency care, and, for girls, obstetric-gynecologic settings. Many girls also receive services in family planning clinics [17], and the use of school-based health centers is growing [18]. During early adolescence and for boys throughout adolescence, teenagers seek care primarily for respiratory, dermatologic, and musculoskeletal complaints. For girls in middle and late adolescence, the leading reason for a visit is an obstetric-gynecologic examination, particularly for pregnancy [19]. Because of the emphasis on providing obstetric-gynecologic services for adolescent girls, and because in many states adolescents may receive family-planning services without parental consent, parents may be unaware that their adolescent daughter has attended the clinic or sought medical care.

In general, adolescents tend to underutilize primary care services and to overutilize emergency services [19–23]. About half of adolescents' visits to emergency services are for nonurgent reasons, and these visits result in hospitalization only about 5% of the time [23]. Even teenagers who frequently use primary care services (eg, girls with gynecologic complaints) tend to overutilize emergency services [24]. These frequent users of primary care (of all ages) are more likely than their counterparts to have mental health problems. For example, Mehl-Madrona [24] found that 63% of persons who use primary care services frequently received psychiatric diagnoses, in comparison with 14% of those who use primary care less frequently. Kramer and Iliffe [14] found that psychiatric and behavioral complaints were significantly more common among adolescents who had four or more visits to a primary care provider during a year than among other adolescents in the practice; and the same pattern was found for younger children aged 7 to 12 years [25].

Underutilization of primary care is especially common among minority adolescents. An analysis of the National Ambulatory Medical Care Survey data [19] showed over-representation of white teenagers (78.5% of visits and 67.6% of population) and under-representation of blacks and Hispanics (8.3% and 9.3% of visits and 15.5 and 13.1% of population, respectively). Part of the reason for underutilization may relate to insurance coverage. As teenagers approach the age of 21 years, the percentage of the population covered by public insurance tends to decrease (from 24.7% to 15.7%), and the percentage without insurance coverage increases (from 12.7% to 19.7%). The decline in the number of primary care visits during adolescence, therefore, may be associated with the increased lack of insurance coverage.

Thus, primary care represents a major point of contact for youth, and mental health problems are more likely to be detected in frequent users of primary care clinics. For mental health services to reach a broader population of youth, particularly adolescents and minority youth, outreach to emergency services, urgent care, and obstetric-gynecologic settings is needed. The increased emphasis on developing school-based and school-linked health centers may also help increase the number of youth who are seen in primary care settings, because these centers bring the services to a setting where most youth are easily accessible.

Detection of depression among primary care patients

Current data suggest that primary care is a major point of contact for most youth but is not currently a major source of mental health care. Although the pediatric office has been described as a de facto mental health service [26], especially under managed care, current studies indicate that pediatricians identify mental health needs in only a small subgroup of the youth who need services [27–33]. Horwitz et al [30] found that problems with "feelings" (including depression) were identified in only 3% of patients. Kramer and Garralda [31] found that 38.2% of youth seen in primary care settings met criteria for a mental disorder, and 20% met criteria for a depressive disorder according to the Schedule for Affective Disorders and Schizophrenia for School-Age Children (K-SADS-III-R) diagnostic interview [34]. However, these disorders were frequently unrecognized and untreated, with primary care physicians recognizing the presence or possible presence of psychiatric disorders in only 12% of youth. Thus, primary care physicians demonstrated a low level of sensitivity (21%) as compared with incidence based on the K-SADS-III-R.

Primary care providers were somewhat better at detecting associated psychological factors. These factors were identified in 31% of youth, representing a sensitivity of 51% against K-SADS-III-R incidence. Specificity was higher (91% for detection of psychiatric disorder and 79% for associated psychological factors) because primary care providers were not likely to falsely identify psychiatric disorder or problems when they were not detected on the K-SADS-III-R.

Several potential barriers to detection of depression or other mental health problems during primary care visits have already been mentioned. Compared with specialty mental health visits, most pediatric visits are brief, lasting about 10 minutes for children [35]. Perhaps because of the variation in types of providers caring for adolescents (pediatricians, adolescent medicine specialists, and family practitioners), data on visit lengths for adolescents are mixed. One study in the United Kingdom indicates that visits with general practitioners are shorter for adolescents than for other age groups [36]; and a study conducted in the United States indicates that the average visit for adolescents lasts about 16 minutes [19]. Even if the provider spends 16 minutes with the youth, the short visit limits the time for screening and reduces the likelihood that mental health problems will be detected. Within the context of the typical brief primary care visit, youth may not disclose their difficulties, and parents may fail to voice concerns about a child's mental health problems. If primary care providers do detect a mental health problem, additional time is required to address the problem, and this time may not be allotted in the schedule. An absence of resources for treating mental health problems and a lack of on-site mental health specialists may also raise barriers to mental health treatment, further decreasing the provider's motivation to detect problems. Youth referred to specialty mental health care may not follow up with these referrals because of stigma or other barriers to initiating care.

Despite these potential barriers, primary care providers do vary in terms of their attention to mental health problems. For instance, Kramer and Iliffe [14] found that detection was best for the small subset of youth with severe functional impairment. Kelleher et al [37] found that the best predictor of whether a provider detects symptoms of behavior disorder is continuity of care, specifically, whether the providers saw their own patients. Horwitz et al [30] found that physicians are more likely to detect psychosocial problems during well-child than during acute-care visits, when the physician knows the child well, when the child is male, and when parents are unmarried. Female physicians are less likely to view psycho-social care as burdensome, tend to spend more time with patients, and are more likely to see younger, Hispanic or black, and socioeconomically disadvantaged children. Male physicians tend to see pediatric patients with higher symptom counts. After these and other variables in caseloads, attitudes, and practice patterns were controlled, no differences were found between male and female physicians in rates of detection and care for childhood psychosocial problems [38]. Specialists in adolescent medicine tend to spend more time with their patients and are more inclined to treat mental health problems when detected[1].

Primary care visits, therefore, seem to offer a potential means for improving care for depression, but this potential seems to be underused. This underutilization may arise in part because youth typically present to primary care with physical symptoms; only 2% of youth present with psychological complaints [14]. Moreover, although self- and parent-report scales have been shown to be feasible screening tools in primary care settings, they are imperfect and are inferior to the more comprehensive diagnostic evaluations with multiple informants typically completed in specialty care settings. Thus, the goal within the primary care setting is to identify screening instruments that will detect most of the youth who would benefit from further evaluation and services. These instruments can improve detection while reducing the time needed for questioning during primary care visits. Youth can then be triaged: youth whose problems can be treated through primary care can be identified, and youth whose difficulties require specialty mental health services can be referred to specialty care.

A variety of self-report scales exist for assessing depression in children and adolescents. There are limited data, however, on the usefulness of these scales in primary care settings. Because of the high rates of health problems and the asso-ciation between health problems and depression among youth receiving primary care services [27], screening tools that separate depressive symptoms from the physical symptoms that are common in primary care populations are useful. The Beck Depression Inventory for Primary Care [39] allows this distinction and has shown usefulness with youth [40]. Although current practices in specialty care emphasize the value of assessments using multiple informants (youth, parent, teacher, other observers), the constraints of primary care settings often make this approach impractical. For example, many adolescents come to primary care clinics without their parents and at times come to clinics without their parents' knowledge for sensitive concerns such as pregnancy or pregnancy prevention. Moreover, adolescents tend to be better reporters than their parents of internalizing symptoms such as depression, underscoring the value of self-report scales as screening tools in primary care settings [41]. The authors have found that adolescents can complete a screening questionnaire, including the Center for Epidemiological Studies-Depression Scale (CES-D) [42], while waiting to see the primary care provider [27]. A useful strategy may be to begin with a self-report questionnaire concerning depression and to follow up with parent and other assessment measures when indicated. Other more general questionnaires such as the Pediatric Symptom Checklist [43], Child Behavior Checklist [44], or Youth Symptom Inventory [45], among others, can be used to obtain reports from parents regarding a broader set of mental health symptoms. Similar self-report scales can be used with youth to assess the broad range of comorbid symptoms and disorders that tend to be associated with depression in youth.

The presentation of depression in primary care populations

Mirroring results in adult studies such as that by Wittchen et al [46], the presentation of adolescent depression in primary care tends to be comorbid with physical health problems. Among the initial 2006 youths screened for depression in the authors' ongoing Youth Partners in Care study (YPIC) [27], only 34.2% of the screener-positive sample (n = 478) reported that their health was "excellent" or "very good," whereas 58.2% in the screener-negative sample described their health this way. Screener-positive youth reported 1.00 chronic health problems (SD, 1.5), on average, whereas screener-negative youth reported 0.35 health problems (SD, 0.7). These findings indicate that depression in adolescents is associated with a greater number of health problems. Prospective analyses suggest that functional impairment and disease are risk factors for future major depressive disorder and that major depressive disorder is a risk factor for future functional impairment and disease [47].

Considerable psychiatric comorbidity can be expected as well. Kramer and Garralda [31] identified comorbid psychiatric disorders in 42% of adolescents with disorder in their primary care sample. Although Kramer and Garralda did not report specific patterns of comorbidity, the most common comorbid disorders reported in samples of depressed youth are anxiety disorders, disruptive behavior disorders, and substance-use disorders. Data from our ongoing study show many psychiatric issues among the adolescents in primary care settings [27]. Examination of preliminary data shows that roughly 28% of youth reported externalizing behavior problems in the clinical range, 62% reported anxiety symptoms in the moderate to severe range, 40.6% reported symptoms of posttraumatic stress disorder, and 34% reported a disordered eating symptom. Thirty-one percent reported some alcohol use, and the average frequency of use was 4.7 days during the previous month. Fourteen percent reported marijuana use, at an average frequency of 8.1 days during the previous month. Eight percent reported use of other drugs, at a frequency of 8.3 days during the previous month.

An important issue in developing treatment strategies for youth in primary care settings involves assessing the severity of illness and impairment. There are minimal data on this issue, and ratings may differ across settings and provider specialties. Data from Kramer and Garralda [31] suggest relatively low levels of impairment among depressed youth detected in primary care settings.

Current practice patterns in primary care

A survey of primary care providers indicates that primary care physicians are most likely to use referral (65%) or counseling (61%) for the management of depression in children [48]. Perhaps because of their experience in treating adult depression, family physicians more frequently prescribe antidepressant medications (18%, versus 9% of primary care physicians). In contrast, pediatricians are more likely to refer depressed youth to specialty care (77% versus 48%). Physicians who are more comfortable with managing depression and are more confident in the effectiveness of antidepressant drugs are also more likely to treat depression in youth with medication [48].

Counseling is not a uniform component of primary care. Estimates suggest that roughly half (50.4%) of primary care visits include counseling, with somewhat higher rates of counseling during obstetric-gynecologic visits (65.1%) than during visits with internists (34.8%) [19]. A survey of adolescents attending community health and private clinics showed that they are not particularly amenable to receiving preventive counseling during their primary care visits [49]. Fewer than 20% of youth reported that they would be willing to talk about depression. There was, however, some indication that receptivity to counseling increases with repetition. Youth were more receptive to primary care counseling if they had been counseled on the topic in an earlier visit or felt the counseling was relevant to their situation. Girls were also found to be more willing to talk about depression than boys. Receptivity to counseling was similar for well visits and acute-care visits.

Outcome data for youth identified as depressed in primary care settings are urgently needed. In adults, quality of care in managed primary care settings has been described as moderate to poor, with resultant poor outcomes [50–52]. In a large sample of almost 2000 patients screened in primary care and followed for 3.5 years, Ormel et al [53] found that 80% of patients recovered from their disorder when a binary outcome measure was employed. When a more detailed outcome measure was used, however, fewer than half of the patients with a disorder showed full recovery. Most patients initially presenting with definite disorders showed improving but continuing symptoms. More data are needed on the outcomes of youth treated for depression in primary care settings, and the care for depression among youth in primary care settings probably needs to be improved. Because of the high rate of comorbid physical health problems in this population, outcomes and response to treatments may be somewhat different in youth whose depressions are detected through primary care services than in youth identified through specialty care.

Where do youth receive mental health care?

Despite the promise of primary care settings for recognizing and treating depression in youth, current research indicates that a relatively small proportion of youth currently receive mental health care through primary care services. Instead, most youth receive care through the schools or the specialty mental health sector. Focusing on youth who receive services and present with both a mental health diagnosis and impairment, Burns et al [54] found that roughly 11% received services through the general health sector. In contrast, 70% of these youth received services from schools, and the school system was the sole provider of services for nearly half of children with serious emotional disturbances. Services were provided through the specialty mental health sector for 40% of these youth, and smaller numbers of youth received services through child welfare agencies (about 16%) and the juvenile justice sector (about 4%). Because these data are based on parent reports, these figures may underestimate the level of mental health care provided through primary care services. These data do, however, emphasize the untapped potential of primary care and show that children frequently receive services through more than one sector (eg, school plus primary care, school plus specialty care, primary care plus specialty care). These data also suggest a different pattern of care for youth as compared with adults. Research involving adults indicates that depression is one of the most common conditions seen in the primary care setting, with a prevalence of 5% to 9% for major depression and 6% for dysthymic disorder [55]. Roughly half of adults receiving mental health care visit only general medical clinicians, and roughly half of all visits related to antidepressant use occur within the primary care setting [52].

Models for treating depression within primary care settings?

Four major models have guided efforts to improve care for depression in the primary care setting. One model emphasizes provider training and increased management by primary care providers. In general, this approach has not been highly successful. Some data suggest that brief provider education programs may be associated with changes in subjective outcomes, such as provider confidence and knowledge. There is, however, little evidence of improvements in objective provider behavior or in outcomes for children treated by these providers [56].

One exception is a pioneering study conducted by Kramer et al [32] who evaluated an intervention designed to improve detection and management of depression within the primary care setting. These investigators developed a provider-education program and a management guide for adolescent depression that can be used during a primary care consultation. The management guides include (1) a study manual that presents a step-by-step guide to screening for depression and implementing an intervention within a primary care consultation, (2) desktop aids that can be used easily during the visit to review the essential steps of the depression screening and provide prompts regarding the intervention, and (3) a computer template that provides a series of prompts to guide the provider through the screening.

The provider-education program included two 1-hour training sessions by child psychiatrists. These sessions included didactic teaching, case discussion, a video vignette, and role-playing. The first session focused on the evaluation and screening of adolescents using the management guides. The second session focused on treatment. Two monthly review meetings supplemented initial training sessions. Provider training emphasized the need to shift the focus from the presenting complaint (which was usually physical) to questions about the youth's feelings and psychologic status, leading to diagnostic screening for depressive disorder. If a depressive disorder was detected, the recommended management strategy involved giving the youth feedback by naming the problem using a diagnosis, explaining depression, linking the problem with known recent stressors, giving information about prognosis and treatment, providing an informational pamphlet about depression, and complimenting the youth for sharing his or her difficulties. Providers were next taught to identify and suggest coping strategies such as mobilizing help, identifying a confidant, scheduling activity, and self-reinforcement. Providers were encouraged to end the visit by emphasizing the likely resolution of symptoms and inviting the youth back for further treatment.

An initial study evaluating this approach revealed that detection of depression could be improved through the combination of provider training and the screening guides (desktop aids and computer template). Moreover, 99% of the adolescents who received the intervention felt that it was helpful, and 77% felt that the provider was interested in their moods and feelings. Given other reports suggesting that provider education alone has little effect, the screening guides probably represent a particularly important component of the intervention.

A second model for treating depression within the primary care setting is to employ specialty mental health providers within the primary care system. There are few adequately controlled evaluations of this approach, and extant evidence is ambiguous [56]. When the literature on treatment of the broad range of mental health problems in the primary care setting is reviewed, some data suggest that treatments such as cognitive behavior therapy are associated with reductions in the number of primary care visits. Few studies, however, were randomized, and the two large-scale studies that were randomized failed to find a marked effect of specialty mental health treatment on child health [57,58].

An ongoing study by Mufson and colleagues funded by the Substance Abuse and Mental Health Services Administration [59] evaluates the effects of inter-personal psychotherapy for adolescent depression when provided by mental health workers in school-based health clinics. School-based social workers were randomly assigned to provide either interpersonal therapy or the usual care. Social workers providing interpersonal therapy received training from the study staff in this treatment, which has demonstrated efficacy in the clinical literature [59,60]. Although it is likely that interventions that are effective in specialty mental health settings will show comparable effects in primary care settings when delivered by comparable providers with similar patients, controlled trials such as that being conducted by Mufson and colleagues are needed to demonstrate the efficacy of specialty mental health treatment within primary care settings [55].

The third model is the consultation-liaison strategy, in which the specialty mental health provider supports primary care management rather than assuming responsibility for the patient. Again, there are few data on this approach. One study by Neira-Munoz and Ward [61] compared eight intervention practices and eight control practices and found the rate of specialty referrals was lower in the consultation-liaison clinics than in the control clinics. Significance tests were not reported, however. Specialty referrals from the consultation clinics were also more likely to be rated as "appropriate," and the consultation-liaison service was rated highly by the general practitioners. Only a small percentage of primary care providers, however, felt that their knowledge and skills had improved, raising questions about the impact of the consultation-liaison service.

A fourth model is the collaborative care model. This model has contributed to major advances in the treatment of depression in adult primary care populations. Much of this work has involved quality-improvement programs that emphasize interventions designed to increase rates of appropriate care through a combination of training, system restructuring, and resources that promote improved care. Collaborative care refers to a team-based disease-management program in which (1) nonphysicians play a major role in patient assessment, education, treatment, and monitoring, and (2) mechanisms are developed for improving partnerships between primary care and specialty mental health care providers [62]. This approach addresses some of the major barriers to improving care for depression in the primary care setting, such as inadequate resources for assessment and treatment, insufficient time during the primary care visit, and limited access to specialty services and treatments with demonstrated effectiveness.

Several groups have demonstrated the usefulness of the collaborative care model for the treatment of depression in adults [63–65]. Current data indicate that this approach can yield improvements in clinical functioning, quality of life, and increased employment stability [65] in a cost-effective manner [66]. As adapted for use in treating depression by Katon et al [63], by Von Korff and Tiemens [67], and by Wells et al [65], the collaborative care model has the following components:

1. Case finding and outreach to patients at risk for chronic disease
2. Empowerment and support of the patient in using self-management techniques to achieve sustainable, appropriate care
3. Provider education and decision-making support based on evidence-based practice guidelines
4. Structural changes in the delivery of care to involve a collaborative team, with defined roles and accountabilities, to support depression care at each step

5. Use of information systems to support proactive follow up and tracking of outcomes
6. Use of nonphysician providers who support the initiation of and adherence to evidence based treatments and assist with linkages between primary care and specialty mental health services
7. Access to specialty mental health consultation for complex patients with complex disorders who are difficult to treat or treatment resistant
8. Effective coordination with community services

In general, adult studies of interventions implementing most of the components of the model have shown positive effects on quality of care and outcomes [63,65,68].

A critical component of the collaborative care model seems to be the use of ancillary, nonphysician staff, such as a care manager or depression nurse specialist, to assist with patient evaluation and management. Studies that have included ancillary staff to support care of depression but exclude other components of the model have shown improved outcomes [69,70]. More negative findings have been reported from studies eliminating the use of ancillary staff and relying instead on such components as provider education, patient education and activation, and reduced co-payments [71,72]. Thus, although additional research is needed, extant studies involving adults underscore the importance of providing ancillary staff to provide the requisite resources for delivering appropriate care for depression within primary care practices.

Two studies are currently being conducted to test the collaborative care model for treating depression among adolescents in the primary care setting. An ongoing study, Youth Partners in Care (YPIC) [27], is modeled after the Partners in Care Study conducted by Wells et al [65]. YPIC is being conducted in five different health care organizations ranging from managed care settings, to academic health centers, to public sector clinics. The approach features aggressive case finding, with screening of youth between the ages of 13 and 22 years conducted in primary care clinics while youth are waiting to see their providers. The screening is based on responses to a brief self-report questionnaire that contains the CES-D [42] and screening items for major depression and dysthymic disorder from the Composite International Diagnostic Interview (CIDI) [73]. Youth are considered as having a positive screening if they met either of the following criteria: (1) a CES-D score of 24 or greater, or (2) a CES-D score of 16 or greater, endorsed screener items for major depressive disorder or dysthymic disorder during the past year, and depressive symptoms lasting 1 week or more during the past month from the CIDI. Youth screening positive for depression based on these criteria are enrolled in the study.

After completing a baseline assessment, youth are randomly assigned (within providers) to either a quality improvement (QI) intervention or to the usual care. The QI intervention is designed centrally by the study but is adapted for the needs of each participating clinic and is implemented by participating clinics with study support. Major components of the QI intervention include:

1. An expert leader team at each site who designs the intervention implementation plan for the site, oversees intervention implementation, and provides expert consultation to participating providers
2. Care managers who support the primary care provider with on-site patient evaluation, education, treatment, monitoring, and linkage with specialty mental health services
3. Cognitive behavior therapists at each site who are trained to deliver rigorous cognitive behavior therapy for depression
4. Training for primary care providers in the evaluation and management of depression
5. Reduced co-payments for mental health services delivered through primary care

For patients, the QI intervention begins with an invitation to come to the clinic for an initial visit with the care manager. The purposes of this initial visit are to evaluate patient and family needs, to educate the patient and family about treatment options, and to develop a treatment plan (eg, cognitive behavior therapy, medication management, combined cognitive behavior therapy and medication, referral and linkage with services, or follow up by the care manager). This treatment plan is reviewed and approved by the primary care provider, and efforts are made to schedule a visit for the primary care provider to review the treatment plan with the youth and family members and to obtain their approval. The care manager follows the patient during the 6-month intervention period and coordinates care with the primary care provider. Patients in the control arm receive treatment as usual, except that providers have received training on the evaluation and management of depression.

The study is still in progress, and it is too early to examine clinical outcomes. The authors' experience and preliminary data support the feasibility of depression screening within primary care settings, but practices vary in their ability to support the screening efforts. It is clear that if practice-wide screening were adopted, most practices would need additional resources to ensure that patients complete the screening instruments and that the assessment data are evaluated and made available to primary care providers. It would also be essential to have practice assistants or nurses available who are trained to oversee screening, who have time allotted to the job of collecting and coordinating screening assessments, and who are responsible for this process.

Screening for depression using self-report instruments seems to yield a high false-positive rate. The authors' preliminary data suggest that fewer than half the youth with positive screenings meet criteria for a depressive disorder based on a diagnostic interview completed at a subsequent assessment. Thus, it is likely that screening using instruments such as those used in YPIC (CES-D, CIDI) will identify a relatively large pool of youth, only a subgroup of whom will meet criteria for depression. It is, therefore, critical that screening results be viewed and interpreted with caution. Providers need to be aware that a positive screening suggests the value of further evaluation or monitoring but does not indicate clinical depression. Moreover, discussions with youth and parents must consider the potential negative consequences of labeling a distress reaction or a "bad day" as a clinical problem.

The authors also have preliminary data on intervention implementation from their first study site. These data must be viewed as tentative because they are based on a subset of the sample and only a single site. This site is an academic medical center and includes a general adolescent medicine clinic as well as satellite pediatric clinics. The preliminary data support the feasibility of the intervention at this site. Most of the youth (82%) received an initial evaluation from the care manager, although this evaluation was conducted by telephone in a subgroup of youth (14% of youth receiving initial evaluations).

Reaching out to youth by telephone was a crucial component of the intervention. Although some youth were eager for care, some patients and families were not motivated to seek care because they did not perceive a problem, because of perceived stigma, or because of practical barriers to coming in for a visit. Extra efforts were needed to develop relationships through telephone contacts. When it became apparent that the youth needed care, repeated telephone contacts were used to educate youth and parents about service options and to increase motivation to enter treatment by coming in for a visit with the care manager or with the primary care provider. On the other hand, when it became apparent that the youth was doing well and that treatment was not indicated, telephone follow-ups were used to monitor patient progress and to support the positive steps that the youth was making.

Preliminary data for this initial site indicate that most of the youth assigned to the QI intervention received some treatment: 41% received psychosocial treatment only (including some cognitive behavior therapy or follow-up by the care manager), 38% received antidepressant medications, and 20% received no treatment. A total of 47% received some cognitive behavior therapy for depression. Although these preliminary data are promising, they must be viewed with caution. Results may differ when more children are enrolled in the study; results may not be the same across sites; data on differences in rates of care between the QI and usual care arms are not yet available; and the association between receiving care and outcome remains unknown.

Another approach to collaborative care is illustrated by a study conducted by Clarke et al [74], also funded by the Agency for Health Care Research and Quality. This study, named the Study to Test Effective Approaches to Depression in Youth (STEADY), focuses on a collaborative care model that has previously been shown to be effective for increasing medication adherence and reducing depressive symptoms in adults [63]. Unlike YPIC, which screens youth within the clinic, the study by Clarke and colleagues enrolls only youth whose depression has been detected through primary care and who are receiving antidepressant medication treatment from their primary care provider. Thus, they target a more narrowly defined group: those who have been determined to need and want treatment within the primary care setting. Following enrollment and completion of the baseline assessment, youth are randomly assigned to receive either usual care or the collaborative care intervention. Major components of the collaborative care intervention include:

1. The blending of primary care and mental health services, so that cognitive behavior therapy sessions often occur before or after a medication visit and are combined with a brief consultation with the primary care provider
2. Regular feedback to primary care providers after each cognitive behavior therapy session concerning life stresses, medication side effects, or other complications
3. Cognitive behavior therapists who work collaboratively with the patient and primary care provider to develop, implement, and modify, when needed, a treatment plan that includes both cognitive behavioral and pharmacologic components
4. Provider education about depression management using established guidelines

Youth receiving the collaborative care intervention receive five to nine sessions of individual cognitive behavior therapy for depression during the acute treatment phase, followed by six follow-up telephone contacts and up to six in-person continuation sessions over the course of a 12-month continuation phase. The cognitive behavior therapy used in this study is flexible and emphasizes two modules: (1) behavioral activation and increasing pleasant activities, and (2) cognitive restructuring. Medication is reviewed regualarly, and interventions are designed to improve medication adherence.

Summary

This article emphasizes the promise of efforts to improve care for depression within the primary care setting. These efforts, however, face a number of potential obstacles. We have reviewed the literature on the detection and treatment of depression among youth in primary care settings and argue that primary care offers underutilized potential for reaching out to youth and improving access to high-quality care for depression. Much work remains to be done before this potential can be realized. The recommendations below highlight crucial directions for future research and clinical efforts:

1. Traditional primary care practices offer an opportunity to identify and reach youth who need care for depression. To reach youth who do not present in typical primary care settings, outreach is needed to emergency services, urgent care, and obstetric-gynecologic settings. The increased emphasis on developing school-based and school-linked health centers may also prove helpful for increasing the number of youth who are seen in primary care because these centers bring the services to a setting that is easily accessible to most youth.

2. Strategies for improving detection of depression in primary care settings must be developed and tested. Given the constraints of primary care visits, these strategies must be relatively brief and not require extensive primary care provider time. Use of nonphysicians such as practice assistants, nursing staff, or associated mental health workers will be needed to support physician efforts. Furthermore, although brief self-report instruments may be useful in identifying a broad group of youth who may benefit from care, available instruments are likely to lead to overidentification and will require additional screening and triage of youth to appropriate services. Some identified youth may not require or want care; others may require further evaluation; others can be treated through primary care resources; and others will have complex conditions that require specialty consultation or referral.

3. Low rates of detection and evidence-based treatment for depression in primary care settings underscore the urgent need to understand the barriers to care within primary care settings and to develop interventions that reduce potential barriers and improve access to high-quality care.

4. Detection efforts within primary care settings are likely to yield a somewhat different population than the population of youth identified in specialty mental health clinics or schools. Notably, physical health problems are likely to be more common in primary care populations. The limited extant data also suggest that, as in most non–primary care samples of depressed youth, youth with depression seen in primary care settings are likely to present with a number of comorbid mental health conditions. Thus, there is a need to test extant treatments within primary care settings, and adaptations may be required to meet the needs of youth seen through primary care.

5. Motivation for treatment is likely to be lower for youth identified through primary care than for those seen in specialty care, particularly when youth have not identified themselves as requiring treatment. Strategies need to be developed and tested to enhance motivation and to target treatment efforts at those youth who are most likely to benefit from services.

6. The confidential nature of the patient-provider relationship, particularly in primary care settings where youth have sought care for sensitive issues (eg, pregnancy, birth control), underscores the need to develop effective strategies for working with families and mobilizing parents to support treatment and recovery. In primary care settings, parents may be less likely to be aware of youth problems, and youth may be reluctant to disclose difficulties to their parents.

7. Research is needed to identify service-delivery strategies that are practical in real-world settings and are associated with improved quality of care and outcomes in children and adolescents treated for depression in primary care settings.

8. Collaborative models of service delivery seem to be promising. These models build on the strengths of primary care settings and relationships and support primary care providers with resources that enable them to expand

their diagnostic and treatment targets to include depression and other mental health problems The recent and ongoing studies reviewed in this article provide some examples of these models. Future research is needed to clarify the effectiveness, costs, and benefits of this approach.

References

[1] American Medical Association. AMA's program on child and adolescent health. In: Guidelines for adolescent preventive services (GAPS) recommendations. Chicago: American Medical Association; 2001.

[2] Office of Disease Prevention and Health Promotion. Healthy people 2010: Understanding and improving health. Washington, DC: US Dept of Health and Human Services; 2000.

[3] Office of the Surgeon General. Mental health: a report of the Surgeon General. Rockville (MD): US Dept of Health and Human Services; 1999.

[4] Lewinsohn PM, Hops H, Roberts RE et al. Adolescent psychopathology: I. prevalence and incidence of depression and other DSM-III-R disorders in high school students. J Abnorm Psychol 1993;102:133–44.

[5] Murray CJ, Lopex AD. The global burden of disease: a comprehensive assessment of mortality and disability from disease, injuries, and risk factors in 1990 and projected to 2020. Boston, MA: The Harvard School of Public Health on behalf of the World Health Organization and the World Bank; 1996.

[6] Asarnow J, Jaycox LH, Tompson M. Depression in youth: psychosocial interventions. Journal of Child Clinical Psychology 2001;30:33–47.

[7] Birmaher B, Brent DA, Benson RS. Summary of the practice parameters for the assessment and treatment of children and adolescents with depressive disorders. J Am Acad Child Adolesc Psychiatry 1998;37:1234–8.

[8] Harrington R, Whittaker J, Shoebridge P. Psychological treatment of depression in children and adolescents. A review of treatment research. Br J Psychiatry 1998;173:291–8.

[9] Hughes CW, Emslie GJ, Crimson ML, et al. Texas consensus conference panel on medication treatment of childhood major depressive disorder. J Am Acad Child Adolesc Psychiatry 1999; 38:1442–54.

[10] Wells KB, Kataoka SH, Asarnow JR. Affective disorders in children and adolescents: addressing unmet need in primary care settings. Biol Psychiatry 2001;49:1111–20.

[11] Emslie GJ, Rush AJ, Weinberg WA, et al. A double-blind, randomized, placebo-controlled trial of fluoxetine in children and adolescents with depression. Arch Gen Psychiatry 1997;54:1031–7.

[12] Jensen PSBV, Vitiello B, Hoagwood K et al. Psychoactive medication prescribing practices for U.S. children: gaps between research and clinical practice. J Am Acad Child Adolesc Psychiatry 1999;38:557–65.

[13] Office of the Surgeon General. Mental. health: culture, race, and ethnicity–a supplement to mental health: a report of the Surgeon General. Rockville (MD): US Dept of Health and Human Services; 2001.

[14] Kramer T, Iliffe S. Which adolescents attend GP? Br J Gen Pract 1997;47:327.

[15] Gans JE, McManus MA, Newacheck PW. Adolescent health care: use, costs, and problems of access, vol 2. Chicago (IL): American Medical Association; 1991.

[16] Monheit A, Cunningham PJ. Children without health insurance. Future Child 1992;2:154–70.

[17] Frost JJ. Family planning clinic services in the United States, 1994. Fam Plann Perspect 1996; 28:92–100.

[18] Kaplan DW, Brindis C, Naylor KE et al. Elementary school-based health center use. Pediatrics 1998;101:E12.

[19] Ziv A, Boulet JR, Slap GB. Utilization of physician offices by adolescents in the United States. Pediatrics 1999;104:35–42.

[20] Lehmann CU, Barr J, Kelly PJ. Emergency department utilization by adolescents. J Adolesc Health 1994;15:485–90.

[21] Melzer-Lange M, Lye PS. Adolescent health care in a pediatric emergency department. Ann Emerg Med 1996;27:633–7.

[22] Wood DL, Hayward RA, Corey CR, et al. Access to medical care for children and adolescents in the United States. Pediatrics 1990;86:666–73.

[23] Ziv A, Boulet JR, Slap GB. Emergency department utilization by adolescents in the United States. Pediatrics 1998;101:987–94.

[24] Mehl-Madrona LE. Frequent users of rural primary care: comparisons with randomly selected users. J Am Board Fam Pract 1998;11:105–15.

[25] Garralda ME, Bowman FM, Mandalia S. Children with psychiatric disorders who are frequent attenders to primary care. Eur Child Adolesc Psychiatry 1999;8:34–44.

[26] Tarnowski K. Disadvantaged children and families in pediatric primary care settings: I. broadening the scope of integrated mental health service. J Clin Child Psychol 1991;20:351–9.

[27] Asarnow JR, Jaycox L, Rea M, et al. Quality improvement for depression among adolescents in primary care. Presented at the 47th Annual Meeting of the American Academy of Child and Adolescent Psychiatry. New York, NY. October 24–29, 2000.

[28] Briggs-Gowan MJ, Horwitz SM, et al. Mental health in pediatric settings: distribution of disorders and factors related to service use. J Am Acad Child Adolesc Psychiatry 2000;39:841–9.

[29] Costello EJ, Edelbrock C, Costello AJ, et al. Psychopathology in pediatric primary care: a new hidden morbidity. Pediatrics 1988;82:415–24.

[30] Horwitz SM, Leaf PJ, Leventhal JM et al. Identification and management of psychosocial and developmental problems in community-based, primary care pediatric practices. Pediatrics 1992;89:480–5.

[31] Kramer T, Garralda ME. Psychiatric disorders in adolescents in primary care. Br J Psychiatry 1998;173:508–13.

[32] Kramer T, Gledhill J, Garralda ME, et al. Identification and management of adolescent depression in primary care: feasibility and efficacy. Presented at the 9th Meeting of the International Society for Research on Child and Adolescent Psychopathology. Barcelona, Spain, 1999

[33] Lavigne JV, Arend R, Rosenbaum D et al. Mental health service use among young children receiving pediatric primary care. J Am Acad Child Adolesc Psychiatry 1998;37:1175–83.

[34] Ambrosini PJ, Metz C, Prabucki K et al. Videotape reliability of the third revised edition of the K-SADS. J Am Acad Child Adolesc Psychiatry 1989;28:723–8.

[35] Chang G, Warner V, Weissman MM. Physicians' recognition of psychiatric disorders in children and adolescents. American Journal of Diseases of Children 1988;142:736–9.

[36] Jacobsen L, Wilkinson C, Owen P. Is the potential of teenage consultations being missed?: a study of consultation times in primary care. Fam Pract 1994;11:296–9.

[37] Kelleher KJ, Childs GE, Wasserman RC, et al. Insurance status and recognition of psychosocial problems. A report from the Pediatric Research in Office Settings and the Ambulatory Sentinel Practice Networks. Arch Pediatr Adolesc Med 1997;151:1109–14.

[38] Scholle SH, Gardner W, Harman J, et al. Physician gender and psychosocial care for children: attitudes, practice characteristics, identification, and treatment. Med Care 2001;39:26–38.

[39] Beck AT, Guth D, Steer RA, et al. Screening for major depression disorders in medical inpatients with the Beck Depression Inventory for Primary Care. Behav Res Ther 1997;35:785–91.

[40] Winter LB, Steer RA, Jones-Hicks L, et al. Screening for major depression disorders in adolescent medical outpatients with the Beck Depression Inventory for Primary Care. J Adolesc Health 1999;24:389–94.

[41] Edelbrock C, Costello AJ, Dulcan MK, et al. Parent child agreement on child psychiatric symptoms assessed via structured interview. J Child Psychol Psychiatry 1986;27:181–90.

[42] Radloff L. The CES-D scale: a self report depression scale for research in the general population. Applied Psychological Measurement 1977;1:385–401.

[43] Jellinek MS, Murphy JM, Little M, et al. Use of the Pediatric Symptom Checklist to screen for

psychosocial problems in pediatric primary care: a national feasibility study. Arch Pediatr Adolesc Med 1999;153:254–60.

[44] Achenbach TM. Manual for the child behavior checklist / 4–18 and 1991 profile. Burlington (VT): Department of Psychiatry, University of Vermont; 1991.

[45] Gadow KDSJ. Adolescent Symptom Inventory-4: norms manual. Stony Brook (NY): Checkmate Plus; 1998.

[46] Wittchen HU, Lieb R, Wunderlich U, et al. Comorbidity in primary care: presentation and consequences. J Clin Psychiatry 1999;60:29–36; discussion 37–28.

[47] Lewinsohn PM, Seeley JR, Hibbard J et al. Cross-sectional and prospective relationships between physical morbidity and depression in older adolescents. J Am Acad Child Adolesc Psychiatry 1996;35:1120–9.

[48] Rushton JL, Clark SJ, Freed GL. Primary care role in the management of childhood depression: a comparison of pediatricians and family physicians. Pediatrics 2000;105:957–62.

[49] Steiner BD, Gest KL. Do adolescents want to hear preventive counseling messages in outpatient settings? J Fam Pract 1996;43:375–81.

[50] Sturm R, Wells KB. How can care for depression become more cost-effective? JAMA 1995; 273:51–8.

[51] Wells KB, Schoenbaum M, Unutzer J, et al. Quality of care for primary care patients with depression in managed care. Arch Fam Med 1999;8:529–36.

[52] Wells KB, Sturm R. Sherbourne CD, Meredith LS. Caring for depression. Cambridge (MA): Harvard University Press; 1996.

[53] Ormel J, Oldehinkel T, Brilman E, et al. Outcome of depression and anxiety in primary care. A three-wave 3 1/2-year study of psychopathology and disability. Arch Gen Psychiatry 1993; 50:759–66.

[54] Burns BJ, Costello EJ, Angold A, Tweed D, Stangl D, Farmer EMZ, et al. Children's mental health services use across service sectors. Health Aff 1995;14:147–59.

[55] Katon W, Schulberg H. Epidemiology of depression in primary care. Gen Hosp Psychiatry 1992;14:237–47.

[56] Bower P, Garralda E, Kramer T, et al. The treatment of child and adolescent mental health problems in primary care: a systematic review. Fam Pract 2001;18:373–82.

[57] Cooper PML. The impact of psychological treatments of postpartum depression on maternal mood and infant development. In: Murray PC, editor. Postpartum depression and child development. New York (NY): Guilford Press; 1997.

[58] Nicol R, Stretch D, Fundudis T. Preschool children in troubled families. Chichester (UK): John Wiley & Sons; 1993.

[59] Mufson L. Effectiveness study of IPT-A in school-based health clinics. Presented at the 47th Annual Meeting of the American Academy of Child and Adolescent Psychiatry, in. New York, NY. October 24–29, 2000.

[60] Rossello J, Bernal G. The efficacy of cognitive-behavioral and interpersonal treatments for depression in Puerto Rican adolescents. J Consult Clin Psychol 1999;67:734–45.

[61] Neira-Munoz EWD. Child Mental Health Services: Side by side. Health Serv J 1998;108:26–7.

[62] Rubenstein LV, Jackson-Triche M, Unutzer J, et al. Evidence-based care for depression in managed primary care practices. Health Aff (Millwood) 1999;18:89–105.

[63] Katon W, Von Korff M, Lin E, et al. Collaborative management to achieve treatment guidelines. Impact on depression in primary care. JAMA 1995;273:1026–31.

[64] Von Korff M, Gruman J, Schaefer J, et al. Collaborative management of chronic illness. Ann Intern Med 1997;127:1097–102.

[65] Wells KB, Sherbourne C, Schoenbaum M et al. Impact of disseminating quality improvement programs for depression in managed primary care: a randomized controlled trial. JAMA 2000; 283:212–20.

[66] Schoenbaum M, Unutzer J, Sherbourne C et al. Cost-effectiveness of practice-initiated quality improvement for depression: results of a randomized controlled trial. JAMA 2001;286: 1325–30.

[67] Von Korff M, Tiemens B. Individualized stepped care of chronic illness. West J Med 2000; 172:133–7.
[68] Katon W, Robinson P, Von Korff M et al. A multifaceted intervention to improve treatment of depression in primary care. Arch Gen Psychiatry 1996;53:924–32.
[69] Hunkeler EM, Meresman JF, Hargreaves WA, et al. Efficacy of nurse telehealth care and peer support in augmenting treatment of depression in primary care. Arch Fam Med 2000;9:700–8.
[70] Simon GE, VonKorff M, Rutter C, et al. Randomised trial of monitoring, feedback, and management of care by telephone to improve treatment of depression in primary care. BMJ 2000;320: 550–4.
[71] Brown J, Shye D, McFarland BH, et al. Controlled trials of CQI and academic detailing to implement a clinical practice guideline for depression. Jt Comm J Qual Improv 2000;26:39–54.
[72] Thompson C, Kinmonth AL, Stevens L, et al. Effects of a clinical-practice guideline and practice-based education on detection and outcome of depression in primary care: Hampshire Depression Project randomised controlled trial. Lancet 2000;355:185–91.
[73] Composite International Diagnostic Interview (CIDI) Core Version 2.1 interviewer's manual. Geneva: World Health Organization; 1997.
[74] Clarke G, DeBar L, Lynch F, et al. CBT for depressed adolescents receiving SSRIs in HMO primary care. Presented at the 47th Annual Meeting of the American Academy of Child and Adolescent Psychiatry, New York, NY. October 24–29, 2000.

Child Adolesc Psychiatric Clin N Am
11 (2002) 499–518

CHILD AND
ADOLESCENT
PSYCHIATRIC
CLINICS

Etiology and genetics of early-onset mood disorders

Richard D. Todd, PhD, MD*, Kelly N. Botteron, MD

Division of Child Psychiatry, Department of Psychiatry, Washington University School of Medicine,
660 South Euclid Avenue, Box 8134, St. Louis, MO 63110, USA

Although major depressive disorder and bipolar affective disorder are recognized as common, impairing, and frequently chronic illnesses by the mental health community, it is not generally recognized that mood disorders represent a significant fraction of the burden of disease on a worldwide basis. As detailed in the Global Burden of Disease study (a 5-year effort sponsored in part by the World Bank and the World Health Organization), major depressive disorders in adults, as defined by International Classification of Disease Version 9 (ICD-9-CM), ranked second in disease incidence, fourth in disease prevalence, fourth in hospital days, and third in disability-adjusted life years (one disability-adjusted life year is defined as the loss of one year of healthy life to disease) [1]. The disability and the social and economic loss associated with childhood- and adolescent-onset mood disorder can be expected to be higher per affected individual, because early-onset illness occurs during important developmental periods, is frequently recurrent, and frequently persists into adulthood. Suicide, the most serious outcome of depression, ranks among the top three causes of death for children aged 5 to 14 years and youth aged 15 to 24 years [2]. A recent analysis of the relationship between National Institutes of Health research funding and estimates of the burden of 29 diseases found that, with respect to disability-adjusted life years, depression is the most underfunded disease [3].

This article reviews what is currently known regarding the etiology and familial and genetic nature of early-onset mood disorders and the relationship of early-onset illness to adult illness. The primary focus is on epidemiology and genetic and imaging studies. This article updates and expands two recent reviews of early-onset mood disorders [4,5]. In this article, the term *early-onset* refers to an index episode occurring in childhood or early adolescence.

This work was supported in part by MH52813 (RDT) and MH01292 (KNB) from the National Institutes of Health, the Charles A Dana Foundation (RDT), and the National Alliance for Research on Schizophrenia and Affective Disorders (KNB)

* Corresponding author.

E-mail address: toddr@psychiatry.wustl.edu (R.D. Todd).

Behavioral genetics of major mood disorders in adults

A variety of family, twin, and adoption studies have demonstrated significant genetic influences on susceptibility to major depressive disorder and to bipolar affective disorder (manic depressive illness). The heritability of manic-depressive illness has generally been thought to be much higher than that of depression, although recent data suggest that this difference is partially explained by the poor reliability (temporal stability) of a lifetime diagnosis of mild major depression [6]. Compared with cross-sectional analyses, analyses of longitudinal data increase heritability estimates for major depression from about 40% to 70% [7–9]. The latter figure is comparable to that for manic-depressive disorder. Similar uncorrected heritabilities for major depressive disorder have been reported for population-based samples of women (0.4) [8] and men (0.4) [10,11] and for clinic-based samples of men and women (0.5) [10,12]. Twin studies indicate that depression seems equally heritable in men and women with largely overlapping genetic risk factors [10,12]. These studies have found little evidence for common environmental effects in the transmission of mania or depression. As described later, the authors find similar cross-sectional and longitudinal heritabilities for childhood- and adolescent-onset depression.

Familiality and continuity of early-onset mood disorder with adult illness

Family and twin studies suggest that early-onset mood disorders are also heritable [9,11,13–21], although there is debate about whether relatives of depressed prepubertal children have a higher risk for recurrence of depression [22,23]. In a prospective family study, Weissman et al [24] have shown that offspring who have adolescence-onset major depressive disorder have a high risk of recurrence of major depressive disorder and continuity of illness into adulthood. If there is a family history of major depressive disorder, both childhood- and adolescence-onset cases of major depressive disorder are likely to be recurrent and to continue in adulthood [24–26]. Similarly, Pine et al [27] have demonstrated that the reporting of symptoms of depression in adolescence prospectively predicts cases of major depressive disorder in young adulthood even in the absence of a depressive episode in adolescence. Hence, most studies agree that adolescence- (and perhaps childhood-) onset major depressive disorder (or symptoms of depression) is likely to be recurrent and to continue into adulthood. Childhood-onset depression may also progress to bipolar affective disorder in a substantial minority of cases [28–31]. This finding is in keeping with the high prevalence of major depressive disorder among the child and adolescent offspring of bipolar parents [18,19].

Little has been published regarding estimates of the heritability of early-onset depression or bipolar disorder in twins. Thapar and McGuffin [32] estimated the heritability of depressive symptom scores at 79% for a sample of 8- to 16-year-old twins. When the sample was split by age, significant genetic effects were found only for the 11- to 16-year-olds. In a separate epidemiologically based study the authors estimated the heritability of depressive symptoms in children. As part of a population-based twin study, they analyzed Child Behavior Checklist (CBCL) subscales [33] of a random sample of 286 pairs of male twins and 206 pairs of female twins aged 8 to 12 years [34]. Previous studies have demonstrated a close correspondence between major depressive disorder (as defined by the criteria in *The Diagnostic and Statistical Manual of Mental Disorders*–4th edition [DSM–IV]) and anxious/depressed subscale scores in children and adolescents [33,35]. The heritability of anxious/depressed behavior was 0.61 (95% confidence interval [CI], 0.48–0.71) for girls and 0.65 (95% CI, 0.55–0.73) for boys in this sample. Part of the discrepancy between these two twin studies may be the limited number of young twin pairs in the study by Thapar and McGuffin [32]. Early segregation analyses also suggested significant heritability for early-onset major depressive disorder and bipolar disorder [17].

Comorbidity as a subtyping approach to familial mood disorders

As recently reviewed by Spencer et al [36] and by Wozniak et al [37], individuals with early-onset bipolar disorder frequently meet criteria for attention deficit hyperactivity disorder (ADHD), conduct disorder, and oppositional defiant disorder. In a case-series study of childhood- versus adolescence-onset mania, Wozniak et al [37] found that cases of pediatric- and adolescence-onset mania had similar rates of bipolar symptoms and mixed-symptom episodes. The patterns of comorbidity differed substantially, however. In particular, whereas almost all pediatric-onset cases qualified for a diagnosis of ADHD, only half the adolescent onset cases had comorbid ADHD. Biederman and colleagues have extended these analyses of bipolar disorder to the familiality of comorbid conditions, reviewed in Spencer et al [36]. Faraone et al [38] presented evidence for the cofamiliality of bipolar disorder and ADHD in families identified through a boy who was comorbid for these two conditions. Recently, these findings have been replicated in families identified through girls with ADHD [39]. Based on these two studies, these researchers conclude that ADHD with bipolar disorder represents a familially distinct form of illness that may be related to what others have termed childhood-onset bipolar disorder. At the 2001 Annual Meeting of the American Academy of Child and Adolescent Psychiatry, the same group presented data supporting the possible existence of other distinct familial subtypes of early-onset bipolar disorder comorbid with conduct disorder [40,41] and comorbid with anxiety disorders [42]. These studies await replication from other research groups using similar or complementary analytic approaches.

Molecular genetics of major depressive disorder and bipolar affective disorder

Although a variety of linkage studies and candidate gene analyses have been published for bipolar affective disorder [43], fewer studies have been published for major depressive disorder. Hence, at present there are no compelling genetic linkage locations for major depressive disorder. The authors recognize that the genetic overlap between manic depressive illness and major depressive disorder, does suggest that testing of the reported linkage locations and candidate gene associations found in manic depressive illness be conducted in populations with major manic depressive disorder.

One exception is the serotonin transporter gene (5-HTT), in which a functionally significant polymorphism has been associated with major depressive disorder [44,45]. Two new studies suggest that 5-HTT is associated with certain components of depression rather than with major depressive disorder itself [46,47]. These results should be interpreted cautiously, however, because previous studies have demonstrated significant differences in allele frequencies as a function of ethnicity [48]. No similar analyses of early-onset depression have been published.

As discussed previously, many genomic surveys investigating possible genetic linkage in bipolar affective disorder have been published [43], and these surveys agree in some respects. No similar studies have been reported for families of patients with early-onset major depressive disorder. Undoubtedly, such families are included in existing linkage studies but no information has been presented in sufficient detail to assess evidence of linkage to early-onset cases per se. Sampling in adults has also suggested a wide variety of candidate genes for bipolar affective disorder. Only two studies have reported candidate genes for early-onset cases. These studies involved the serotonin transporter gene (5-HTT), and the catecholamine-O-methytransferase (COMT) gene [49,50]. In the study of the serotonin transporter gene, 46 complete trios consisting of a subject with early-onset bipolar affective disorder and both parents were genotyped for functional polymorphisms of the serotonin transporter promoter region. In the COMT study, 52 complete trios were genotyped for high- and low-activity alleles. No evidence for biased transmission of alleles was found for either gene. These initial studies do not support the association of these functional polymorphisms with early-onset bipolar affective disorder. The small sample sizes, however, preclude any firm conclusion about the role of these polymorphisms in early-onset bipolar disorder.

Prefrontal–subcortical limbic circuits in affective disorders

Increasing evidence from several lines of research suggests that specific prefrontal–subcortical limbic regions are highly interconnected in the neuronal circuits that are important in both normal affect regulation and in disorders of affective regulation such as major depressive disorder or bipolar disorder. The existence of such circuitry is supported by converging evidence from investigations of neurophysiology, cognitive functioning, lesion analysis, postmortem neuropathology, patterns of neuroanatomic connectedness, and animal models of depression or stress response. Space limitations prohibit a thorough review of this large body of literature, but readers are referred to several pertinent reviews [51–56]. Functional imaging measures, studies of specific physiologic or cognitive functions, postmortem neuropathologic studies, chemical or spectroscopic imaging, and structural imaging studies provide a remarkable convergence of support for the critical role of specific regions of the brain in modulating normal affective expression and show consistent corresponding differences between individuals with affective disorders and controls. A simplified schematic of the hypothesized neural network is illustrated in Fig. 1. In humans with affective disorders, functional and structural imaging studies have provided the greatest support for alterations in the function and structure of certain regions in these prefrontal-striatal-limbic circuits. These studies have shown alterations in specific prefrontal regions illustrated in Fig. 1 such as the ventral medial prefrontal cortex (VMPFC), the orbital frontal cortex (OFC), cingulate, amygdala and highly interconnected limbic portions of the striatum and mediodorsal thalamus. Many, but not all, studies of persons with affective disorders are also reported to show differences in other, more dorsal neocortical regions, including but not limited to the dorsal and lateral regions of the prefrontal cortex, the dorsal and posterior regions of the cingulated, and the posterior parietal cortex.

Only a limited number of imaging studies have been reported in children or adolescents with major depression or bipolar affective disorder. Recent reports suggest functional and structural differences that are consistent with this circuit model and are compatible with results from investigations in adults.

A brief review of a few representative adult studies provides some background for interpretation of the reported child and adolescent studies. Functional imaging studies in adults with positron emission tomography (PET) and functional MR imaging (fMR imaging) demonstrate that regions of the ventral medial and orbital frontal cortex, the subcallosal cingulate, ventral anterior cingulate, and amygdala are consistently identified as critical and necessary components of this circuit for affective regulation. Specifically, increased cerebral blood flow or metabolism in the ventral medial prefrontal cortex and portions of anterior cingulate has been consistently reported in adults with clinically ascertained depression [57–59]. Increased flow has also been reported in the amygdala, including alterations in amygdalar activity in relation to the induction of rapid-eye-movement (REM) sleep [60,61] A recent study designed explicitly to examine interactions in regional activity through examination of major depression and treatment response and through induction of sadness in nondepressed controls demonstrated strong reciprocal interactions with changes in blood flow in limbic and paralimbic regions (such as the anterior cingulate and insula) and neocortical regions (right dorsal lateral prefrontal cortex [DLPFC] and right parietal) in persons with depression and in controls [62]. Other PET studies of mood induction in normal individuals have consistently indicated that the ventral medial and orbital prefrontal cortex and the amygdala are involved in affective expression [63–65].

Subcortical and thalamic changes are also reported in functional imaging studies. Some studies have reported reduced flow in the medial caudate

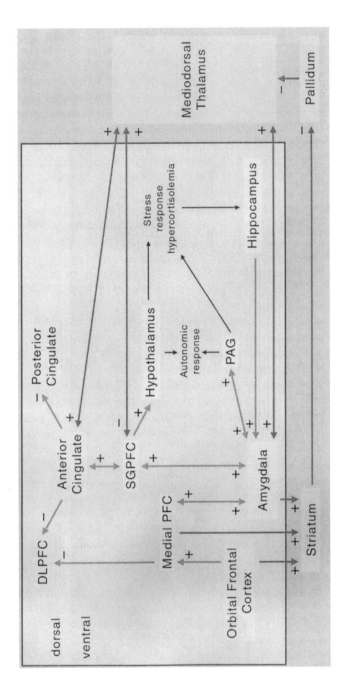

Fig. 1. Simplified model of circuitry for depression. Excitatory (+) and inhibitory (−) inputs are indicated. DLPPC, dorsal lateral prefrontal cortex; SGFPC, subgenual prefrontal cortex; PAG, periaquaductal gray matter; medial PFC, medial prefrontal cortex.

[57,62,66]. Alterations in medial dorsal thalamic activity have also been consistently reported as a state-type change [57,67]. Specific neurologic diseases of the striatum, such as Parkinson's disease, Huntington's disease, and strokes affecting the caudate, are associated with high rates of secondary depression. Positron emission tomographic studies of secondary depression in these disorders have reported decreased metabolic activity in the caudate and orbital frontal cortex [62,68].

Although many conflicting results have been reported for structural brain changes in adults with affective disorders, recent critical reviews by the authors [67,69,70] and others [71] indicate that major depression is associated with specific neuromorphometric differences in some regions of this circuit (see Fig. 1). The number of reported structural imaging studies in affective disorders is severalfold less than those reported in schizophrenia, and many technical considerations limit the interpretation of many studies conducted more than 8 or 10 years ago. Nevertheless, a meta-analysis of earlier and more recent studies [72] shows increases in lateral and third ventricular volume, reduction in caudate volume, and possibly a reduction or change in lateralization in total prefrontal lobe volume. Recent advances in MR imaging technology and image analysis have allowed more precise volumetric definition of smaller, more anatomically relevant regions than was possible even 7 or 8 years ago. Using these improved methods, several studies have reported that structures in the ventral medial prefrontal-striatal-pallidal-thalamic circuit may be reduced or increased in volume in adults with a history of major depressive disorder or bipolar affective disorder. Decreases in core amygdala volume [73] or changes in amygdala lateralization [74] have been reported in some persons with depression, although other investigators have reported no differences [75,76]. Several studies have also reported reduced hippocampal volume in persons with major depression [74,76,77] or in persons with depression who did not respond to treatment [78], whereas other investigators have found no difference between persons with major depression and controls [79,80].

Imaging studies of early-onset major depressive disorder

Few published MR imaging studies of children and adolescents with major depressive disorder have been published [81]. In a retrospective analysis of MR imaging scans obtained clinically on hospitalized children and adolescents, Steingard et al [81 reported that this group of children had decreased frontal lobe volume and increased lateral ventricular size in comparison with hospitalized psychiatric controls. In a pilot study of an epidemiologically ascertained sample of adolescent and young-adult women with adolescent-onset depression (30 participants with depression and 18 controls) the authors demonstrated a significant reduction in left subgenual prefrontal cortex (SGPFC) volume [82]. This finding was consistent with their earlier demonstration of a highly significant reduction in the left SGPFC in both primary major depressive disorder and in manic depressive disorder in middle-aged adults. This change in adults is associated with decreased metabolic activity in depression but with increased activity in mania [83]. This region of the subcallosal cingulate is part of the hypothesized prefrontal-limbic circuits and is also part of the ventromedial prefrontal cortex system that Damasio [51] believes to be responsible for mediating autonomic responses to emotional experiences. There was no significant correlation between volume reduction and length of illness as measured by number of recurrences or age of onset (RD Todd et al, unpublished data, 2000). This finding has been replicated in individuals with first-episode psychosis with affective disorder [84,85]. Together these findings suggest some continuity in structural anatomy between early-onset and adult-onset mood disorders.

Hippocampal changes in structure and function have been reported in some but not in other studies in adults. No results have been published of studies in children or adolescents with depression or bipolar disorder. As illustrated, the hippocampus has afferent and efferent connections to these circuits; however, it may not be a necessary component for affective functioning. For example, hippocampal lesions have not been associated with affective dysfunction. The hippocampus, however, is known to be a region that is sensitive to excitotoxicity and hypercortisolemic damage [86–88] and has been reported to be reduced in volume in several (but not all) MR imaging studies of persons with major depression. Therefore, the hippocampus may be a suitable region for further investigation of potential neurodegenerative changes related to proposed excitotoxic mechanisms resulting from hypercortisolemia associated with repeated or prolonged episodes of depression.

In studies published to date, the ventral medial prefrontal limbic regions (orbital frontal, ventral medial prefrontal, subgenual cortex, and amygdala) are more consistently reported as critical in affective function and disorder and may be more primary in the pathophysiology of mood disorders. Other regions such as the dorsal lateral prefrontal cortex, posterior cingulate, parietal cortex, basal ganglia, and thalamus may be more secondarily involved in familial early-onset affective disorders. The proposed primary affective circuitry cannot explain all the symptomatology of affective disorders, such as inattention, poor concentration, or other cognitive deficits. Such symptoms undoubtedly involve interactions with the more dorsal cingulate, dorsal prefrontal, and parietal regions [62]. Alterations in the proposed circuitry may be sufficient to explain changes in approach-withdrawal behaviors, assessment of affective or reward valence of stimuli, hypothalamic-pituitary-adrenal (HPA) axis dysregulation, and, possibly, severity or chronicity. The ventral medial prefrontal cortex and amygdala are highly interconnected with the hypothalamus and brainstem regions that are important in the regulation of stress response [89]. Although the specific findings of HPA axis dysfunction are somewhat different in children and adolescents than in adults, studies in childhood and adolescent mood disorders have reported significant alterations in parameters of HPA dysfunction, such as alterations in growth hormone regulation [90,91] and cortisol dysregulation. Several authors have recently reviewed the complex and somewhat conflicting literature related to neuroendocrine studies in early-onset mood disorders [92,93].

Imaging studies of early-onset bipolar disorder

A few neuroimaging studies in childhood and adolescent bipolar affective disorder have been published. All have been small in scale and reported as pilot studies [94–96]. Botteron et al [94] reported a loss of normal prefrontal lobe asymmetry in a sample of eight 8- to 16-year-olds with mania in comparison with five age-matched controls. This study also reported a 25% rate of significant deep white matter hyperintensities, consistent with a number of studies in adults. Although such studies are preliminary, several presentations at recent meetings of the American Academy of Child and Adolescent Psychiatry suggest there is continuity between early- and later-onset bipolar disorder with respect to at least some biologic findings. Structural imaging studies of adults with bipolar affective disorder have reported enlarged ventricles, decreased volume of temporal lobes and thalamus, abnormalities in the size of the amygdala, and increased frequencies of deep white matter hyperintensities. New data on 42 boys with early-onset bipolar disorder demonstrated smaller total cerebral cortex and thalamus volumes as well as decreased size of the hippocampus and the right amygdala [97]. There were also suggestions that there may be unique anatomic brain changes in pediatric bipolar disorder. Taking a different approach, DelBello [98] reported imaging studies of asymptomatic children who are the offspring of bipolar disorder parents. Using structural MR imaging he found that children at risk for bipolar disorder demonstrated structural changes similar to those found in children and adults with bipolar disorder, suggesting that the structural abnormalities may be present before the onset of symptomatology and that similar abnormalities are present across the age span.

A few brain chemistry studies have been reported. Using proton magnetic resonance spectroscopy in the same high-risk group of children, DelBello [98] found evidence for decreased N-acetylaspartate (NAA) and creatine (CR) in cerebellar regions and increased levels of myoinositol (MI) in orbital frontal gray matter, as has been reported for adult patients with bipolar disorder. In a small sample of 11 persons with early-onset bipolar disorder and 11 normal controls Davanzo et al [99] found a trend in patients with early-onset bipolar disorder towards higher MI/CR ratios in the anterior cingulate region during the manic phase. This ratio was significantly reduced following acute lithium treatment. Castillo et al [100] found no difference in NAA or choline (Cho) in the same regions in a group of 10 prepubertal patients with bipolar disorder and in controls. They did find elevated levels of glutamate and glutamine and lipids in frontal lobes. Though not definitive, these studies suggest that many of the neurobiologic abnormalities found in adult patients with bipolar disorder also exist in childhood-onset illness and in children at risk for the development for bipolar disorder. There are suggestions that there may also be specific abnormalities in pediatric-onset cases.

Lateralization of functional and structural changes

A substantial body of literature [53,101,102], which because of space considerations cannot be reviewed in any detail here, demonstrates that there are lateralized differences in affective processing in both normal expression and affective disorders. Since the late 1800s it has been noted that left-sided cerebral lesions are commonly associated with depressive reactions, and right-sided lesions are associated with more activated, disinhibited, or maniclike states. Numerous studies of depression following stroke and other lesions have demonstrated this lateralized association. Robinson et al conducted a number of studies examining this lateralization and reported an increased risk for secondary major depressive disorder with left frontal lesions, the risk increasing with the proximity of the lesions to the frontal pole (reviewed in [103]). Similar results were found for major depressive disorder resulting from traumatic brain injury [103] and multiple sclerosis [104]. Several authors have also reported an association with right or bilateral ventral medial or orbital frontal lesions and disinhibited behavior or maniclike syndromes and a loss of usual autonomic reactivity [105,106]. Lesions involving bilateral ventral medial frontal cortex are also associated with similar syndromes. There are few studies or reports of individuals with left ventral medial lesions. Davidson and others hypothesized that in general the left prefrontal lobe is important in approach and exploratory behavior [101,107], whereas the right prefrontal lobe is more specialized for withdrawal behavior or negative affect. Because the number of studies completed to date is small, and all involve only a small number of participants, it is unclear if differences in structural lateralization in many regions are associated with major depressive disorder. The findings of Drevets et al [83], which have subsequently been replicated by Hirayasu et al [84] and by Botteron et al [82], demonstrate reduced left subgenual prefrontal cortical volume.

Neuropathology of cortical differences seen on MR imaging

In neuropathologic studies of the SGPFC, Drevets et al [57,108] have found decreased gray matter volume and decreased glial cell counts but normal neuron cell counts in tissue from the brains of depressive and manic depressive patients. Using unbiased stereologic sampling methods, the agranular portion of the subgenual part of Brodman's area 24 (Sg24, which roughly corresponds to the area of SGPFC measured on MR scans) was reduced in volume by about 20% in brains from patients with major depressive disorder and those with manic depressive disorder. Glial cell density (cells/mm^3) was reduced by 40% to 50% in both disorders compared with controls. No differences in neuron number were seen. There were no changes in glial number or density in somatosensory area 3b. In a different series, Rajkowska et al [109] have reported similar glial findings in prefrontal areas. In this study, some areas also had modest decreases in neuronal size. The reductions in volume and glial cell number in region Sg24 were greater for brains from patients who had an affected first-degree relative [83,108]. This finding is similar to the imaging study of Hirayasu et al [84,85], who report decreases in left SGPFC volume in depressive patients only if there is a positive family history for depression. The authors' original study primarily used probands of families with multiple incidences of affective disorder [83].

Selective glial cell loss has not been previously reported for any CNS disorder. Most neurodegenerative diseases or brain injuries result in glial proliferation. In the context of previous family and genetic studies the current neuropathologic results, although based on only a few postmortem samples, suggest that reduced glial cell number may be a transmissible neurodevelopmental process. Alternatively, reduced glial cell number may reflect the effects of exposure to psychotropic drugs or alcohol or to other illness-related processes in genetically predisposed individuals. Reduced SGPFC volume may be a marker for a glial pathophysiology of depression and could represent an "endo" phenotype for clinical and genetic studies of the affective disorders. Of note, astrocytes (a major class of glial cells present in the SGPFC) are known to express both serotonin receptors and transporters. As discussed previously, serotonin pathway components have been proposed as candidate genes for the affective disorders because of the known effects of antidepressant medications.

In summary, imaging and neuropathologic studies have focused attention on ventral and medial prefrontal limbic circuits as the core neural substrates of mood disorders. Changes in these circuits associated with mania and major depressive disorder are frequently lateralized and are more commonly seen in familial cases of mania and major depressive disorder. The authors have replicated some of these findings in adolescence-onset major depressive disorder. Together these findings suggest that the clinical and morphologic features of mood disorders may be mediated by the same genetic factors.

Genetics of brain morphometry

Studies in mammals and other organisms demonstrate that there are important genetic and environmental components to the development of CNS structures. For example, in a recent special issue of the journal *Cerebral Cortex* the effects of 52 individual genes on cortical development were reviewed [110]. Similarly, changes in sensory input to specific cortical areas can result in differences in brain cortical folding patterns [80]. Although some clinical syndromes have been related to gross changes in brain structure, and specific hypotheses can be put forward for genes that are homologous to those found in flies, worms, or rodents, little is known about the specifics of the genetic control of brain structure in humans. Less is known about the heritability of individual variations in specific brain structures.

Most studies that address the familiality or genetics of brain volume or regional brain volume differences in humans have been small studies of normal twin pairs or the study of discordant twins with schizophrenia and unaffected family members of schizophrenic patients [111,112]. These studies suggest that certain imaging abnormalities associated with psychosis are familial, whereas others may result from illness. Because monozygotic twins are genetically identical, brain volume differences in twins discordant for schizophrenia have been interpreted as being caused by environmental effects such as sequelae of illness or as indicating an environmental effect operating on predisposing genes which do not cause imaging abnormalities per se [113].

Small studies of normal twins have examined the familiality of regional cortical surface areas or gyral patterns. Each study has examined a small sample size and has used a different methodologic approach. Biondi et al [114] reported clear similarity in the qualitative analysis of gyral patterns in monozygotic twins, with six expert raters correctly matching twin pairs based on cortical surface reconstructions. Bartley et al [115] examined 10 monozygotic and 9 dizygotic pairs reporting strong heritability for total brain volume but little genetic contribution to gyral patterns based on two-dimensional gyral representations. Tramo et al [116] compared regional cortical areas in 10 monozygotic twin pairs and in 20 unrelated adults and found a much stronger resemblance between twin pairs than between unrelated pairs. Although these studies offer tantalizing suggestions of significant heritabilities, limitations in the sample sizes and study designs limit conclusions to the observation that certain neuroanatomic features, including surface area and gyral patterns, are familial.

Several new twin studies of brain morphometry have been published recently. Carmelli et al [117] reported on the heritability of cross-sectional areas in MR imaging scans of a group of 85 elderly male twin pairs who were part of a longitudinal study of risk factors for cardiovascular disease. Univariate analyses estimated the contributions of additive genetic factors, shared environmental factors, and unique environmental factors to variations in morphometric measures. The additive genetic contributions to corpus callosum and lateral ventricular cross-sectional areas were both 0.79 with no contribution of shared environment. Pennington et al [118] reported on the heritability of cortical and noncortical volume factors (derived from factor analysis of volume data from 13 brain regions) in a group of 18 control twin pairs and 48 twin pairs in which at least one twin had a reading disability. Correlations for both factors and for both brain hemispheres were higher in the monozygotic pairs than in the dizygotic pairs. LeGoualher et al [119] also applied principal component analysis to the shape of the central sulcus in a group of 10 monozygotic and 10 dizygotic twin pairs and found monozygotic twins to be more similar. Although the nature and size of the samples preclude firm conclusions, the results of these studies are compatible with moderate to marked heritabilities for cortical and subcortical brain volume.

The authors know of no similar family or twin studies of brain morphometry for major depressive disorder or bipolar disorder in childhood or adolescence.

Assessing prevalence and heritability of early-onset mood disorders in the general population: preliminary results

As reviewed elsewhere [5], there are few epidemiologically based prevalence studies for early-onset mood disorders. As part of an ongoing epidemiologically based adolescent female twin study of alcohol and substance abuse in which both twin interviews or a parent interview have been completed, the authors have currently identified 276 individuals who had a DSM–IV major depressive disorder based on self-reporting or on parental report if no self-reported data were available. This total included 186 twins from pairs that were discordant at initial assessment. Based on this single cross-sectional assessment, the authors observe probandwise concordance rates of 39% for monozygotic female pairs and concordance of 25% rates for dizygotic female pairs (13.6% lifetime prevalence of depression), yielding an additive genetic heritability estimate of 53% [120]. A subgroup of twins was re-interviewed 1 to 3 years later as part of an imaging study. When these data are combined with the original interview data in a common pathway analysis, the heritability of major depressive disorder increases to 65% (95% CI, 45%–85%) [120]. Less than one third of these cases of depression had come to clinical attention, and fewer than 10% had received antidepressant medications. The average length of an episode of major depression was 28.0 ± 31.2 weeks (range, 2–104 weeks, median 12 weeks), and 38.5% of participants reported one or more recurrent episodes (the number of previous episodes was not recorded). The median age of onset of first episode was 16 years (range, 5–19 years) with only 2.8% of participants reporting onset before 11 years of age.

In summary, depression in general-population samples of child, adolescent, and young-adult twins is significantly heritable in both boys and girls (0.50–0.65). Given the length of episodes and degree of recurrence, major depressive disorder detected in adolescents and young adults in the authors' two twin samples is clinically significant and largely untreated. This finding is consistent with economic-impact studies demonstrating that untreated depression in adults is a larger public health problem than many other psychiatric or medical disorders [1,3].

In a birth records–based twin study of female ADHD in the state of Missouri the authors have found evidence for the presence of multiple, genetically independent forms of ADHD that overlap only partially with DSM–IV ADHD subtypes [121]. Although conduct disorder was rare, and mania was not assessed in this sample, there was little evidence for transmission of anxiety or depressive symptoms or diagnoses with most of these ADHD subtypes [122]. In contrast, oppositional defiant disorder was cotransmitted with two ADHD subtypes [54]. In a companion birth records–based study of ADHD including female, male, and opposite-sex twin pairs in Missouri, the authors did assess mania (RD Todd, et al, submitted). In the first 600 twin pairs aged 7 through 17 years who have completed full diagnostic evaluations (including 175 random control families) there were two cases of mania and two cases of hypomania (lifetime diagnoses). One case of mania occurred in the 175 random control families (1 of 350 twins, 0.3%), consistent with findings that mania is uncommon in this age group. One case of mania and the two cases of hypomania occurred in the presence of ADHD (0.7% of ADHD cases), consistent with an increased prevalence of mania comorbid with ADHD. The low comorbidity rate of mania with ADHD in this sample suggests that this is not a common genetic subtype of ADHD or bipolar disorder in the general population.

How do estimates of heritability of early-onset mood disorders and regional brain volumes relate?

Preliminary univariate and bivariate genetic analyses of some regional brain volumes and depression have been completed with 32 of the adolescent or young adult female twin pairs described previously. All analyses were conducted using the statistical package Mx [123]. Models were compared using maximum likelihood estimation. The best-fitting univariate models for different brain volumes included additive genetic (a^2) and unique environment (e^2) terms but no common environment (c^2). As described previously, the common pathway model for the transmission of current and past depressive episodes gave a heritability of 65% for the MR imaging sample [120]. Simple heritabilities for brain volume ranged as follows: total brain volume, 0.52; total prefrontal lobe volume, 0.25; total SGPFC volume, 0.30. Heritabilities were similar for right and left prefrontal lobe and SGPFC [124]. Bivariate analysis of the effect of regional brain volume on heritability of depression demonstrated significant correspondence of the genetic contribution to total SGPFC volume with that for depression, with little sharing of genetic factors between prefrontal lobe volume and depression (although confidence intervals at the estimated genetic correlations were broad because of the limited sample size) [125,126]. A larger sample is required to estimate these parameters accurately and to conduct multivariate analyses.

Summary

Most studies dealing with the familiality and genetics of mood disorders have been limited to adults, but several studies suggest that there is continuity between childhood- and adolescence-onset depression and mania and adult illness. More direct estimates of the heritability of depressive symptoms or episodes in children and adolescents indicate that the genetic contributions may be greater than 50%. A number of functional and structural imaging studies have identified particular circuitry as being involved in the generation of emotion and mood disorders. Imaging studies of twins have suggested that regional brain volume and characteristics of brain shape are heritable. A potentially important new avenue of research will be the correlation of the genetics of brain structure or function with the genetics of mood disorders. Preliminary studies of adolescent and young adult twins suggest a significant correspondence between the genetic contributions to some regional brain volumes and early-onset mood disorders.

References

[1] Murray CJ, Lopez AD. Evidence-based health policy – lessons from the Global Burden of Disease Study. Science 1996;274:740.

[2] Center for Disease Control and Prevention. Deaths and death rates for the 10 leading causes of death in specified age groups, by Hispanic origin, race for non-Hispanic population, and sex. United States 2000. National Vital Statistics Reports 2000;48:37.

[3] Gross CP, Anderson GF, Powe NR. The relation between funding by the National Institutes of Health and the burden of disease. N Engl J Med 1999;340:1881.

[4] Todd RD, Botteron KN. Family, genetic, and imaging studies of early-onset depression. Child Adolesc Psychiatric Clin North Am 2001;10:375.

[5] Todd RD. Genetics of early onset bipolar affective disorder: are we making progress? Curr Psychiatry Rep 2002;4:141.

[6] Rice JP, Rochberg M, Endicott J, et al. Stability of psychiatry diagnoses: an application to the affective disorders. Arch Gen Psychiatry 1992;49:824.

[7] Kendler KS, Neale MC, Kessler RC, et al. A longitudinal twin study of 1-year prevalence of major depression in women. Arch Gen Psychiatry 1993;50:843.

[8] Kendler KS, Neale MC, Kessler RC, et al. A population-based twin study of major depression in women. Arch Gen Psychiatry 1992;49:257.

[9] Kendler KS, Neale MC, Kessler RC, et al. The lifetime history of major depression in women: reliability and heritability. Arch Gen Psychiatry 1993;50:863.

[10] Kendler KS, Prescott CA. A population-based twin study of lifetime major depression in men and women. Arch Gen Psychiatry 1999;56:39.

[11] Lyons MJ, Eisen SA, Goldberg J, et al. A registry-based twin study of depression in men. Arch Gen Psychiatry 1998;55:468.

[12] Bierut LJ, Heath AC, Bucholz KK, et al. Major depressive disorder in a community-based twin sample – are there different genetic and environmental contributions for men and women? Arch Gen Psychiatry 1999;56:557.

[13] Kovacs M, Devlin B, Pollock M, et al. A controlled family history study of childhood-onset depressive disorder. Arch Gen Psychiatry 1997;54:613.

[14] Kutcher SP, Marton P. Affective disorders in first-degree relatives and adolescent bipolar, unipolar and normal controls. J Am Acad Child Adolesc Psychiatry 1991;30:75.

[15] Orvaschel HH. Early onset psychiatry disorder in high risk children and increased familial morbidity. J Am Acad Child Adolesc Psychiatry 1990;29:184.

[16] Rice J, Reich T, Andreasen NC, et al. The familial transmission of bipolar illness. Arch Gen Psychiatry 1987;44:441.

[17] Todd RD, Neuman R, Geller B, et al. Genetic studies of affective disorders: should we be starting with childhood onset probands? J Am Acad Child Adolesc Psychiatry 1993;32:1164.

[18] Todd RD, Reich W, Petti T, et al. Psychiatric diagnoses in the child and adolescent members of extended families identified through bipolar affective disorder probands. J Am Acad Child Adolesc Psychiatry 1996;35:664.

[19] Todd RD, Reich W, Reich T. Prevalence of affective disorder in the child and adolescent offspring of a single kindred: a pilot study. J Am Acad Child Adolesc Psychiatry 1994;33:198.

[20] Weissman MM, Gershon ES, Kidd KK, et al. Psychiatric disorders in the relatives of probands with affective disorders. Arch Gen Psychiatry 1984;41:13.

[21] Williamson DE, Ryan ND, Birmaher B, et al. A case-control family history study of depression in adolescents. J Am Acad Child Adolesc Psychiatry 1995;34:1596.

[22] Harrington R, Rutter M, Weissman M, et al. Psychiatric disorders in the relatives of depressed probands. I. comparison of prepubertal, adolescent and early onset cases. J Affect Disord 1997; 42:9.

[23] Neuman RJ, Geller B, Rice JP, et al. Increased prevalence and earlier onset of mood disorders among relatives of prepubertal versus adult probands. J Am Acad Child Adolesc Psychiatry 1997;36:466.

[24] Weissman MM, Wolk S, Goldstein RB, et al. Depressed adolescents grown up. JAMA 1999; 12:1707.

[25] Weissman MM, Wolk S, Wickramaratne P, et al. Children with prepubertal-onset major depressive disorder and anxiety grown up. Arch Gen Psychiatry 1999;56:794.

[26] Wickramaratne PJ, Warner V, Weissman NM. Selecting early onset MDD probands for genetic studies: results from a longitudinal high-risk study. Am J Med Genet 2000;96:93.

[27] Pine DS, Cohen E, Cohen P, et al. Adolescent depressive symptoms as predictors of adult depression: moodiness or mood disorder? Am J Psychiatry 1999;156:133.

[28] Birmaher B, Ryan ND, Williamson DE, et al. Childhood and adolescent depression: a review of the past 10 years. Part I. J Am Acad Child Adolesc Psychiatry 1996;35:1427.

[29] Geller B, Fox LW, Clark KA. Rate and predictors of prepubertal bipolarity during follow-up of 6- to 12-year-old depressed children. J Am Acad Child Adolesc Psychiatry 1994;33:461.

[30] Geller B, Zimerman B, Williams M, et al. Reliability of the Washington University in St. Louis Kiddie Schedule for Affective Disorders and Schizophrenia (WASH-U-KSADS) mania and rapid cycling sections. J Am Acad Child Adolesc Psychiatry 2001;40:450–5.

[31] Strober M, Lampert C, Schmidt S, et al. The course of major depressive disorder in adolescents: I. recovery and risk of manic switching in a follow-up of psychotic and nonpsychotic subtypes. J Am Acad Child Adoles Psychiatry 1993;32:34.

[32] Thapar A, McGuffin P. A twin study of depressive symptoms in childhood. Br J Psychiatry 1994; 165:259.

[33] McConaughy SH, Achenbach TM. Comorbidity of empirically based syndromes in matched general population and clinical samples. J Child Psychol Psychiatry 1994;35:1141.

[34] Hudziak JJ, Rudiger LP, Neale MC, et al. A twin study of inattentive, aggressive and anxious/depressed behaviors. J Am Acad Child Adolesc Psychiatry 2000;39:469.

[35] Achenbach TM. Integrative guide for the 1991 CBCL/4–18, YSR and TRF profiles. Burlington (VT): Department of Psychiatry, University of Vermont; 1991.

[36] Spencer TJ, Biederman J, Wozniak J, et al. Parsing pediatric bipolar disorder from its associated comorbidity with the disruptive behavior disorders. Biol Psychiatry 2001;49:1062.

[37] Wozniak J, Biederman J, Richards JA. Diagnostic and therapeutic dilemmas in the management of pediatric-onset bipolar disorder. J Clin Psychiatry 2001;62:10–5.

[38] Faroane SV, Biederman J, Mennin D, et al. Attention deficit hyperactivity disorder with bipolar disorder: a familial subtype? J Am Acad Child Adolesc Psychiatry 1997;36:1378–87.

[39] Faraone SV, Biederman J, Monuteaux MC. Attention deficit hyperactivity disorder with bipolar in girls: further evidence for a familial subtype? J Affect Disord 2001;64:19.

[40] Faraone SV. Comorbidity of juvenile bipolar disorder with antisocial behavior disorders. In: Proceedings of the 48th Annual Meeting of the American Academy of Child and Adolescent Psychiatry. Honolulu: Hilton Hawaii Village; 2001:29A.

[41] Faraone SV, Biederman J, Mennin D, et al. Bipolar and antisocial disorders among relatives of ADHD children: parsing familial subtypes of illness. Am J Med Genet 1998;81:108.

[42] Wozniak J. Comorbidity of juvenile bipolar disorder with multiple anxiety disorders. In: Proceedings of the 48th Annual Meeting of the American Academy of Child and Adolescent Psychiatry. Honolulu: Hilton Hawaii Village; 2001:29D.

[43] Prathikanti S, McMahon FJ. Genome scans for susceptibility genes in bipolar affective disorder. Annals of Medicine 2001;33:257.

[44] Du LS, Faludi G, Palkovits M, et al. Frequency of long allele in serotonin transporter gene is increased in depressed suicide victims. Biol Psychiatry 1999;46:196.

[45] Furlong RA, Ho L, Walsh C, et al. Analysis and meta-analysis of two serotonin transporter gene polymorphisms in bipolar and unipolar affective disorders. Am J Med Genet 1998;81:58.

[46] Kim DK, Lim SW, Lee S, et al. Serotonin transporter gene polymorphism and antidepressant response. Neuroreport 2000;11:215.

[47] Russ MJ, Lachman HM, Kashdan T, et al. Analysis of catechol-O-methyltransferase and 5-hydroxytryptamine transporter polymorphisms in patients at risk for suicide. Psychiatry Today 2000;93:73.

[48] Gelernter J, Kranzler H, Cubells JF. Serotonin transporter protein (SLC6A4) allele and haplotype frequencies and linkage disequilibria in African- and European-American and Japanese populations and in alcohol-dependent subjects. Human Genet 1997;101:243.

[49] Geller B, Cook Jr EH. Ultradian rapid cycling in prepubertal and early adolescent bipolarity is not in transmission disequilibrium with val/met COMT alleles. Biol Psychiatry 2000;47:605.

[50] Geller B, Cook EH. Serotonin transporter gene (HTTLPR) is not in linkage disequilibrium with prepubertal and early adolescent bipolarity. Biol Psychiatry 1999;45:1230.

[51] Damasio AR. Descarte's error: emotion, reason, and the human brain. New York: Grosset/Putnam; 1995.

[52] Drevets WC, Todd RD. Depression, mania and related disorders. In: Guze SB, editor. Adult psychiatry. St. Louis (MO): Mosby; 1997. p. 99.

[53] Liotti M, Tucker DM. Emotion in asymmetric corticolimbic networks. In: Davidson RJ, Hugdahl H, editors. Brain asymmetry. Cambridge, MA: The MIT Press; 1995. p. 389.

[54] Mayberg HS. Limbic-cortical dysregulation: a proposed model of depression. J Neuropsychiatry Clin Neurosci 1997;9:471.

[55] Starkstein SE, Robinson RG. Depression and frontal lobe disorders. In: Miller BL, Cummings JL, editors. The human frontal lobes: functions and disorders. New York: Guilford Press; 1999. p. 537.

[56] Swerdlow NR, Koob GF. Dopamine, schizophrenia, mania and depression: toward a unified hypothesis of cortico-striato-pallido-thalamic function. Behav Brain Sci 1987;10:197.

[57] Drevets WC. Onghr D, Price JL: Neuroimaging abnormalities in the subgenual prefrontal cortex implications for the pathophysiology of familial mood disorders. Mol Psychiatry 1998;3:220.

[58] Ketter TA, Kimbrell TA, George MS, et al. Baseline cerebral hypermetabolism associated with carbamazepine response, and hypometabolism with nimodipine response in mood disorders. Biol Psychiatry 1999;46:1364.

[59] Mayberg HS, Brannan SK, Mahurin RK, et al. Cingulate function in depression: a potential predictor of treatment response. Neuroreport 1997;8:1057.

[60] Ho AP, Gillin JC, Buchsbaum MS, et al. Brain glucose metabolism during non-rapid eye movement sleep major depression. A positron emission tomography study. Arch Gen Psychiatry 1996;53:645.

[61] Nofzinger EA, Nichols TE, Meltzer CC, et al. Changes in forebrain function from waking to REM sleep in depression: preliminary analyses of [18F]FDG PET studies. Psychiatry Res 1999;91:59.

[62] Mayberg HS, Loitti M, Brannan SK, et al. Reciprocal limbic-cortical function and negative mood: converging PET findings in depression and normal sadness. Am J Psychiatry 1999;156:675.

[63] George MS, Ketter TA, Parekh PI, et al. Brain activity during transient sadness and happiness in healthy women. Am J Psychiatry 1995;152:341.

[64] Paradiso S, Johnson DL, Andreasen NC, et al. Cerebral blood flow changes associated with attribution of emotional valence to pleasant, unpleasant, and neutral visual stimuli in a PET study of normal subjects. Am J Psychiatry 1999;156:1618.

[65] Teasdale JD, Howard RJ, Cox SG, et al. Functional MRI study of the cognitive generation of affect. Am J Psychiatry 1999;156:209.

[66] Elliott R, Baker SC, Rogers RD, et al. Prefrontal dysfunction in depressed patients performing a complex planning task: a study using positron emission tomography. Psychol Med 1997;27:931.

[67] Botteron KN, Figiel GS. The neuromorphometry of affective disorders. In: Krishnan KRR, Doraiswamy M, editors. Brain imaging in clinical psychiatry. New York: Dekker; 1997. p. 145.

[68] Mayberg HS, Starkstein SE, Peyser CE, et al. Paralimbic frontal lobe hypometabolism in depression associated with Huntington's disease. Neurology 1992;42:1791.

[69] Drevets W, Botteron KN. Neuroimaging in psychiatry. In: SB Guze, editor. Adult psychiatry. St Louis (MO): Mosby; 1996. p. 53.

[70] Krishnan K, Boyko OB, Botteron KN, et al. Imaging in psychiatric disorders. In: Greenberg JO,

editor. Neuroimaging: a comparison to Adams and Victor's principles of neurology 2nd edition. New York: McGraw-Hill; 1999. p. 273.

[71] Soares JC, Mann JJ. The anatomy of mood disorders review of structural neuroimaging studies. Biol Psychiatry 1997;41:86.

[72] Jeste DV, Lohr JB, Goodwin FK. Neuroanatomical studies of major affective disorders. Br J Psychiatry 1988;153:444.

[73] Sheline YI, Gado MH, Price JL. Amygdala core nuclei volumes are decreased in recurrent major depression. Neuroreport 1998;9:2023.

[74] Mervaala E, Fohr J, Kononen M, et al. Quantitative MRI of the hippocampus and amygdala in severe depression. Psychol Med 2000;30:117.

[75] Ashtari M, Greenwald BS, Kramer-Ginsberg E, et al. Hippocampal/amygdala volumes in geriatric depression. Psychol Med 1999;29:629.

[76] Bremner JD, Narayan M, Anderson ER, et al. Hippocampal volume reduction in major depression. Am J Psychiatry 2000;157:115.

[77] Sheline YI, Sanghavi M, Mintun MA, et al. Depression duration but not age predicts hippocampal volume loss in medically healthy women with recurrent major depression. J Neurosci 1999;19:5034.

[78] Pillay SS, Renshaw PF, Bonello CM, et al. A quantitative magnetic resonance imaging study of caudate and lenticular nucleus gray matter volume in primary unipolar major depression: relationship to treatment response and clinical severity. Psychiatry Res 1998;84:61.

[79] Coffey CE, Wilkinson WE, Parashos IA, et al. Quantitative cerebral anatomy of the aging human brain: a cross-sectional study using magnetic resonance imaging. Neurology 1992; 42:527.

[80] Vakili K, Pillay SS, Lafer B, et al. Hippocampal volume in primary unipolar major depression: a magnetic resonance imaging study. Biol Psychiatry 2000;47:1087.

[81] Steingard RJ, Renshaw PF, Yurgelun-Todd D, et al. Structural abnormalities in brain magnetic resonance images of depressed children. J Am Acad Child Adolesc Psychiatry 1996;35:307.

[82] Botteron KN, Raichle ME, Drevets WC, et al. Volumetric reduction in left subgenual prefrontal cortex in early onset depression. Biol Psychiatry 2002;51:342.

[83] Drevets WC, Price JL, Simpson JR, et al. Subgenual prefrontal cortex abnormalities in mood disorders. Nature 1997;386:824.

[84] Hirayasu Y, Shenton ME, Salisbury DF, et al. Subgenual cingulate cortex volume in first-episode psychosis. Am J Psychiatry 1999;156:1091.

[85] Hirayasu Y, Shenton ME, Salisbury DF, et al. Subgenual prefrontal cortex reduction in first episode affective psychosis. Biol Psychiatry 1998;43:97S.

[86] Sapolsky RM, Krey LC, McEwen BS. Prolonged glucocorticoid exposure reduces hippocampal neuron number: implications for aging. J Neurosci 1985;5:1222.

[87] Sapolsky RM, Krey LC, McEwen BS. The neuroendocrinology of stress and aging: the glucocorticoid cascade hypothesis. Endocr Rev 1986;7:284.

[88] Sapolsky RM, McEwen BS. Why dexamethasone resistance? Two possible neuroendocrine mechanisms. In: Schatzberg AF, Nemeroff CB, editors. The hypothalamic pituitary-adrenal axis: physiology, pathophysiology and psychiatric implications. New York: Raven Press; 1988. p. 155.

[89] Lopez JF, Akil H, Watson SJ. Neural circuits mediating stress. Biol Psychiatry 1999;46:1461.

[90] Coplan JD, Wolk SI, Goetz RR, et al. Nocturnal growth hormone secretion studies in adolescents with or without major depression re-examined: integration of adult clinical follow-up data. Biol Psychiatry 2000;47:594.

[91] Dahl RE, Birmaher B, Williamson DE, et al. Low growth hormone response to growth hormone-releasing hormone in child depression. Biol Psychiatry 2000;48:981.

[92] Birmaher B, Heydl P. Biological studies in depressed children and adolescents. Int J Neuropsychopharmacol 2001;4:149.

[93] Kaufman J, Martin A, King RA, et al. Are child-, adolescent-, and adult-onset depression one and the same disorder? Biol Psychiatry 2001;49:980.

[94] Botteron KN, Vannier MW, Geller B, et al. Preliminary study of magnetic resonance imaging

characteristics in 8- to 16-year-olds with mania. J Am Acad Child Adolesc Psychiatry 1995; 34:742.

[95] Dasari M, Friedman L, Jesberger J, et al. A magnetic resonance imaging study of thalamic area in adolescent patients with either schizophrenia or bipolar disorder as compared to healthy controls. Psychiatry Res 1999;91:155.

[96] Friedman L, Findling RL, Kenny JT, et al. An MRI study of adolescent patients with either schizophrenia or bipolar disorder as compared to healthy control subjects. Biol Psychiatry 1999; 46:78.

[97] Frazier JA. Anatomic brain magnetic resonance imaging (MRI) in pediatric bipolar disorder (BPD). In: Proceedings of the 48th Annual Meeting of the American Academy of Child and Adolescent Psychiatry. Honolulu: Hilton Hawaii Village; 2001;21D.

[98] DelBello MP. Neurobiological characterization of children at risk for bipolar disorder (BPD). In: Proceedings of the 48th Annual Meeting of the American Academy of Child and Adolescent Psychiatry. Honolulu: Hilton Hawaii Village; 2001;21C.

[99] Davanzo P, Thomas A, Yue K, et al. Decreased anterior cingulate myo-inositol/creatine spectroscopy resonance with lithium treatment in children with bipolar disorder. Neuropsychopharmacology 2001;24:359.

[100] Castillo M, Kwock L, Courvoisie H, et al. Proton MR spectroscopy in children with bipolar affective disorder: preliminary observations. AJNR Am J Neuroradiol 2000;21:832.

[101] Davidson RJ, Abercrombie H, Nitschke B, et al. Regional brain function, emotion and disorders of emotion. Curr Opin Neurobiol 1999;9:228.

[102] Sackeim HA, Greenberg MS, Weiman AL, et al. Hemispheric asymmetry in the expression of positive and negative emotions. Arch Neurol 1988;39:210.

[103] Robinson RG, Chemerinski E, Jorge R. Pathophysiology of secondary depressions in the elderly. J Geriatr Psychiatry Neurol 1999;12:128.

[104] George MS, Kellner CH, Bernstein H, et al. A magnetic resonance imaging investigation into mood disorders, multiple sclerosis: a pilot study. J Nerv Ment Dis 1994;182:410.

[105] Bechara A, Damasio H, Damasio AR, et al. Emotion, decision making and the orbitofrontal cortex. Cereb Cortex 2000;10:295.

[106] Damasio AR, Tranel D, Damasio H. Individuals with sociopathic behavior caused by frontal damage fail to respond autonomically to social stimuli. Behav Brain Res 1990;41:81.

[107] Henriques JB, Glowacki JM, Davidson RJ. Reward fails to alter response bias in depression. J Abnorm Psychol 1994;103:460.

[108] Önghr D, Drevets WC, Price JL. Glial reduction in the subgenual prefrontal cortex in mood disorders. Proc Natl Acad Sci U S A 1998;95:13290.

[109] Rajkowska G, Miguel-Hidalgo JJ, Wei J, et al. Morphometric evidence for neuronal and glial prefrontal cell pathology in major depression. Biol Psychiatry 1999;45:1085.

[110] Rubenstein JLR, Rakic P. Genetic control of cortical development. Cereb Cortex 1999;9:521.

[111] Frangou S, Murray RM. Imaging as a tool in exploring the neurodevelopment and genetics of schizophrenia. Br Med Bull 1996;52:587.

[112] Sharma T, Du Boulay G, Lewis S, et al. The Maudsley family study I: structural brain changes on magnetic resonance imaging in familial schizophrenia. Prog Neuropsychopharmacol Biol Psychiatry 1997;21:1297.

[113] Suddath RL, Christison GW, Torrey EF, et al. Anatomical abnormalities in the brains of monozygotic twins discordant for schizophrenia (published erratum appears in N Engl J Med 1990;322:1616). N Engl J Med 1990;322:789.

[114] Biondi A, Nogueira H, Dormont D, et al. Are the brains of monozygotic twins similar? A three-dimensional MR study. AJNR Am J Neuroradiol 1998;19:1361.

[115] Bartley AJ, Jones DW, Weinberger DR, et al. Genetic variability of human brain size and cortical gyral patterns. Brain 1997;120:257.

[116] Tramo MJ, Loftus WC, Thomas CE, et al. Surface area of human cerebral cortex and its gross morphological subdivisions: In vivo measurements in monozygotic twins suggest differential hemisphere effects of genetic factors. J Cogn Neurosci 1995;7:292.

[117] Carmelli D, Sullivan EV, Swan GE, et al. Evidence for heritability of brain structure in elderly male twins [abstract 298]. In: Proceedings of the World Congress on Psychiatric Genetics. Monterey, CA: International Society on Psychiatric Genetics; 1999

[118] Pennington BF, Sullivan EV, Swan-Filipek PA, et al. A twin MRI study of size variations in human brain. J Cogn Neurosci 2000;12:223.

[119] LeGoualher G, Argenti AM, Duyme M, et al. Statistical sulcal shape comparisons: application to the detection of genetic encoding of the central sulcus shape. Neuroimage 2000;11:564.

[120] Todd RD, Heath AC, Botteron KN, et al: Heritability of adolescent onset major depressive disorder: a longitudinal perspective. Mol Psychiatry 1999;4;(Suppl 1):169.

[121] Todd RD, Rasmussen ER, Neuman RJ, et al. Familiality and heritability of subtypes of ADHD in a population sample of female twins. Am J Psychiatry 2001;158:1891.

[122] Neuman RJ, Heath AC, Hudziak JJ, et al. Latent class analysis of ADHD and comorbid symptoms in a population sample of adolescent female twins. J Child Psychol Psychiatry 2001; 42:933.

[123] Neale MC. Mx: statistical modeling. Department of Psychiatry, Virginia Commonwealth University, Richmond, VA; 1997;4.

[124] Todd RD, Heath AC, Raichle ME, et al. Heritability of human brain morphometry. Mol Psychiatry 1999b;4:S27.

[125] Botteron KN, Raichle ME, Heath AC, et al. An epidemiological twin study of prefrontal neuromorphometry in early onset depression. Biol Psychiatry 1999;45:S188.

[126] Botteron KN, Sternhell K, Heath A, et al. Genetic analysis of major depression and prefrontal lobe volume. Mol Psychiatry 1999;4:S22.

CHILD AND
ADOLESCENT
PSYCHIATRIC
CLINICS

Child Adolesc Psychiatric Clin N Am
11 (2002) 519–532

Affective neuroscience and the study of normal and abnormal emotion regulation

Robinder K. Bhangoo, MD*, Ellen Leibenluft, MD

Pediatrics and Developmental Neuropsychiatry Branch, National Institute of Mental Health, Room 4N-208, NIMH Building 10, 10 Center Drive, MCS 1255, Bethesda, MD 20892, USA

The study of emotional processes and their neural components is referred to as affective neuroscience [1]. Although most research in affective neuroscience has been done in animals [2] and control human subjects [1,3], work now being done in clinical populations should increase the understanding of the pathophysiology of mood disorders. Some of the studies performed in control populations have focused on the normal development of the regulation of emotion. For example, researchers have learned a great deal about how and when children typically are able to regulate their own emotional experiences. This knowledge about the normative development of the regulation of emotions is a necessary prerequisite to understanding the pathology of children who exhibit mood dysregulation, either chronically or in the context of well-demarcated episodes of mania or depression. Thus, studying the sequence of neural events that culminates in the effective regulation of emotions can identify vulnerable periods of development that, if disrupted, could result in emotional dysregulation.

This article introduces the basic concepts of affective neuroscience and demonstrates how they can be applied to research on the normal development of the regulation of emotion. The discussion focuses on the biologic mechanisms mediating emotional processes and the regulation of emotion. The development of such mechanisms is influenced by endogenous and environmental factors. The most important environmental influences are the relationships with caregivers. This article describes techniques that can be used to identify the neural circuitry underlying the regulation of emotions and to study how such circuitry functions differently in patients with bipolar and other mood disorders than in control subjects. The techniques described here are not, however, designed to distinguish endogenous from environmental influences on the development of these neural mechanisms or, indeed, on the development

---

* Corresponding author
E-mail address: bhangoor@intra.nimh.nih.gov (R.K. Bhangoo).

of the regulation of emotion. Such questions, although undoubtedly of great importance, are outside the scope of this discussion. Thus, studies identifying physiologic processes associated with affective modulation are reviewed, and the authors discuss methods that can be used to study the abnormal development and the presentation of the dysregulation of emotions from the perspective of affective neuroscience. In particular, this article highlights research techniques of particular relevance to the study of childhood bipolar disorder.

Emotion and mood

The essential components of affective neuroscience are the concepts of emotion and mood. There are many definitions of these abstract concepts, although most agree that emotions represent responses evoked by salient environmental stimuli. The purpose of the emotional reaction is to facilitate an appropriate response. For simplicity, emotional reactions and motivated actions are considered either positive or negative [3]. In negative situations, the organism's safety and integrity are jeopardized. The corresponding negative emotions, such as fear or disgust, bias the individual to withdraw or avoid the situation. In positive situations, the organism is safe and in the presence of stimuli, such as food, children, or a mate, with which the organism should interact to ensure its own survival or propagation. Positive emotions, such as happiness or lust, motivate the organism to approach these stimuli. An emotion's association with either approach or avoidance behavior is called its valence; positive-valence emotions are associated with approach behavior, whereas negative-valence emotions are associated with avoidance behavior. The emotion of anger has received relatively little attention from researchers and has been difficult to fit into this paradigm. Although anger is considered a negative emotion, it is also associated with approach behavior, because anger is often associated with fighting. Therefore, anger is a negative-valenced emotion that can be associated with both approach and avoidance behavior.

Researchers have also recognized that emotional reactions, both positive and negative, have varying degrees of intensity. The level of emotional intensity, experienced by the organism as physiologic activation, serves as an indicator of its propensity for action. For example, in situations that are life-threatening the organism has a strong sympathetic response that signals and prepares the organism for "fight or flight." Likewise, positive feelings of high intensity, such as strong sexual attraction, prepare and propel an organism toward a potential and suitable mate. The level of emotional intensity is termed "arousal" [3]. Thus, whereas the valence assigns a directional component of action, arousal assigns a level of urgency to that action.

The two components of emotion, valence and arousal, can be used to characterize emotions and to depict these emotions graphically. By plotting valence on the ordinate and arousal on the abscissa, one can create an emotion circumplex (Fig. 1). This graphic representation allows each emotion to be considered in gradations of valence and arousal. For example, high arousal/ positive emotions, such as sexual excitement, are plotted in the upper right quadrant, and high arousal/negative emotions, such as fear, are plotted in the lower right hand quadrant.

Thus far, the discussion has been limited to the concept of emotion, which has received considerable attention in the literature. In contrast, the concept of mood has proven more difficult to define and to study. Mood is considered to be a longer-lasting state than emotion and is not necessarily evoked by an environmental stimulus. Thus, by definition, it would be more difficult to evoke mood, as opposed to emotion, in an experimental laboratory. Although mood and emotion are related concepts, they differ in how easily and quickly they can change: emotions are easily evoked by environmental stimuli and are of brief duration; moods are more durable. Although generally considered stable, moods can change quickly in some individuals, however. Although moods are less likely than emotions to be precipitated by a discrete environmental stimulus, changes in mood can be precipitated by major life events.

Some researchers have suggested that the relationship between emotions and moods is bidirectional. For example, Ekman proposed that moods can be brought about by what he called "dense emotional experiences." That is, recurrent experiences of the same emotion at a high intensity, in the absence of opposing

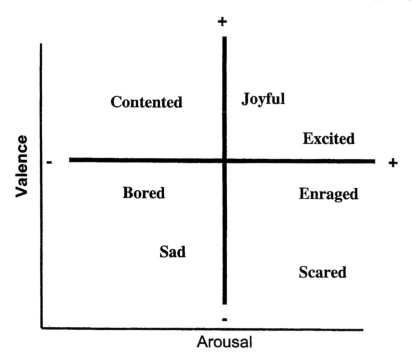

Fig. 1. Emotion circumplex.

emotions, can precipitate a sustained mood of the same valence [4]. Conversely, a prevailing mood of a given valence can predispose an individual to experience a similarly valenced emotion. Examples of such related emotions and moods are fear and anxiety. Both emotions and moods become dysfunctional when they occur in inappropriate contexts or when their intensity exceeds the needs of the situation. A recurrent, high-intensity dysfunctional emotion, if occurring without intervening functional emotions, could result in a dysfunctional mood, or mood disorder.

Psychopathology other than mood disorders also can occur when an individual experiences unstable and highly reactive emotions that are out of proportion to the precipitating situation. Such emotional lability can occur in the setting of a mood disorder, such as bipolar disorder or depression, and is often the chief complaint in children with mood and behavioral difficulties. Emotion instability can also present in individuals with developmental disabilities, such as Down syndrome [5]. Indeed, infants and young children typically show inconsistent regulation of emotions and exhibit some degree of emotion lability in the form of crying and tantrums. Such emotional lability may be more adaptive for young children than for individuals with developmental disabilities, because the normal infant's lability may be more consistently related to a negative stimulus and therefore serve as a means of communicating the child's needs to the caregiver. This lability is outgrown, in most cases, as the maturing child develops alternative forms of communication. Thus, the regulation of emotions undergoes a complex, normal developmental process which is related to other areas of development but which can be disrupted, leading to mood and behavioral problems.

Emotional regulation and normal development

The regulation of emotion is an individual's ability to respond to his or her life experiences with a range of socially acceptable emotions that flexibly permit or delay reactions as the situation requires [6]. In other words, the regulation of emotion is the ability to manage arousal or to modulate the intensity of emotional reactions [7]. The regulation of emotion is influenced by a number of neural structures, including the autonomic nervous system and the frontal cortex. Excitatory systems, such as the sympathetic nervous system, are functional at birth, but the corresponding inhibitory structures, such as the parasympathetic nervous system and the prefrontal cortex, continue to develop after birth [8]. Therefore, newborns cannot dampen their internal excitatory experiences and are largely dependent on adult caregivers to regulate their emotions [6,9]. Parents use cues from the child, such as crying or smiling, to initiate soothing, distracting, or stimulating behavior [10].

Between the ages of 7 and 15 months, myelination occurs in the limbic and cortical association areas, allowing maturation of the inhibitory cortical areas [11]. In primates, inhibitory neural projections descending from the prefrontal cortex to subcortical (excitatory) structures also develop during this period [12].

It is believed that such development in human infants contributes to a child's ability to regulate his or her own affective experiences. The period during which this process occurs corresponds approximately to critical periods of infant development, such as Mahler's practicing period [11]. In humans, improved affect regulation can be observed when infants more effectively use gaze aversion and self-soothing mechanisms. Studies with temperamentally difficult children have shown a decreased use of these tactics and an increased likelihood for negative emotional reactions [6].

As children enter the preschool years, they show an enhanced ability to regulate emotions, and episodes of negative emotional expression, such as tantrums and crying, decrease in intensity and duration. Several factors contribute to this increased inhibitory control. As mentioned previously, inhibitory cortical and parasympathetic structures provide a dampening effect over subcortical and sympathetic structures. In addition, maturation of the frontal lobes allows the development of executive function and specifically of effortful control. Effortful control refers to the ability of an organism to inhibit a dominant response to perform a subdominant response [13]. The processes involved in effortful control include the ability to sustain the focus of attention over prolonged periods of time and the ability to delay reactions. The ability to sustain attention is correlated with self-control measures and with other measures of affective and behavioral style. For example, children capable of highly sustained attention at 12 months have been described as more quiet and inactive at 24 and 36 months than children who had shorter attention spans at 12 months [13].

A particularly marked increase in executive attention occurs during the third year of life [14] and is demonstrated by an increased ability to filter out extraneous stimuli and to maintain attention on an intended task. As reported by Rothbart and Posner [14], children were given a variant of the Stroop task involving the presentation of a picture stimulus on either side of a screen. They were asked to press whichever one of two keys matched the stimulus, regardless of the side that the key was on. The matching key was either on the same side as the stimulus (compatible trial), or on the opposite side (incompatible trial). Children younger than 3 years tended to duplicate the preceding response but showed improved accuracy for the compatible trials versus the incompatible ones. By the end of the third year, children performed with high accuracy during both compatible and incompatible trials, although reaction time was slower for the incompatible trials. This study demonstrates that the older children are able to inhibit an incorrect response, an element of effortful control.

Because control involves the ability to focus executive attention, to shift set, and to exert inhibitory control, effortful control facilitates the child's ability to diminish negative affect (and, indirectly, aggressive behavior) by shifting attention away from negative cues [14]. The ability to shift attention away from a negative stimulus or toward a positive stimulus is called attentional control. By directing attention away from a negative stimulus, attentional control dampens high levels of arousal; conversely, maintaining attention on positive stimuli can sustain prosocial behavior [15]. A child's degree of attentional control seems to correlate with his or her ability to cope with emotional demands. For example, a study of 4- to 6-year-old boys with good attentional control showed that they tended to deal with anger by using verbal, nonhostile methods rather than aggressive behavior. The children with high attentional control were also rated as having better social skills by their teachers and were chosen as playmates more often by their peers than were children with low attentional control [15].

Another major factor in affect regulation is the development of language skills, which progresses during the toddler and preschool years. As children develop verbal skills, they are better able to think and to talk about their emotions and can communicate more effectively with their caregivers, enhancing social contact [6]. Enhanced linguistic skills also allow children to express their feelings verbally rather than behaviorally. The ability to seek assistance from adults can further increase the child's repertoire of self-regulating techniques.

Development of language also provides a form of internal inhibition called verbal self-control [10]. Verbal self-control consists of using the symbolic capacity of language to control unconditioned reflexes and conditioned responses. Rothbart and Posner have hypothesized that the development of verbal self-control depends on the maturation of the hippocampus and prefrontal cortex [10]. Thus, verbally coded internal descriptions of reward or punishment could trigger activation or inhibition systems, allowing children to respond appropriately in a variety of situations.

Regulation of emotion progresses through childhood as cognitive and language skills continue to develop. For example, a study of children between the ages of 6 and 10 years demonstrated that children older than 6 years were more likely to follow display rules in suppressing emotional displays in certain situations [16]. Saarni describes display rules as occurring when children develop the cognitive capacity to understand that some emotions should not be expressed externally and that others must be exaggerated [16]. These rules become more complex as the child matures [16]. Visuospatial skills and the increasing ability to abstract also allow the growing child to perceive emotion in others and to modify behavior accordingly. As children approach adolescence, their verbal skills and social environment expand, and they have more opportunities and experiences to develop enhanced self-regulatory methods.

As this discussion indicates, a number of neural systems interact and contribute to the development of emotion regulation. Disruption in one or more of these systems (eg, language delays or deficiencies in executive functioning or attention) can lead to emotional dysregulation. In fact, children with bipolar disorder often present with developmental delays in these areas, and further study is needed to characterize developmental disruptions in this clinical population more thoroughly. A better understanding of the relationship between the regulation of emotion and cognitive skills, notably attentional control and executive functioning, could help elucidate the high comorbidity between bipolar disorder and attention deficit hyperactivity disorder (ADHD). Language and learning disabilities can also contribute to emotion dysregulation and may provide a possible area of intervention. A better understanding of the role of these facilitators in the development of affective regulation would allow the development of new strategies to help children with bipolar disorder, and with other psychopathologies of mood and emotion, maintain emotional control.

Physiologic correlates of emotion and emotional regulation

Prefrontal cortex

Two neural systems described as key facilitators of affective regulation are the prefrontal cortex and the parasympathetic nervous system. One line of research exploring the role of the prefrontal cortex in the regulation of emotion has posited that the neural processing of emotions is, to some extent, lateralized. According to this hypothesis, emotions with positive or approach valences are associated with greater left frontal activation, and emotions involving negative or with-drawal valences are associated with greater right frontal activation [17,18]. This hypothesis has been supported by lesion [19–22], electroencephalogram (EEG) [23,24] and neuroimaging [25] studies in clinical populations and by EEG [26–28] and neuroimaging [29] studies in control populations.

Measurements of EEG activity are used to assess prefrontal function, and suppression of the alpha frequency is used as a measure of activation. Studies assessing anterior activation have demonstrated an association between frontal activation and affective style. Davidson et al [18] have hypothesized that individuals with greater left frontal activity tend to display more approach behaviors and positive affect, whereas those with greater right frontal activity tend to demonstrate avoidance behavior and negative affect in response to negative stimuli. For example, Davidson and Rickman found that toddlers and very young children with relatively greater right-sided activation demonstrated more behavioral inhibition and wariness in laboratory-based paradigms [30]. In a study of college-student controls, those with greater left frontal asymmetry received higher scores of behavioral activation on the Behavioral Activation System/Behavioral Inhibition System (BAS/BIS) scales, self-reporting measures that assess individual differences in the strength of the behavioral activation and inhibition systems [31]. Conversely, greater right frontal asymmetry was associated with higher scores of behavioral inhibition [28]. Studies of fron-tal asymmetry as a marker for affective style demonstrate that it is a stable trait [28,32,33] that predicts response to a valenced emotional stimulus [26,27]. In adults, decreased left anterior activity is seen in depressed and remitted pa-tients [23,24]. In infants and children, increased right anterior activation is seen in 10-month-olds demonstrating a marked response to maternal separation [34] and in 4-year-olds with social withdrawal [35].

Although frontal asymmetry maintains stability, it is possible that the typical lateralization patterns prevail during intense emotional experiences, regardless of the individual's resting asymmetry. Lateralization of emotional processes accord-ing to valence could also facilitate regulation of emotion. For example, left frontal activation associated with positive valence and approach behavior would enable an individual to explore the environment and seek out social contact [36]. Similarly, right frontal activation associated with negative emotions and withdrawal behavior removes the individual from potentially dangerous situations, facilitating the dampening of negative emotions. There also is inhibitory interaction between the two hemispheres, so that the individual is more likely to remain in a state of homeostasis, expressing both positive and negative emotions when appropriate.

Although asymmetrical frontal activation seems to correlate with differences in emotional valence, generalized frontal activation in response to emotional stimuli represent increased emotional intensity or arousal [37]. In a study of infants aged 12 to 21 months, researchers examined EEGs taken before and after the infant's mother left the room and in other conditions of varying emotional intensities. The baseline situation (mother in room) and the situation of maternal separation were designated as situations of low and high emotional intensity, respectively. During the high-intensity experience, the children expressed intense emotional responses accompanied by significant activation in both frontal hemispheres, which was more pronounced than the subtle asymmetrical differences [37].

In another EEG study of infant distress on maternal separation using a scale that assesses bodily changes and distress vocalization, researchers noted a correlation between global frontal activation, measured at baseline and during the separation, and higher ratings of distress during separation (correlation between baseline measures and subsequent distress: for right side, $r = -0.48$; for left side, $r = -0.49$; $P < 0.05$; correlation between EEG and distress measures during separation: for right side, $r = -0.72$; for left side, $r = -0.69$; $P < 0.005$; negative correlations were obtained because decreased alpha power was used as a measure of increased frontal activation) [38]. No significant differences, however, were noted between left-side and right-side activation, perhaps because the children generally experienced significant amounts of anger (as assessed by the Ekman's Facial Action Coding System [EM-FACS]) [39]. As mentioned previously, although anger is considered a negative emotion, it also is associated with approach behaviors, and therefore the laterality pattern with which it is associated is unclear. It is also possible that the degree of prefrontal asymmetry observed in response to emotional stimuli may diminish with extreme levels of arousal.

Autonomic nervous system

The autonomic nervous system, composed of the sympathetic and parasympathetic nervous systems, is also involved in the processing of emotional stimuli and in emotional expression. Activation of the sympathetic nervous system, which can be seen as a measure of arousal, occurs in response to anxiety-provoking situations and results in increased heart rate, respiration, and sweat gland activity. As early as the nineteenth century, scientists noted a connection between sympathetic activity and certain emotional states, as documented in

Tarchanoff's observation, "The recall of something arousing fear, fright, joy, or strong emotions of any sort also produced electric currents in the skin" [40].

As opposed to the excitatory nature of the sympathetic nervous system, the parasympathetic nervous system acts in an inhibitory capacity. The two counter-balanced systems, acting together, provide homeostasis in the cardiac, respiratory, gastric, and muscular systems, among others. Parasympathetic fibers run from the brain stem with cranial nerve X to effector organs in the head, thorax and abdomen. The muscles of facial expression (ie, smiling and frowning) are controlled by the facial nerve, cranial nerve VII. In studies measuring the electromyographic (EMG) activity of corrugator (frown) and zygomatic (smile) muscles in adults viewing pictures developed as standardized emotional stimuli, researchers noted significant correlations between ratings of emotional valence and EMG activity. Namely, corrugator EMG activity was negatively correlated with pleasantness ratings (r = − 0.90), and zygomatic EMG activity was positively correlated (r = 0.56) [3]. Cranial nerve VII is known to have parasympathetic involvement. Indeed, the source nuclei of the facial nerve lie so close to the regulatory center of the vagus nerve that cranial nerve VII is sometimes included as part of the vagus complex [41].

The vagus nerve, or cranial nerve X, is important in the area of emotion perception and expression. This myelinated nerve with both motor and sensory components has many target organs, including the heart, and the influence of the parasympathetic system on the heart and other organs is described as vagal tone. Although variations in vagal tone have been associated with gastric problems and asthma [42], the measure of vagal tone primarily involves the heart. Vagal tone is assessed by calculating the amplitude of respiratory sinus arrhythmia (RSA) or the spontaneous changes in heart rate associated with respiration. Respiratory sinus arrhythmia reflects the rhythmic increases in heart rate seen with inspiration and corresponding decreases with expiration; these fluctuations result from the influence of respiratory mechanisms in the brain stem on the vagal efferents to the sinoatrial node of the heart. These efferents are attenuated by the brain stem during inspiration and are reinstated during expiration [42].

Vagal tone is hypothesized to be a measure of an individual's tendency to be hypo- or hyperreactive, because baseline measures of vagal tone may predict how an individual's autonomic nervous system will respond to stressors [41]. Studies have demonstrated that higher levels of vagal tone are associated with greater variability in heart rate [41] and may indicate more organized neural control. This higher level of neural control would allow a faster and larger parasympathetic response to sympathetic arousal, facilitating the appropriate response to environmental stimuli by providing increased physiologic reaction to stress [42]. Neonatal studies of resting vagal tone have shown that infants with lower vagal tone, and therefore lower variability in heart rate, did not have as much reduction in vagal tone during bottle feeding as those with higher baseline vagal tone. The reduction in vagal tone during stress, such as feeding, may reflect the body's need to decrease the vagal control of the heart to facilitate increased metabolic demands. The infants who did not have as marked a reduction in vagal tone may exhibit inadequate physiologic responses to stressors [43]. For example, studies indicate that premature infants, who have lower vagal tones than full-term infants [44], also respond to stressors, such as gavage feedings [45] and circumcision [46] with increased behavioral reactivity and pitch of crying. Thus, vagal tone may be a useful measure of behavioral and physiologic reactivity. Proper functioning of neural control over heart rate variability may also allow a rapid and effective response to a stimulus and a rapid return to baseline. Thus, there is some evidence that increased vagal tone facilitates the maintenance of physiologic homeostasis. Specifically, in 3-month-old infants, there was a significant association between resting vagal tone and ability to be soothed [47].

In addition, longitudinal studies have demonstrated the ability of vagal tone measurementss (ie, RSA) to predict future behavioral regulation. For example, in a study of 41 very low birth weight infants, heart rate and RSA were measured using weekly electrocardiograms from 48 hours after birth until discharge. The mean gestational age was 28 weeks (range, 24–33 weeks), and the mean birth weight was 930 g (range, 500–1325 g). An increase was seen in mean RSA between 33 and 35 weeks of gestation [48], perhaps indicating a maturational shift resulting from increased myelination in vagal nerve fibers. Three years later, the children were assessed on various behavioral measures. On follow up, RSA measurements predicted behavioral development, with higher mean RSA values being associated with greater social competence as measured on the California Preschool Social Competency Scale (CPSCS), with more efficient mental processing as measured on the Kaufman Assessment Battery for Children, Mental Processing Composite Scale, and with better gross motor skills as measured on the Revised Denver Prescreening Questionnaire for Motor Abilities. A subsample of the same population was assessed a second time 3 to 5 years later using the Kaufman Assessment Battery for Children and a parent-completed Child Behavior Checklist (CBCL). The RSA maturation score, assessed during the 33- to 35-week gestation period, correlated significantly with social competence scores on the CBCL ($r = 0.54$), and accounted for 50% of the variance when factors of socioeconomic status (SES) and medical risk were removed [43]. Thus, neuronal self-regulatory mechanisms, which are present and can be assessed early in life, may be related to later behavioral abilities. Further studies are needed to assess the normal development of RSA and vagal nerve fibers and the implications of this development for regulatory capacities.

Potential applications of affective neuroscience to research on childhood-onset bipolar disorder

The parents of children with bipolar disorder often describe chronic histories of low frustration levels, severe emotional reactions, and behavioral problems. These complaints are not unique to bipolar disorder, however, because many psychiatric disorders in children involve abnormal regulation of emotion. Like children with bipolar disorder, those with depression, anxiety disorders, posttraumatic stress disorder, or developmental disabilities may manifest emotional dysregulation in the form of exaggerated reactions to negative stimuli. In addition, some children do not fit the full criteria of bipolar disorder because of the absence of cardinal manic symptoms, such as grandiosity, decreased need for sleep, or increased goal-directed activity, but share with the bipolar children the symptoms of hyperarousal, chronic abnormal baseline mood, and extreme responses to frustration. It is therefore important to compare the physiologic and behavioral responses of control children, those with classic bipolar disorder, and those with severe emotional dysregulation, perhaps resulting from other psychiatric illnesses, to frustrating and other negative stimuli. It is also possible that children with bipolar disorder are unique in having an increased responsiveness to positive emotional stimuli. Increased responsiveness to positive emotional stimuli could underlie the propensity to develop the positive-valence, high-arousal, state of mania.

Therefore, one approach to understanding the pathophysiology of emotional dysregulation involves exposing children to standardized emotional stimuli, such as film clips and computer games which the children win or lose. The authors are currently studying the responses of children and adolescents with bipolar disorder to such positively and negatively valenced emotional stimuli to test the hypothesis that the patients will have more pronounced physiologic and behavioral reactions to negative emotional stimuli than do controls. The physiologic processes that are being measured are heart rate (including RSA), skin conductance (a measure of arousal), evoked-response potential, and startle eyeblink magnitude (an index of emotional valence). If these physiologic studies find meaningful differences between patients and controls, similar methodology could be used in neuro-imaging studies. Imaging studies could provide information on differences between patients and controls in the neural activation in frontal and subcortical areas, including limbic areas such as the hippocampus, dorsal striatum, ventral pallidum, medial prefrontal cortex, amygdala, and nucleus accumbens [49]. Neuroimaging also might help clarify the pathophysiologic basis of various forms of emotional dysregulation seen in different psychiatric illnesses. For example, it may be that different neurocircuitry is involved when an autistic child displays irritability because of inflexibility than when a bipolar child has an irritable rage. Longitudinal physiologic studies might also provide information on the development of affective regulation in both clinical and control populations, perhaps demonstrating areas of abnormal or delayed development.

Summary

Affective neuroscience allows investigators to study the biologic basis of psychologic phenomena such as emotion and mood. Understanding the components of emotion, valence, and arousal and their physiologic correlates is the starting point for studies that quantify emotional and physiologic reactions. This information could provide insight into the biologic foundations of numerous psychiatric conditions. Understanding the normal development of emotions and regulation of emotion will provide new avenues of research into the complex problem of severe mood disorders.

References

[1] Davidson RJ, Irwin W. The functional neuroanatomy of emotion and affective style. Trends Cogn Sci.1999;3:11–21.

[2] LeDoux J. Fear and the brain: where have we been, and where are we going? [see comments] Biol Psychiatry 1998;44:1229–38.

[3] Lang PJ, Bradley MM, Cuthbert BN. Emotion, motivation, and anxiety: brain mechanisms and psychophysiology. Biol Psychiatry 1998;44:1248–63.

[4] Ekman P. Moods, emotions, and traits. In: Ekman P, Davidson RJ, editors. The nature of emotion: fundamental questions. New York (NY): Oxford University Press; 1994. p. 56–8.

[5] Cicchetti D, Ganiban J, Barnett K. Contributions from the study of high-risk populations to understanding the development of emotion regulation. In: Garber J, Dodge K, editors. The development of emotion regulation and dysregulation. Cambridge, UK: Cambridge University Press; 1991. p. 15–48.

[6] Cole P, Michel M, Teti L. The development of emotion regulation and dysregulation: a clinical perspective. Monographs of the Society for Research in Child Development 1994; 240(59):73–100.

[7] Fox N. Temperament and regulation of emotion in the first years of life. Pediatrics 1998;102: 1230–5.

[8] Thompson R. Emotion and self-regulation. Nebraska Symposium on Motivation. Lincoln, Nebraska: University of Nebraska Press; 1990. p. 367–467.

[9] Kraemer G, Ebert M, Schmidt D, et al. Strangers in a strange land: psychobiological study of infant monkeys before and after separation from real or inanimate mothers. Child Dev 1991; 62:548–66.

[10] Rothbart M, Posner M. Temperament and the development of self-regulation. In: Harlage L, Telzrow C, editors. The neuropsychology of individual differences, a developmental perspective. New York (NY): Plenum Press; 1985. p. 93–123.

[11] Shore A. Affect regulation and the origin of the self. Hillsdale (NJ): Lawrence Erlbaum; 1994.

[12] Johnson T, Rosvold H, Galkin T, et al. Postnatal maturation of subcortical projections from the prefrontal cortex in the rhesus monkey. J Comp Neurol 1976;166:427–44.

[13] Rothbart M, Bates J. Temperament. In: Damon W, Eisenberg N, editors. Handbook of child psychology, vol.3: social, emotional and personality development. 5th edition. New York (NY): Wiley; 1998. p. 105–76.

[14] Rothbart M, Posner M. Developing mechanisms of self-regulation. Dev Psychopathol 2000; 12:427–41.

[15] Eisenberg N, Fabes R, Nyman M, et al. The relations of emotionality and regulation to children's anger-related reactions. Child Dev 1994;65:109–28.

[16] Saarni C. Children's understanding of display rules for expressive behaviors. Dev Psychol 1979; 15:424–9.

[17] Gray JA. Three fundamental emotion systems. In: Ekman P, Davidson RJ, editors. The nature of emotion: fundamental questions. New York (NY): Oxford University Press; 1994. p. 243–7.

[18] Davidson RJ, Jackson DC, Kalin NH. Emotion, plasticity, context and regulation: perspectives from affective neuroscience. Psychol Bull 2000;126:890–909.

[19] Robinson RG, Boston JD, Starkstein SE, et al. Comparison of mania and depression after brain injury: causal factors. Am J Psychiatry 1988;145:172–8.

[20] Starkstein SE, Bryer JB, Berthier ML, et al. Depression after stroke: the importance of cerebral hemisphere asymmetries. J Neuropsychiatry Clin Neurosci 1991;3:276–85.

[21] Starkstein SE, Robinson RG. Mechanism of disinhibition after brain lesions. J Nerv Ment Dis 1997;185:108–14.

[22] Morris PL, Robinson RG, Raphael B, et al. Lesion location and poststroke depression. J Neuropsychiatry Clin Neurosci 1996;8:399–403.

[23] Henriques JB, Davidson RJ. Regional brain electrical asymmetries discriminate between previously depressed and healthy control subjects. J Abnorm Psychol 1990;99:22–31.

[24] Henriques JB, Davidson RJ. Left frontal hypoactivation in depression. J Abnorm Psychol 1991; 100:535–45.

[25] Drevets WC. Functional neuroimaging studies of depression: the anatomy of melancholia. Annu Rev Med 1998;49:341–61.

[26] Tomarken AJ, Davidson RJ, Henriques JB. Resting frontal brain asymmetry predicts affective responses to films. J Pers Soc Psychol 1990;59:791–801.

[27] Wheeler RE, Davidson RJ, Tomarken AJ. Frontal brain asymmetry and emotional reactivity: a biological substrate of affective style. Psychophysiology 1993;30:82–9.

[28] Sutton SK, Davidson RJ. Prefrontal brain asymmetry: a biological substrate of the behavioral approach and inhibition systems. Psychological Science 1997;8:204–10.

[29] Sutton SK, Ward RT, Larson CL, et al. Asymmetry in prefrontal glucose metabolism during appetitive and aversive emotional states: an FDG-PET study [abstract]. Psychophysiology 1997; 34:S89.

[30] Davidson RJ, Rickman M. Behavioral inhibition and the emotional circuitry of the brain: stability and plasticity during the early childhood years. In: Schmidt LA, Schulkin J, editors. Extreme fear and shyness: origins and outcomes. New York (NY): Oxford University Press; 1999. p. 67–87.

[31] Carver C, White T. Behavioral inhibition, behavioral activation, and affective responses to impending reward and punishment: the BIS/BAS scales. J Pers Soc Psychol 1994;67:319–33.

[32] Tomarken AJ, Davidson RJ, Wheeler RW, et al. Psychometric properties of resting anterior EEG asymmetry: temporal stability and internal consistency. Psychophysiology 1992;29:576–92.

[33] Tomarken AJ, Davidson RJ, Wheeler RE, et al. Individual differences in anterior brain asymmetry and fundamental dimensions of emotion. J Pers Soc Psychol 1992;62:676–87.

[34] Davidson RJ, Fox NA. Frontal brain asymmetry predicts infants' response to maternal separation. J Abnorm Psychol 1989;98:127–31.

[35] Fox NA, Rubin KH, Calkins SD, et al. Frontal activation asymmetry and social competence at four years of age. Child Dev 1995;66:1770–84.

[36] Fox N. Dynamic cerebral processes underlying emotion regulation. Monographs of the Society for Research in Child Development 1994;240(59):152–66.

[37] Dawson G. Frontal electroencephalographic correlates of individual differences in emotion expression in infants: a brain systems perspective on emotion. Monographs of the Society for Research in Child Development 1994;240(59):135–51.

[38] Thompson R, Lamb M. Individual differences in dimensions of socioemotional development in infancy. In: Plutchik R, Kellerman H, editors. Emotion: theory, research and experience, vol. 2: emotions in early development. New York (NY): Academic Press; 1984. p. 87–114.

[39] Ekman P, Friesen W. EM-FACS coding manual. San Francisco (CA): Consulting Psychologists Press; 1984.

[40] Tarchanoff J. Galvanic phenomena in the human skin during stimulation of the sensory organs and during various forms of mental activity. Pflugers Archiv fur die gesamte Physiologie des Menschen und der Tiere 46, 1890;46:46–55.

[41] Porges S, Doussard-Roosevelt J, Maita AK. Vagal tone and the physiological regulation of emotion. Monographs of the Society for Research in Child Development 1994;240(59):167–86.

[42] Porges S. Vagal tone: an autonomic mediator of affect. In: Garber J, Dodge K, editors. The development of emotion regulation and dysregulation. Cambridge (UK): Cambridge University Press; 1991. p. 111–28.

[43] Doussard-Roosevelt J, McClenny B, Porges S. Neonatal cardiac vagal tone and school-age developmental outcome in very low birth weight infants. Dev Psychobiol 2001;38:56–66.

[44] Porges S. Vagal tone: a physiological marker of stress vulnerability. Pediatrics 1992;90:498–504.
[45] DiPietro J, Porges S. Vagal responsiveness to gavage feeding as an index of preterm stress. Pediatr Res 1991;29:231–6.
[46] Porter F, Porges S, Marshall R. Newborn pain cries and vagal tone: parallel changes in response to circumcision. Child Dev 1988;59:495–505.
[47] Huffman L, Bryan Y, del Carmen R, et al. Autonomic correlates of reactivity and self-regulation at twelve weeks of age. Rockville (MD): National Institute of Mental Health; 1992.
[48] Doussard-Roosevelt J, Porges S, Scanlon J, et al. Vagal regulation of heart rate in the prediction of developmental outcome for very low birth weight preterm infants. Child Dev 1997;68:173–86.
[49] Swerdlow NR, Caine SB, Braff DL, et al. The neural substrates of sensorimotor gating of the startle reflex: a review of recent findings and their implications. J Psychopharmacol 1992;6: 176–90.

Child Adolesc Psychiatric Clin N Am
11 (2002) 533–553

CHILD AND
ADOLESCENT
PSYCHIATRIC
CLINICS

Children of parents with bipolar disorder
A population at high risk for major affective disorders

Sheilagh Hodgins, PhD*, Brigitte Faucher, MSc,
Anica Zarac, Mark Ellenbogen, PhD

*Department of Psychology, Université de Montréal, C.P. 6128, Succ. Centre Ville Montréal,
Québec H3C 3J7, Canada*

Children of parents who suffer from bipolar disorder (BD) are largely invisible, despite the fact that they constitute a population at very high risk for either major depression (MD) or BD in late adolescence and adulthood and for multiple disorders in childhood. In the United States, it is estimated that about one third of persons with BD receive treatment. Even when parents with BD are treated, little attention is paid to their offspring. A Canadian study illustrates the current situation. The study was conducted at a large university hospital in which the child psychiatry department had been actively promoting services for the children of adults receiving psychiatric care. A random sample of 100 adults being treated for MD or BD was recruited. Of these adults, 47 had 138 children. Of the 47 patients who had children, 19 reported that at least one of their children had received some type of mental health service. Only 4 of the 19 patients reported that the treating psychiatrist inquired about their children, and in only 1 case was the child referred for assessment [1]. This population of high-risk offspring thus remains invisible, most receive no care, and very few participate in prevention programs despite the fact that such programs have been proven to have positive effects, at least in the short term [2].

There are four important reasons to study the offspring of persons with BD. First, many of them will develop either MD or BD in adulthood; studying their development from conception to adulthood may help identify the processes by which genetic and nongenetic factors interact to cause these disorders. Second, it

---

This work was supported by a grant from the Fonds de recherche en santé du Québec.
* Corresponding author.
E-mail address: sheilagh.hodgins@umontreal.ca (S. Hodgins).

is important to identify critical periods during development when specific interventions would have the effect of delaying onset, attenuating the course, or even preventing BD and MD. Third, a proportion of these children are experiencing considerable difficulty in childhood and need care. Finally, the children who are having difficulty are likely creating stress in the family, which in turn can trigger episodes of mania and depression in the ill parent [3].

Prevalence of bipolar disorder

Recent results from a United States epidemiological investigation suggest that 1.6% of men and women suffer from BD [4]. The lifetime prevalence of BD varies across countries and across ethnic groups within the same countries [5,6]. The ratio of bipolar to major depressive disorder also varies across nations and ethnic groups. Although most studies report similar prevalence among men and women [7], there is some evidence of higher rates among women than men [8–10]. Younger birth cohorts and samples in the United States [11], Germany [12], the Netherlands [13], Hungary [14], and New Zealand [15] show high rates of BD even in adolescence. For example, in a New Zealand cohort born 1971 to 1972, in the year between the subjects' 20th and 21st birthdays, 2.0% met criteria for BD [15]. By contrast, among the 11,017 persons born in two provinces of Finland in 1966, there were only five cases with a confirmed diagnosis of BD by age 31 [16]. In Denmark, among all persons born 1965 through 1967, lifetime prevalence ranged from 0.07% in men to 0.13% in women [5]. Methodological features of these investigations fail to explain the observed differences [5,6,17].

The mean age of onset of BD also varies widely across time periods and countries. A number of studies have reported a median age of onset for bipolar 1 disorder between 17 and 19 years of age [18–20]. The highest rates of onset for both males and females are reported to be between 15 and 19 years of age [14,21,22]. Investigations of cohorts and samples of subjects born since 1968 in the United States [11,23], New Zealand [15], Hungary [14], and the Netherlands [13] documented rates of bipolar 1 disorder by the early 20s that are as high or higher than those reported for adults. By contrast, in a Finnish study of all first admissions for BD in the entire country in 1994, only 2% were under age 20 and another 14% under age 30 [24]. No methodological artifacts have been identified to explain these differences in age of onset [25–28]. It has been proposed that they reflect a birth cohort effect [28–31]. In the United States, it is generally agreed that half of all cases of BD are identified before age 20 [19].

In the United States, it is estimated that about one third of persons with BD receive treatment [19,32]. Of those who do receive treatment, most relapse despite state-of-the-art pharmacotherapy [33,34]. Most persons with BD also present low levels of psychosocial functioning between acute episodes and according to one study, reduced cognitive functioning [35]. Researchers from the United States National Collaborative Project on Depression have concluded that "The psychosocial impairment associated with mania and major depression extends to essentially all areas of functioning and persists for years, even among individuals who experience sustained resolution of clinical symptoms" [36]. Poor psychosocial functioning in the early stages of the disorder is associated with poor long-term outcome [37]. Among persons with BD, the risk of suicide is 30 times greater than that for the general population [38], and premature mortality is elevated even among those who are treated [39]. Rates of comorbid personality disorders, especially antisocial personality disorder [40], vary from 41% to 55% [41,42]. Rates of drug abuse or dependence are also elevated compared with the rates in the general population where the persons with BD live [43]. Often not mentioned are the elevated rates of criminal convictions among persons with BD. For example, in the New Zealand study described above, 31.6% of the young adults with mania had a criminal record [15]. All of these correlates of BD may negatively impact on the offspring.

In summary, although BD affects approximately 1.6% of men and women in the United States, half before they reach their 20th birthday, the prevalence and age of onset vary across countries and across ethnic groups within the same countries. These differences could result from genetic factors [44] or nongenetic environmental factors acting to trigger a genetic vulnerability. Given the chronicity of BD, the associated problems (especially suicide, personality disorders, and substance misuse), and the low levels of psychosocial functioning, studies of the children of persons with this disorder are warranted.

Childhood and adolescent disorders of adults with BD

Studies that have collected information about childhood and adolescence from adults with BD concur in suggesting that various symptoms and problems were present long before the disorder and that adjustment and disruptive behavior disorders are common [45]. In a study of all first admissions for psychosis in a defined catchment area in the state of New York, 69% of the BD patients were found to have a history of childhood disorders, 21% had a history of behavior disorders, and 48% had histories of other disorders. BD patients with a history of behavior disorders in childhood were more often male, abused drugs and alcohol, were poorly educated, had an earlier age of onset of affective symptoms, and had poorer functioning both before and after the onset of BD [46,47]. Given that patients and their families have provided information after the patient fell ill and that only those individuals who develop BD are studied, such retrospective findings tend to overestimate the prevalence of childhood problems among those who develop BD, and by design, do not take into account that many children with the same problems do not develop BD (eg, see Meyer et al, who discussed the differences when findings from a prospective longitudinal study are analyzed retrospectively [48]). Retrospective studies, however, are cost-effective, feasible, and conducted in a relatively short time; furthermore, they provide rich information for the development of hypotheses that can be tested in prospective investigations.

Offspring of persons with BD: disorders in adulthood

Men and women with BD have as many if not more children than the general population [49]. These BD offspring (BDO) are at increased risk for both MD and BD compared with the general population. This conclusion is based on the results of studies reporting higher rates of MD and BD among the biological relatives of persons with BD than among the relatives of persons with no mental disorder [50–53]. Many more of the relatives of BD patients are diagnosed with MD than BD. The opposite, however, is usually not observed; BD is rarely reported among the relatives of persons with MD. Similar proportions of male and female relatives of persons with BD are diagnosed with BD, while twice as many women as men meet criteria for MD. One study of the adult offspring of BD parents indicates that almost one in two develop either MD or BD [52].

The family aggregration of BD and MD is due largely to genetic factors. Twin studies, one adoption study, and molecular genetic studies have all consistently indicated that a hereditary factor plays a role in the development of both BD and MD [50–52,54–58]. The twin studies [54,55,58] indicate that while the hereditary factor associated with BD is more powerful than that associated with MD, neither is sufficient to cause the disorder. For both BD and MD, nongenetic factors interact with the inherited vulnerability to determine the disorder. Little is known about how these inherited factors act to cause the disorder or about the nongenetic factors that are involved.

Several investigations indicate that adults with BD mate disproportionately with persons with affective disorders [59]. This means that a subgroup of BDO have increased genetic risk for BD and MD due to having two affected parents, but also due to being raised by two adults coping with disorders.

Presently, there is no biological marker for either the genes associated with the major affective disorders nor for the disorders [60]. This situation has three important consequences. For research, it means that the severity of family history of affective disorders is the only feasible indicator available for assessing genetic risk for a major affective disorder among children. For adults with BD, it means that while they may know that one or another of their children will develop BD or MD, they do not know which one. For adolescents being raised by a parent with BD, it means wondering, and perhaps fearing, the onset of mania or depression.

Offspring of parents with BD: disorders in childhood and adolescence

Cross-sectional studies

In 1994, we conducted a meta-analysis of all published studies that compared diagnostic assessments of children of parents suffering from bipolar disorder and children of parents with no mental disorder [61,62]. A number of methodological features of these investigations are important to consider. (1) The samples of children examined may not be representative of the population of children of parents with BD. They or their parents may have been more disturbed or distressed, and consequently were more easily recruited into studies. (2) Many of these studies did not examine other characteristics of the BD parent that may be associated with offspring problems, such as personality traits and disorders and substance misuse. (3) We included in our meta-analysis only studies with comparison groups of parents with no mental disorder or no major mental disorder, some of whom had medical disorders. In most of the studies, these parents did not undergo a diagnostic assessment. It was simply presumed that they had no mental disorder. (4) Most of these studies were cross-sectional in design and thus involved only one assessment of the offspring. (5) The sample sizes, in general, were small and thereby limited the study of the effects of both parent and child gender. (6) The age of the children varied from early childhood to late adolescence making it difficult to identify critical ages when disorders onset.

Of the 973 children in the studies included in the meta-analysis, 52% of those with BD parents and 29% of those with nondisordered parents received a diagnosis. Of the 795 children for whom specific diagnoses were made, 26.5% of those with BD parents but only 8.3% of those with nondisordered parents received a diagnosis of an affective disorder, and 5.4% of those with BD parents and none of those with nondisordered parents received a diagnosis of bipolar disorder. Interestingly, the percentages with major depression were similar among children of BD parents (8.5%) and children of nondisordered parents (7.5%). In addition, 20.6% of the children of BD parents and 20.4% of the children of nondisordered parents received diagnoses for nonaffective disorders. Since the publication of this meta-analysis, to our knowledge, no new study fulfilling the criteria for inclusion has been published.

Two relevant studies have been published subsequently. Chang and colleagues [63] examined 29 boys and 31 girls between the ages of 6 and 18 years, 30 of whom had one parent with BD and 30 had one parent with BD and the other with BD or MD. Diagnoses were made using the Washington University Kiddie SADs by clinicians not blind to parental diagnoses, plus symptom rating scales and teacher and parent rating scales. Of the total sample, 45% received no diagnosis, 15% (8 boys and 1 girl) were diagnosed with BD, 28% were diagnosed with attention deficit hyperactivity disorder (ADHD) (14 boys and 3 girls), 15% were diagnosed with depression (4 boys and 5 girls), and 13% (3 boys and 5 girls) had other diagnoses. Interestingly, 88% of those with BD also received a diagnosis of attention-deficit disorder. Parental diagnosis of ADHD did not distinguish the offspring with ADHD. While the prevalence of disorders did not vary between the offspring with one or two ill parents, those with two ill parents had more severe symptoms, including depressed mood, irritability, mood reactivity, rejection, sensitivity, crying, and social withdrawal. There was no comparison group, and the authors noted that parents of children experiencing difficulty were over-represented in the sample.

In another diagnostic study, BDO participating in a genetic study were examined. To be eligible, the parents had to have had one parent and an adult first-degree relative with BD. Sixteen children of BD parents were examined and compared with 27 children of nondisordered parents (NMDO). Childrens' ages ranged from 6 to 17 years. Bipolar disorder was diagnosed in 4 of the BDO and one of the NMDO. More of the BDO, compared with the NMDO, had anxiety disorders (7 BDO, 4 NMDO), comorbid anxiety-affective disorders (4 BDO, 0 NMDO), and affective disorders (5 BDO, 1 NMDO) [64].

Few studies have examined other characteristics of BDO. One study of offspring between the ages of 10 and 17 reported that two thirds of the BDO and only one third of the NMDO evidenced abnormal personality traits. Among the BDO, three types were identified: (1) high anxiety and depressive reactivity; (2) high depressive reactivity and emotional instability; and (3) hyperthymic [65]. In contrast, another study found that compared with NMDO, BDO sought new experiences and were less inhibited [66]. Similar discrepancies have been observed in studies of cognitive functioning. One study reported greater verbal performance IQ discrepancies among BDO than NMDO due to lower perform-ance than verbal IQ in the BDO [67], while another study reported no differences in IQ between BDO and NMDO [68]. Finally, one study has reported that the offspring of adults with BD may be more autonomically reactive to a mild stressor [69,70]. Although the BDO did not differ from controls in electrodermal activation (EDA) at baseline or during rest periods, they showed significantly higher EDA to a mental arithmetic task and during the instructions for a reaction time task than a control group. Of interest, the BDO group rated themselves as more dysphoric than controls during the mental arithmetic task. Further exam-ination of the BDO sample demonstrated that the heightened autonomic reactivity to mild stress correlated positively with state anxiety (during the mental arithmetic task) and the personality trait of neuroticism; these associations were not found in control subjects [70]. These results suggest an underlying hypersensitivity to mild stress in offspring of bipolar parents; however, we are not aware of any replication of this study in the published literature.

In summary, cross-sectional studies that have compared mental disorders among the offspring of parents with BD and those with no mental disorder, docu-ment elevated rates of disorders among the BD offspring. This conclusion, how-ever, must be tempered by considering the sampling bias that characterizes many of these investigations (eg, families participating because of problems in the children or severity of the parents' disorder or children in large extended families with many relatives with major affective disorders). This same bias, of course, characterizes samples of BDO who are assessed and treated in child psychiatry services. The results taken together, however, do suggest that BD rarely occurs before puberty, that it occurs in families where it is already present, and that many of the offspring experience considerable difficulty in childhood.

Longitudinal prospective investigations.

To identify the nongenetic precursors of a disorder, it is necessary to conduct longitudinal prospective investigations. Such investigations identify precursors of disorders. A longitudinal, prospective investigation can be genetically informed, that is, it can compare the development of individuals who have presumably inherited a vulnerability for a disorder to that of individuals without the vulnerability. In most investigations of this type, the development of offspring of parents with a disorder is compared with that of offspring of nondisordered parents. Thus, the presence of a disorder in the parent is used to index genetic vulnerability in the offspring. Given that the genes associated with the disorder have not yet been identified, this is the best that can be done for the moment; however, it is important to note that among BDO, some will have inherited a genetic vulnerability for BD or MD, while others will not. Presently, there is no way to distinguish BDO who have the vulnerability for a major affective disorder from those who do not. Not surprisingly, given the financial and other difficulties associated with such investigations, few have been undertaken with the children of parents with BD. It must be emphasized, however, that this is the only type of investigation that can uncover the processes that lead to BD and that could be the targets of preventive interventions.

The most innovative and rigorous prospective investigation in this field is being carried out at the National Institute of Mental Health (NIMH) under the direction of Dr. Marion Radke-Yarrow [71]. In 1979, 98 families were recruited, each having one child between the ages of 1.5 and 3.5 years and a second child between the ages of 5 and 8 years. Of the 192 children, 48 had mothers with BD, 84 had mothers with MD, and 60 had mothers with no disorder. So far, the offspring have been assessed five times. When the older siblings were, on average, 6 years old and the younger siblings were 33 months old, the authors concluded that "The general picture for the [BDO] suggest a degree of irritability in both mothers and children that is especially likely to be observed under what are probably high-intensity or stressful circumstances" [72]. This finding is similar to an earlier report by Zahn-Waxler and colleagues [73,74], who examined seven 2-year-old boys of parents with BD. Naturalistic observations and creative laboratory social stressors demonstrated that these toddlers had difficulty modulating hostile impulses, showed maladaptive patterns of aggressive behaviors, and were overly sensitive to stress and less able to cope appropriately. Their mothers were distinguished by anger. These findings are similar to those reported by Gaensbauer (1984) [75] in a sample of 7 male BDO aged between 15 and 18 months. Compared with the NMDO, the BDO were reported to display more negative affect and slower recovery once upset. These kinds of detailed observations of interactions between parents and children contribute valuable information about the possible mechanisms by which environmental factors trigger or add to the genetic vulnerability for MD or BD.

At the fifth assessment of the participants in the longitudinal NIMH study, the younger offspring were between 18 and 25 years old, the older ones between 22 and 27 years old. Almost half (21) of the BDO have been assessed; among them, three have BD, three have BD spectrum diagnoses, three have MD or dysthymia, three have drug abuse or dependence, two have alcohol abuse or dependence, and one has other anxiety disorders. Interestingly, of the three cases of BD, two also have substance use disorders, and of the three cases of MD, one has comorbid substance abuse (Stephanie Meyer, Bethesda, Maryland, personal communication, 2001). While three of the offspring of BD mothers were diagnosed with BD, so were two offspring of mothers with MD. Of the five participants with BD, all but one displayed disruptive behavior problems since early childhood, and among two of them these problems were identified when the subjects were toddlers. The only case of BD that did not have disruptive problems had depression in early childhood and adolescence. Having a mother with either BD or MD and behavior problems in childhood greatly increased the risk of BD; however, the best predictor of BD was the mothers' anger and irritability [48]. This is the only study to have followed offspring into adulthood, to have early childhood measures, and to have made systematic observations of family functioning [76].

This longitudinal NIMH investigation was used to examine a neglected topic: suicide among BDO [77]. Suicidal ideation and attempts were measured four times from age 5 to 18 years. Among the older cohort, but not the younger one, more of the BDO than the NMDO reported suicidal ideations from middle childhood onwards. Suicidal ideations preceded attempts by several years. In the older cohort, the proportions of BDO and of offspring of depressed mothers with suicidal ideation and attempts did not differ. Two significant correlates of suicide ideation were identified, hypomanic symptoms and having a mother with a history of suicide attempts. This confirms previous reports suggesting that among adolescents once BD is present, or about to be, the risk of suicide attempts and completion rises dramatically, and that manic symptoms and rapid cycling often trigger the suicidal behaviors [78]. Comorbid substance misuse and the availability of weapons further increase the risk.

A two-year prospective investigation compared offspring of parents with BD in their early teens with children of mothers who have recurrent MD, medical illnesses, and no disorders. Almost three quarters of the BDO had at least one disorder, and most of them suffered from affective or anxiety disorders [79]. Mothers' ratings on the Child Behavior Checklist (CBCL) did not distinguish the BDO from the offspring of nondisordered women [80,81].

This latter study [79–83] clearly showed that children and young adolescents who have mothers with BD experienced less difficulty than those who have mothers with MD. This is consistent with observations in the Radke-Yarrow et al investigation [83] showing that until midadolescence, the BDO are less impaired than those who have mothers with MD [48]. Several reasons have been offered to explain this difference. For example, mothers with BD, compared with those with MD, experience fewer episodes of depression [80], are exposed to less stress [3], and engage in fewer negative interactions with their children [76,80]. These findings suggest a vicious cycle in which child problems contribute to worsening the course of the mothers' disorder. Radke-Yarrow et al [83] proposed that BDO in childhood may develop certain psychosocial competencies in reaction to maternal disorganization that are lost by early adolescence.

Retrospective studies of adults with BD and some—though not all—cross-sectional studies have found that behavior and attention problems afflict more BDO than NMDO. Such problems were found to precede the onset of both mood disorders and other types of disorders in adulthood in the Stony Brook High Risk Project [84,85]. In this longitudinal, prospective investigation, when the BDO were 18 years old or older, fewer than half were free of mental disorders. Although 45% of those with no behavior problems and 44% of those with no attention problems had no disorder in young adulthood, this was true of only 23% of those with behavior problems and 28% with attention problems. As would be expected, behavior and attention problems were associated with the development of a wide variety of disorders, substance abuse, and low psychosocial functioning, but also with the development of a mood disorder. Chronic stress in the family was found to be associated with adult disorders, and there was some evidence that in childhood the BDO were particularly sensitive to stress, notably marital discord [85].

Conclusion

There are few studies of BDO and even fewer that have prospectively followed them from conception through adulthood. Retrospective reports from adults who have developed BD and the two longitudinal studies [48,84] that have followed BDO into adulthood suggest that early-onset BD is preceded by externalizing problems. Taken together, studies of BDO in childhood and early adolescence suggest that half develop disorders, most often a disruptive behavior disorder, and a few present depression or anxiety problems. Studies of other characteristics of BDO are rare and have included very few children. Results are tantalizing, however, suggesting that even as toddlers BDO are overly sensitive to certain types of stress, have difficulty recovering from stress, and show maladaptive behaviors. Findings about the psychosocial competence of BDO at various stages of development are contradictory. Because only a subgroup of BDO have inherited a genetic vulnerability for MD or BD, and there is no way currently to identify them, the precursors of the adult affective disorders in this population will only be known when the ongoing prospective investigations succeed in following BDO through the period of risk for adult disorders.

A hypothesis of the development of MD and BD among BDO

We are currently conducting a longitudinal prospective investigation comparing the development of 108 BDO to that of 108 NMDO. The sample includes 27 BD mothers, 31 BD fathers, 53 of their spouses who are biological parents of the child, and 10 new partners who are acting as parents to the children. The parents with BD all have clinical diagnoses of BD that were confirmed by research clinicians using the Structured Clinical Interview for DSM-IV. About one quarter of the BD mothers and one third of the BD fathers received diagnoses of substance use disorders, and 26% of the mothers and 45% of the fathers received diagnoses of personality disorders. Among the spouses of the BD parents, one third of the women and two thirds of the fathers met criteria for an affective disorder. The

NMD parents include 92 adults with no history of mental disorders and in whom no disorders were revealed during the diagnostic interview. To be eligible for the study, all parents had to have at least one child between the ages of 5 and 12 years old at the time of recruitment. The BD parents were recruited for the most part from a consumer association and the NMD parents via pediatricians' offices.

BD parents, compared with NMD parents, showed lower levels of psychosocial functioning, lower block design scores (an estimate of performance IQ), higher scores on the personality trait of neuroticism, lower scores on the trait of conscientiousness, greater use of emotional and lesser use of task-centered coping skills, and less social support. They reported providing their children with less support and structure than did the NMD parents, and the BD fathers, in addition, provided less control. The spouses of the BD parents evidenced lower psychosocial functioning than the NMD parents, but higher than that of the BD parents.

We have observed elevated rates of impaired psychosocial functioning among the BDO. At the initial assessment, when the offspring were between the ages of 5 and 12, mental disorders and psychosocial functioning were assessed by clinicians

---

Fig. 1. (a) Generation 1's high neuroticism contributes to the development of emotional coping skills and a lack of task-centered coping skills. (b) Generation 2's high neuroticism is partially heritable. (c) Generation 1's emotional coping skills and lack of task-centered coping skills contribute to the development of high levels of self-generated stress. (d) Generation 1's coping style and high level of stress contributes to the development of inadequate parenting practices, specifically engaging in behaviors that are potentially harmful to the fetus during pregnancy and providing inadequate levels of support and structure to the offspring. (e) Generation 1's coping style and high level of stress contribute to a low level of psychosocial functioning. (f) Generation 1's coping style and high level of stress contribute to a more severe course of bipolar disorder. (g) Stress on Generation 1 influences stress on Generation 2. (h) Generation 2 learns emotional coping skills and fails to learn task-centered coping skills from Generation 1. (i) Generation 1's inadequate parenting practices contribute to, or at least fail to modify Generation 2's high neuroticism. (j) Generation 1's low psychosocial functioning (eg, low family income, low educational attainment) contributes to the development of externalizing problems in Generation 2. (k) Generation 1's inadequate parenting practices (maternal smoking during pregnancy and the provision of insufficient support and structure) contribute to the development of externalizing problems in Generation 2. (l) Generation 2's externalizing problems contribute to the maintenance of inadequate parenting skills in Generation 1. (m) Generation 2's high neuroticism contributes to the development of emotional coping skills and a lack of task-centered coping skills. (n) Generation 2's emotional coping skills and a lack of task-centered coping skills contribute to the development of high levels of self-generated stress. (o) In Generation 2, emotional coping skills, a lack of task-centered coping skills, and self-generated stress contribute to the development of BD. (p) In Generation 2, emotional coping skills, a lack of task-centered coping skills, and self-generated stress contribute to the development of MD. (q) In Generation 2, emotional coping skills, a lack of task-centered coping skills, and self-generated stress contribute to the development of inadequate parenting practices. (r) Generation 2's externalizing problems contribute to increasing the level of stress for Generation 1. (s) Generation 2's externalizing problems contribute to increasing the level of stress for themselves. (t) Generation 2's externalizing problems contribute to the development of bipolar disorder. (u) Generation 2's externalizing problems contribute to the development of inadequate parenting skills. (v) Generation 3's HPA dysfunction and excessive reactions to stress are partially heritable. (w) Generation 2's inadequate parenting practices contribute to the development and maintenance of a dysfunctional hypothalamic pituitary adrenal axis and excessive emotional reactions to stress in Generation 3 as babies.

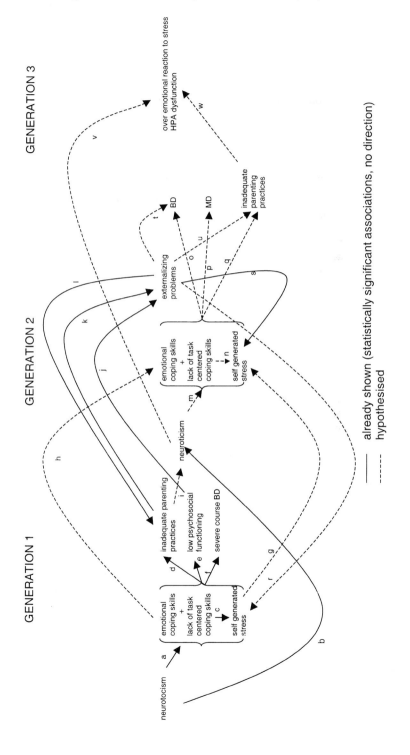

using the Dominic, Child Assessment Scale (CAS) and Child and Adolescent Functioning Scale (CAFAS), and by the mother, father and teacher using the CBCL. While only 11% of the NMDO obtained diagnoses on the CAS, this was true of 27% of the BDO. In addition, only 8% of the NMDO but 30% of the BDO were rated as impaired by at least two informants (child psychiatrist, mother, father, teacher). The BDO who were impaired, in most cases, presented multiple problems whereas the NMDO usually presented only one. On the CBCL, the mean scores of the BDO were just under the clinical cut-off score and were far in excess of those of the NMDO [86].

We hypothesize that BDO are at increased risk for MD and BD in adolescence and adulthood and for other disorders in childhood and adolescence as a result of specific nongenetic factors interacting with an inherited vulnerability (Fig. 1), and that the inherited vulnerability for the major affective disorders is expressed, at least in part, as the trait of neuroticism. Neuroticism is a personality trait expressed as emotional lability, with a susceptibility to negative affects such as fear, anger, sadness, embarrassment, guilt, and disgust [87]. The child who inherits the genes associated with MD or BD inherits a tendency to react emotionally to stressors and daily hassles. The vulnerable child is raised by one or two parents who themselves have high levels of neuroticism, who react emotionally to stress and daily hassles, and who create stress. These parents thus provide their children with an environment that is stressful, chaotic, and unpredictable; furthermore, they model the use of ineffective strategies for dealing with problems. High levels of neuroticism in the parents are also associated with low levels of psychosocial functioning, two aspects of which (low income and low educational attainment) are specifically related to psychosocial functioning in children [88,89]. High levels of neuroticism in the parents are also associated with poor parenting practices, specifically providing insufficient support and structure and engaging in behaviors during the pregnancy that are potentially harmful to the offspring. Poor parenting practices, parents' use of emotional rather than task-centered coping skills, high levels of stress and daily hassles in the family, and poor psychosocial functioning of the parents act together to strengthen the child's inherited tendency to react to problems emotionally rather than instrumentally, to the development in the child of emotional rather than instrumental coping skills, and thereby a tendency to create stress. These characteristics are in turn associated with the development of mental disorders and poor psychosocial functioning.

What is the evidence for such a model? The trait of neuroticism is elevated among parents with BD. The presence of the trait of neuroticism was defined according to the NEO-PI-R manual [87]: T scores above 55 indicate the presence of the trait, T scores between 44 to 54 are normative, and scores less than 44 are lower than the population mean. As seen in Table 1, two thirds of the fathers and mothers with BD were characterized by the trait. Interestingly, the trait also characterized one third of the husbands of women with BD and 27% of the wives of men with BD. (Depending on the analysis, neuroticism was defined as a category or as a continuous variable, the total T score.) We have shown that high levels of neuroticism in the parents are associated with poor psychosocial

Table 1
T scores on neuroticism scale NEO-PI-R obtained by parents

	Men				Women			
	Neuroticism T scores				Neuroticism T scores			
	Low	Normative	High		Low	Normative	High	
Bipolar disorder	10.3%	20.7%	66.7%	X^2 (N=94) = 32.115, P = 0.000	3.8%	26.9%	69.2%	X^2 (N=102) = 24.016, P = 0.000
Partner of a parent with bipolar disorder	33.3%	33.3%	33.3%		43.3%	30.0%	26.7%	
No mental disorder	52.3%	40.9%	6.8%		45.7%	37.0%	17.4%	

NEO-PI-R, NEO Personality Inventory.

functioning as indicated by low global ratings of functioning, low levels of educational attainment, low income, lack of employment stability, poor intimate relations, low levels of social support, and higher verbal aggression in the home [90]. Furthermore, our results indicate that neuroticism is associated with the use of emotional coping skills, the failure to use task centered skills, and an elevated number of negative life events dependent on the person (which we call self-generated stress). High levels of neuroticism are associated with parenting practices. Specifically, during pregnancy, high levels of neuroticism are associated with smoking, which is in turn associated with externalizing problems in middle childhood, and with providing offspring with low levels of support and structure.

In the proposed model, assortative mating confers both genetic and nongenetic risk to the offspring for the development of MD and BD. Genetic risk for the trait of neuroticism is conferred by having two parents who present high levels of neuroticism. Nongenetic risk for MD and BD is increased for offspring of BD parents: (1) when the non-BD parent presents low levels of psychosocial functioning and is thus not able to act as a buffer to protect the children from the negative impact of the BD parent's functioning; (2) when the non-BD parent models an ineffective emotional coping style; (3) when the non-BD parent self-generates stress for him/herself and the family; and (4) when the non-BD parent presents inadequate parenting practices either during pregnancy or childhood. The children with two parents with high neuroticism scores were the most impaired in middle childhood.

The trait of neuroticism has a heritability coefficient of approximately 50% [91,92]. In an investigation of a large unbiased sample of female twins, the genetic liability for depression largely overlapped with that for neuroticism [93,94]. A recent study of monozygotic twins discordant for major depression from this sample has shown that the relationship between neuroticism and MD is likely due to a genetic mechanism and not individual environmental experiences [95]. These results suggest that a shared genetic influence accounts for both MD and neuroticism. Furthermore, prospective studies of first-onset depression [96,97] as well as studies of subjects at high risk for depression [98,99] have shown that high neuroticism is associated with an elevated risk of MD. We have found that the higher the neuroticism score the greater the number of first and second degree relatives with MD or BD and the earlier the age of onset of BD. In our investigation, the number of relatives with MD and BD was not associated with offspring functioning in middle childhood, once we accounted for the parents' neuroticism.

We have shown that high levels of neuroticism are associated with ineffective stress-coping abilities, particularly the use of emotion-focused coping skills and the lack of task-centered skills. Among both the parents and their first-degree relatives who have either BD or MD, we have found that these coping skills are associated with a high level of negative life events that are dependent on the individual's own behavior. This finding confirms the notion that neuroticism mediates the experience of stress [100–103] and leads to the high levels of stress experienced by individuals with BD [104,105]. The high levels of stress have been found to be present before the onset of MD [103] and to trigger acute episodes [33,104]. Further, the greater the stress, measured as negative life events, the greater the number of relatives with MD and BD and the higher the number of negative life events among the relatives [106].

We hypothesize that the well-documented association between a positive family history for MD and elevated numbers of negative life events [105,107] is either mediated or simply reflected by the trait of neuroticism. Inheriting the genes associated with the trait, as well as growing up in a family environment that strengthens the trait, leads to the development of ineffective coping characterized by an inability to effectively resolve problems as they arise. As problems accumulate, individuals create more stress for themselves and for those around them. The extent to which the inherited tendency leads to the development of ineffective coping skills and the self generation of stress depends, we hypothesize, on the coping skills that parents model for their children, the overall level of stress in the family, specific parenting practices, and parents' level of psychosocial functioning.

The role of stress in the pathophysiology of affective disorders is well established, both at the behavioral [108,109] and neurobiological levels [110,111]. Converging evidence indicates that the stress-sensitive hypothalamic–pituitary–adrenal (HPA) axis is compromised in MD [112] and BD [113,114]. A recent study found that compared young adults who had high neuroticism compared with those who had low neuroticism showed a blunted cortisol response to the administration of dexamethasone and corticotropin-releasing hormone, perhaps indicating hypersensitive negative feedback regulation of the axis [115]. This blunting may reflect an adaptation of the HPA axis resulting from the high levels of stress and interpersonal difficulties that individuals high on neuroticism create for themselves. Thus, abnormal adrenocortical function may represent a risk factor for BD and MD.

HPA function also provides a good index of adaptive and competent functioning in children and adolescents. High cortisol levels have been observed in children and adolescents with internalizing disorders [116,117]. Healthy adolescents who exhibited an increase in cortisol in response to a mild naturalistic stressor, compared with subjects who showed either no response or a decreasing cortisol response, reported more depressive and conduct symptoms one year later [118]. HPA functioning during childhood has been shown to be influenced by genetic factors [119], socioeconomic status, daycare [120,121], psychosocial competence [122], repeated stress [123], and parenting [124]. Maternal care and mother–child interaction are critical factors in the development of the HPA axis [120,124–127], suggesting that parenting and the family environment are important determinants of offspring HPA functioning. There also is some evidence in rodents and primates of an interaction between the early environment and genetic vulnerability in producing HPA dysfunction [128,129]. Thus, we propose that HPA functioning, as assessed by cortisol levels during baseline and stressful conditions, will provide an index of adaptation to the environment. We predict that abnormalities in cortisol will be associated with behavioural or emotional problems in adolescence, high stress in the family, and poor parenting.

Clincial implications

Adults with BD who become parents may need help from the time their child is conceived, so as to forego engaging in behaviors during the pregnancy that may be harmful to the fetus, to replace an emotional coping style with one that is task-oriented and includes good problem solving skills, and to learn how to provide their offspring with sufficient structure and support. Learning these skills, it is hoped, would reduce the amount of self-generated stress, and perhaps mothers' anger and negativity.

Given the high prevalence of problems in BDO, all adults with BD should be asked about their children, and those reporting difficulty should be assessed. Those with disorders need appropriate treatment and they may well benefit from an intervention aimed at improving problem solving abilities and decreasing reliance on emotional coping skills. If treatment of the child is effective, this may in turn have positive consequences for the course of the parent's disorder. Present findings suggest, however, that interventions with the child will only be effective if they are accompanied by interventions for the parents, such as those described above, that focus on parents' coping skills and parenting practices.

Research implications

In this era of the genome, it is essential to continue longitudinal prospective investigations that will elucidate the complex interactions over the lifespan of genetic and nongenetic factors [17]. Only these kinds of investigations will identify the processes in childhood that lead to disorder and to mental health. An understanding of the processes and the time during development when they occur will provide the basis for the development of early childhood prevention programs for this high-risk population.

References

[1] Vanharen J, LaRoche C, Heyman M, et al. Have the invisible children become visible? Can J Psychiatry 1993;38:678–80.

[2] Beardslee WR, Gladstone TRG. Prevention of childhood depression: recent findings and future prospects. B Psychiatry 2001;49:1101–10.

[3] Hammen C, Burge D, Adrian C. Timing of mother and child depression in a longitudinal study of children at risk. J Consult Clin Psychol 1991;59:341–5.

[4] Kessler RC, McGonagle KA, Zhao S, et al. Lifetime and 12-month prevalence of DSM-III-R psychiatric disorders in the United States. Results from the National Comorbidity Survey. Arch Gen Psychiatry 1994;51:8–19.

[5] Hodgins S, Ellenbogen M, Munk-Jørgensen P. The prevalence of bipolar disorder in three recent Danish cohorts: further evidence of national variations, submitted for publication.

[6] Kirov G, Murray RM. Ethnic differences in the presentation of bipolar affective disorder. Eur Psychiatry 1999;14:199–204.

[7] Weissman MM, Bland RC, Canino GJ, et al. Cross-national epidemiology of major depression and bipolar disorder. JAMA 1996;276:293–9.

[8] Faravelli C. Guerrini Degl'Innocenti B, Aiazzi L, et al. Epidemiology of mood disorders: a community survey in Florence. J Affect Disord 1990;20:135–41.

[9] Kebede DA. Major mental disorders in Addis Ababa, Ethiopia. II. Affective disorders. Acta Psychiatr Scand 1999;(Suppl 397):18–23.

[10] Lynge I, Munk-Jørgensen P, Mortensen PB. Affective disorders among Greenlandic psychiatric patients. Acta Psychiatr Scand 1999;100:424–32.

[11] Lewinsohn PM, Klein DN, Seeley JR. Bipolar disorders in a community sample of older adolescents: prevalence, phenomenology, comorbidity, and course. J Am Acad Child Adolesc Psychiatry 1995;34:454–63.

[12] Wittchen HU, Nelson CB, Lachner G. Prevalence of mental disorders and psychosocial impairments in adolescents and young adults. Psychol Med 1998;28:109–26.

[13] Verhulst FC, van der Ende J, Ferdinand RF, et al. The prevalence of DSM-III-R diagnoses in a national sample of Dutch adolescents. Arch Gen Psychiatry 1997;54:329–36.

[14] Szádóczky E, Papp ZS, Vitrai J, et al. The prevalence of major depressive and bipolar disorders in hungary. Results from a national epidemiologic survey. J Affect Disord 1998;50:153–62.

[15] Newman DL, Moffitt TE, Caspi A, et al. Psychiatric disorder in a birth cohort of young adults: prevalence, comorbidity, clinical significance, and new case incidence from ages 11–21. J Consult Clin Psychol 1996;64:552–62.

[16] Veijola J, Castle D, Jablenskly A. Low incidence of mania in Northern Finland. Br J Psychiatry 1996;168:520–1.

[17] Rutter M, Pickles A, Murray R, et al. Testing hypotheses on specific environmental causal effects on behavior. Psychol Bull 2001;127:291–324.

[18] Fogarty F, Russell JM, Newman SC, et al. Epidemiology of psychiatric disorders in Edmonton. Mania. Acta Psychiatr Scand 1994;(Suppl 376):16–23.

[19] Weissman MM, Livingston-Bruce ML, Leaf PJ, et al. Affective disorders. In: Robins LN, Regier D, editors. Psychiatric disorder in America. New York: MacMillan/Free Press; 1991. p. 53–80.

[20] Wells JE, Bushnell JA, Hornblow AR, et al. Christchurch psychiatric epidemiology study, part I: methodology and lifetime prevalence for specific psychiatric disorders. Aust N Z J Psychiatry 1989;23:315–26.

[21] Burke KC, Burke JD Jr, Regier DA, et al. Age at onset of selected mental disorders in five community populations. Arch Gen Psychiatry 1990;47:511–8.

[22] Schurhoff F, Bellivier F, Jouvent R, et al. Early and late onset bipolar disorders: two different forms of manic-depressive illness? J Affect Disord 2000;58:215–21.

[23] Lewinsohn PM, Hops H, Roberts RE, et al. Adolescent psychopathology: I. Prevalence and incidence of depression and other DSM-III-R disorders in high school students. J Abnorm Child Psychol 1993;102:133–44.

[24] Räsänen P, Tiihonen J, Hakko H. The incidence and onset-age of hospitalized bipolar affective disorder in Finland. J Affect Disord 1998;48:63–8.

[25] Angst J. Epidémiologie du spectre bipolaire. Encéphale 1995;21:37–42.

[26] Bruce ML, Leaf PJ. Psychiatric disorders and 15-month mortality in a community sample of older adults. Am J Public Health 1989;79:727–30.

[27] Bruce ML, Leaf PJ, Rozal GP, et al. Psychiatric status and 9-year mortality data in the new haven epidemiologic catchment area study. Am J Psychiatry 1994;151:716–21.

[28] Gershon ES, Hamovit JH, Guroff JJ, et al. Birth cohort changes in manic and depressive disorders in relatives of bipolar and schizoaffective patients. Arch Gen Psychiatry 1987;44: 314–9.

[29] Joyce PR, Oakley-Browne MA, Wells JE, et al. Birth cohort trends in major depression: increasing rates and earlier onset in New Zealand. J Affect Disord 1990;18:83–9.

[30] Klerman GL, Lavori PW, Rice J, et al. Birth-cohort trends in rates of major depressive disorder among relatives of patients with affective disorder. Arch Gen Psychiatry 1985;42:689–93.

[31] Lasch K, Weissman M, Wickramaratne P, Bruce ML. Birth-cohort changes in the rates of mania. Psychiatry Res 1990;33:31–7.

[32] Rutz W, von Knorring L, Pihlgren H, et al. An educational project on depression and its consequences: is the frequency of major depression among Swedish men underrated, resulting in high suicidality? Primary Care Psychiatry 1995;1:59–63.

[33] Gitlin M, Swendsen J, Heller TL, et al. Relapse and impairment in bipolar disorder. Am J Psychiatry 1995;152:1635–40.

[34] Harrow M, Goldberg JF, Grossman LS, et al. Outcome in manic disorders. a naturalistic follow-up study. Arch Gen Psychiatry 1990;47:665–71.

[35] Atre-Vaidya N, Taylor MA, Seidenberg MM, et al. Cognitive deficits, psychopathology, and psychosocial functioning in bipolar mood disorder. Neuropsychiatry Neuropsychol Behav Neurol 1998;11:120–6.

[36] Coryell W, Scheftner W, Keller M, et al. The enduring psychosocial consequences of mania and depression. Am J Psychiatry 1993;150:720–7.

[37] Coryell W, Turvey C, Endicott J, et al. Bipolar I affective disorder: predictors of outcome after 15 years. J Affect Disord 1998;50:109–16.

[38] Guze SB, Robins E. Suicide and primary affective disorders. Br J Psychiatry 1970;117:437–8.

[39] Brodersen A, Licht RW, Vestergaard P, et al. Sixteen-year mortality in patients with affective disorder commenced on lithium. Br J Psychiatry 2000;176:429–33.

[40] Skodol AE, Stout RL, McGlashan TH, et al. Co-occurrence of mood and personality disorders: a report from the collaborative Longitudinal Personality Disorders Study (CLPS). Depress Anxiety 1999;10:175–82.

[41] Barbato N, Hafner J. Comorbidity of bipolar and personality disorder. Aust N Z J Psychiatry 1998;32:276–80.

[42] Ücok A, Karaveli D, Kundakçi T, et al. Comorbidity of personality disorders with bipolar mood disorders. Comp psychiatry 1998;39:72–4.

[43] Tohen M, Greenfield SF, Weiss RD, et al. The effect of comorbid substance use disorders on the course of bipolar disorder: a review. Harv Rev Psychiatry 1998;6:133–41.

[44] Bellivier F, Golmard J-L, Henry C, et al. Admixture analysis of age at onset in bipolar I affective disorder. Arch Gen Psychiatry 2001;58:510–2.

[45] Akiskal HS, Downs J, Jordan P, et al. Affective disorders in referred children and younger siblings of manic-depressives. Arch Gen Psychiatry 1985;42:996–1003.

[46] Carlson GA, Bromet EJ, Driessens C, et al. The role of antecedent childhood psychopathology in bipolar disorder intitially presenting with psychosis. 2000. unpublished manuscript.

[47] Carlson GA, Bromet EJ, Sievers S. Phenomenology and outcome of subjects with early- and adults-onset psychotic mania. Am J Psychiatry 2000;157:213–9.

[48] Meyer SE, Ronsaville DS, Gold PW, et al. A prospective study of children at risk for mood disorder. Presented at the meeting of the International Society for Research on Child and Adolescent Psychopathology, Vancouver, British Columbia, 2001.

[49] Oates M. Patients as parents: the risk to children [review]. Br J Psychiatry 1997;170(Suppl): 22–7.

[50] Andreasen NC, Rice J, Endicott J, et al. Familial rates of affective disorder: a report from the National Institute of Mental Health Collaborative Study. Arch Gen Psychiatry 1987;44:461–9.

[51] Gershon ES, Hamovit J, Guroff JJ, et al. A family study of schizoaffective, bipolar I, bipolar II, unipolar, and normal control probands. Arch Gen Psychiatry 1982;39:1157–67.

[52] Pauls DL, Morton LA, Egeland JA. Risks of affective illness among first-degree relatives of bipolar I old-order Amish probands. Arch Gen Psychiatry 1992;49:703–8.

[53] Weissman MM, Fendrich M, Warner V, et al. Incidence of psychiatric disorder in offspring at high and low risk for depression. J Am Acad Child Adolesc Psychiatry 1992;31:640–8.

[54] Allen MG. Twin studies of affective illness. Arch Gen Psychiatry 1976;33:1476–8.

[55] Bertelsen A, Harvald B, Hauge M. A Danish twin study of manic-depressive disorder. Br J Psychiatry 1977;130:330–51.

[56] Gershon ES. Genetics. In: Goodwin FK, Jamison KR, editors. Manic depressive illness. Oxford: Oxford University Press; 1990. p. 373–402.

[57] Mendlewicz J, Rainer JD. Adoption study supporting genetic transmission in manic-depressive illness. Nature 1977;268:327–9.

[58] Torgersen S. Genetic factors in moderately severe mild affective disorders. Arch Gen Psychiatry 1986;43:222–6.

[59] Merikangas KR, Spiker DG. Assortative mating among in-patients with primary affective disorder. Psychol Med 1982;12:753–64.

[60] Lane C, Palmour R. Are there biological markers to indicate risk of affective disorders in children? In: Hodgins S, editor. A critical review of the literature on children at risk for major affective disorders. Ottawa, Canada: Report commissioned by the minister of Health of Canada; 1994. p. 149–95.

[61] Hodgins S, Lapalme M, Laroche C, et al. Évaluation du risque des enfants ayant un parent souffrant de trouble bipolaire. Rapport final—FRSQ/CQRS. Québec, Canada; 1996.

[62] Lapalme M, Hodgins S, LaRoche C. Children of parents with bipolar disorder: a meta-analysis of risk for mental disorders. Can J Psychiatry 1997;42:623–31.

[63] Chang KD, Steiner H, Ketter TA. Psychiatric phenomenology of child and adolescent bipolar offspring. J Am Acad Child Adolesc Psychiatry 2000;39:453–60.

[64] Todd RD, Reich W, Petti TA, et al. Psychiatric diagnoses in the child and adolescent members of extended families identified through adult bipolar affective disorder probands. J Am Acad Child Adolesc Psychiatry 1996;35:664–71.

[65] Grigoroiu-Serbanescu M, Christodorescu D, Totoescu A, et al. Depressive disorders and depressive personality traits in offspring aged 10–17 of bipolar and of normal parents. Journal of Youth and Adolescence 1991;20:135–48.

[66] Nurnberger JI, Hamovit J, Hibbs ED, et al. A high-risk study of primary affective disorder: selection of subjects, initial assessment, and 1- to 2-year follow up. In: Dunner DL, Gershon ES, Barret JE, editors. Relatives at risk for mental disorders. New York: Raven Press; 1988. p. 161–77.

[67] Decina P, Kestenbaum CJ, Farber S, et al. Clinical and psychological assessment of children of bipolar probands. Am J Psychiatry 1983;140:548–53.

[68] Winters KC, Stone AA, Weintraub S, Neale JM. Cognitive and attentional deficits in children vulnerable to psychopathology. J Abnorm Child Psychol 1981;9:435–53.

[69] Zahn TP, Nurnberger JI, Berrettini WH. Electrodermal activity in young adults at genetic risk for affective disorder. Arch Gen Psychiatry 1989;46:1120–4.

[70] Zahn TP, Nurnberger JI, Berrettini WH, et al. Concordance between anxiety and autonomic

nervous system activity in subjects at genetic risk for affective disorder. Psychiatry Res 1991; 36:99–110.

[71] Radke-Yarrow M. Children of depressed mothers: from early childhood to maturity. New York: Cambridge University Press; 1998.

[72] Inoff-Germain G, Nottelmann ED, Radke-Yarrow M. Evaluative communications between affectively ill and well mothers and their children. J Abnorm Child Psychol 1992;20:189–212.

[73] Zahn-Waxler C, Cummings EM, Iannotti RJ, et al. Young offspring of depressed parents: a population at risk for affective problems. In: Cicchetti D, Schneider-Rosen K, editors. Child depression. 1984. p. 81–105.

[74] Zahn-Waxler C, Cummings EM, McKnew DH, et al. Altruism, aggression, and social interactions in young children with a manic-depressive parent. Child Dev 1984;55:112–22.

[75] Gaensbauer TJ, Harmon RJ, Cytryn L, et al. Social and affective development in infants with a manic-depressive parent. Am J Psychiatry 1984;141:223–9.

[76] Hay DF, Vespo JE, Zahn-Waxler C. Young children's quarrels with their siblings and mothers: links with maternal depression and bipolar illness. British Journal of Developmental Psychology 1998;16:519–38.

[77] Klimes-Dougan B, Free K, Ronsaville D, et al. Suicidal ideation and attempts: a longitudinal investigation of children of depressed and well mothers. J Am Acad Child Adolesc Psychiatry 1999;38:651–9.

[78] Brent DA, Perper JA, Moritz G, et al. Suicide in affectively ill adolescents: a case-control study. J Affect Disord 1994;31:193–202.

[79] Hammen C, Burge D, Burney E, et al. Longitudinal study of diagnoses in children of women with unipolar and bipolar affective disorder. Arch Gen Psychiatry 1990;47:1112–7.

[80] Anderson CA, Hammen CL. Psychosocial outcomes of children of unipolar depressed, bipolar, medically ill, and normal women: a longitudinal study. J Consult Clin Psychol 1993;61: 448–54.

[81] Hammen C, Gordon D, Burge D, et al. Maternal affective disorders, illness, and stress: risk for children's psychopathology. Am J Psychiatry 1987;144:736–41.

[82] Kochanska G. Patterns of inhibition to the unfamiliar in children of normal and affectively ill mothers. Child Dev 1991;62:250–63.

[83] Radke-Yarrow M, Nottelmann E, Martinez P, et al. Young children of affectively III parents: a longitudinal study of psychosocial development. J Am Acad Child Adolesc Psychiatry 1992; 31:68–77.

[84] Carlson GA, Weintraub S. Childhood behavior problems and bipolar disorder—relationship or coincidence? J Affect Disord 1993;28:143–53.

[85] Weintraub S. Risk factors in schizophrenia. The Stony Brook High Risk Project. Schizo Bull 1987;13:439–50.

[86] Lalonde N. Comparaison d'enfants de parents souffrant d'un trouble bipolaire avec des enfants de parents sans trouble mental, sur la base de caractéristiques comportementales sociales et émotionnelles. Unpublished thesis. University of Montreal, Montreal, Canada. 1999.

[87] Costa PT, McCrae RR. Revised NEO Personality Inventory (NEO PI-R): professional manual. Baltimore (MD): NIH National Institute on Aging Gerontology Research Center: Laboratory of Personality & Cognition; 1992.

[88] Chase-Lansdale PL, Brooks-Gunn J. Escape from poverty: what makes a difference for children? New York: Cambridge University Press; 1995.

[89] Serbin LA, Cooperman JM, Peters PL, et al. Intergenerational transfer of psychological risk in women with childhood histories of aggression, withdrawal, or aggression and withdrawal. Dev Psychol 1998;34:1246–62.

[90] Ellenbogen MA, Hodgins S. The impact of high neuroticism in parents on psychosocial functioning in children: family environmental and genetic pathways of intergenerational risk, submitted for publication.

[91] Eysenck HJ. Genetic and environmental contributions to individual differences: the three major dimensions of personality. J Pers 1990;58:245–61.

[92] Plomin R, Defries JC, McClearn GE, et al. Behavioral genetics. 3rd edition. New York: WH Freeman; 1997.

[93] Kendler KS, Neale MC, Kessler RC, et al. A longitudinal twin study of personality and major depression in women. Arch Gen Psychiatry 1993;50:853–62.

[94] Kendler KS, Neale MC, Kessler RC, et al. A test of the equal environment assumption in twin studies of psychiatric illness. Behav Genet 1993;23:21–7.

[95] Kendler KS, Gardner CO. Monozygotic twins discordant for major depression: a preliminary exploration of the role of environmental experiences in the aetiology and course of illness. Psychol Med 2001;31:411–23.

[96] Clayton PJ, Ernst C, Angst J. Premorbid personality traits of men who develop unipolar or bipolar disorders. Eur Arch Psychiatry Clin Neurosci 1994;243:340–6.

[97] Hirschfeld RMA, Klerman GL, Lavori P, et al. Premorbid personality assessments of first onset of major depression. Arch Gen Psychiatry 1989;46:345–50.

[98] Lauer CJ, Bronisch T, Kainz M, et al. Pre-morbid psychometric profile of subjects at high familial risk for affective disorder. Psychol Med 1997;27:355–62.

[99] Maier W, Minges J, Lichtermann D, et al. Personality patterns in subjects at risk for affective disorders. Psychopathology 1995;28:59–72.

[100] Kendler KS, Thornton LM, Gardner CO. Genetic risk, number of previous depressive episodes, and stressful life events in predicting onset of major depression. Am J Psychiatry 2001;158:582–6.

[101] Plomin R, Lichtenstein P, Pedersen NL, et al. Genetic influence on life events during the last half of the life span. Psychol Aging 1990;5:25–30.

[102] Saudino KJ, Pedersen NL, Lichtenstein P, et al. Can personality explain genetic influences on life events? J Pers Soc Psychol 1997;72:196–206.

[103] van Os J, Jones PB. Early risk factors and adult person-environment relationships in affective disorder. Psychol Med 1999;29:1055–67.

[104] Hammen C, Gitlin M. Stress reactivity in bipolar patients and its relation to prior history of disorder. Am J Psychiatry 1997;154:856–7.

[105] Kendler KS, Karkowski-Shuman L. Stressful life events and genetic liability to major depression: genetic control of exposure to the environment? Psychol Med 1997;27:539–47.

[106] McGuffin P, Bebbington P. The Camberwell collaborative depression study. III. Depression and adversity in the relatives of depressed probands. Br J Psychiatry 1989;152:775–82.

[107] Silberg JL, Pickles A, Rutter M, et al. The influence of genetic factors and life stress on depression among adolescent girls. Arch Gen Psychiatry 1999;56:225–32.

[108] Benes FM. Developmental changes in stress adaptation in relation to psychopathology. Dev Psychopathol 1994;6:723–39.

[109] Perris H. Life events and personality characteristics in depression. In: Miller TW, editor. Stressful life events. Madison (CT): International Universities Press; 1989. p. 485–98.

[110] Gold PW, Goodwin FK, Churosos GP. Clinical and biochemical manifestations of depression: relation to the neurobiology of stress (part 1). N Engl J Med 1988;319:348–53.

[111] Heim C, Nemeroff CB. The impact of early adverse experiences on brain systems involved in the pathophysiology of anxiety and affective disorders. B Psychiatry 1999;46:1509–22.

[112] Holsboer F. Neuroendocrinology of mood disorders. In: Bloom FE, Kupfer DJ, editors. Psychopharmacology: the fourth generation of progress. New York: Raven Press; 1995. p. 957–69.

[113] Cassidy F, Ritchie JC, Carroll BJ. Plasma dexamethasone concentration and cortisol response during manic episodes. B Psychiatry 1998;43:747–54.

[114] Yehuda R, Boisoneau D, Mason JW, et al. Glucocorticoid receptor number and cortisol excretion in mood, anxiety, and psychotic disorders. B Psychiatry 1993;34:18–25.

[115] McCleery JM, Goodwin GM. High and low neuroticism predict different cortisol responses to the combined dexamethasone-CRH test. B Psychiatry 2001;49:410–5.

[116] Granger DA, Weisz JR, Kauneckis D. Neuroendocrine reactivity, internalizing behavior problems, and control-related cognitions in clinic-referred children and adolescents. J Abnorm Child Psychol 1994;103:267–76.

[117] Kagan J, Reznick JS, Snidman N. Biological bases of childhood shyness. Science 1988;240: 167–71.

[118] Susman EJ, Dorn LD, Inoff-Germain G, et al. Cortisol reactivity, distress behavior, and behavioral and psychological problems in young adolescents: a longitudinal perspective. Journal of Research on Adolescence 1997;7:81–105.

[119] Wüst S, Federenko I, Hellhammer DH, et al. Genetic factors, perceived chronic stress, and the free cortisol response to awakening. Psychoneuroendocrinology 2000;25:707–20.

[120] Dettling AC, Parker SW, Lane S, et al. Quality of care and temperament determine changes in cortisol concentrations over the day for young children in childcare. Psychoneuroendocrinology 2000;25:819–36.

[121] Lupien SJ, King S, Meaney MJ, et al. Child's stress hormone levels correlate with mother's socioeconomic status and depressive state. B Psychiatry 2000;48:976–80.

[122] Gunnar MR, Tout K, de Haan M, et al. Temperament, social competence, adrenocortical activity in preschoolers. Dev Psychobiol 1997;31:65–85.

[123] Coplan JD, Andrews MW, Rosenblum LA, et al. Persistent elevations of cerebrospinal fluid concentrations of corticotropin-releasing factor in adult nonhuman primate exposed to early-life stressors: implications for the pathophysiology of mood and anxiety disorders. Proc Natl Acad Sci USA 1996;93:1619–23.

[124] Gunnar M. Psychoneuroendocrine studies of temperament and stress in early childhood: expanding current models. In: Bates JE, Wachs TD, editors. Temperament: individual differences at the interface of biology and behavior. Washington (DC): American Psychological Association; 1994. p. 175–98.

[125] Carlson M, Earls F. Social ecology and the development of stress regulation. In: Bergman LR, Cairns RB, editors. Developmental science and the holistic approach. Mahwah (NJ): Erlbaum; 2000. p. 229–48.

[126] Field T, Hernandez-Reif M, Seligman S, et al. Juvenile rheumatoid arthritis: benefits from massage therapy. J Ped Psychol 1997;22:607–17.

[127] Gunnar M, Larsen M, Hertsgaard L, et al. The stressfulness of separation among 9-month-old infants: effects of social context variables and infant temperament. Child Dev 1992;63:290–303.

[128] King JA, Edwards E. Early stress and genetic influences on hypothalamic-pituitary-adrenal axis functioning in adulthood. Horm Behav 1999;36:79–85.

[129] Lyons DM, Martel FL, Levine S, et al. Postnatal experiences and genetic effects on squirrel monkey social affinities emotional distress. Horm Behav 1999;36:266–75.

CHILD AND
ADOLESCENT
PSYCHIATRIC
CLINICS

Child Adolesc Psychiatric Clin N Am
11 (2002) 555–578

Somatic treatment for depressive illnesses in children and adolescents

Robert L. Findling, MD*, Norah C. Feeny, PhD,
Robert J. Stansbrey, MD, Denise DelPorto-Bedoya, MA,
Christine Demeter, BA

*Department of Psychiatry, University Hospitals of Cleveland, Case Western Reserve University,
11100 Euclid Avenue Cleveland, OH 44106–5080, USA*

An ever-increasing body of evidence has demonstrated that depressive illnesses are chronic conditions associated with significant human suffering, psychosocial morbidity, and the risk of suicide in children and adolescents. [1,2] As the malignant outcome of pediatric depression has become better understood, the need for identifying safe and effective interventions for these vulnerable young people has also become clearer.

Somatic interventions are commonly considered for adults suffering from major depression or dysthymia. These treatments include pharmacotherapy, electroconvulsive therapy, light therapy, and alternative therapies. Unfortunately, much less is known about these interventions in children and adolescents than in adults with depressive illnesses.

This article briefly reviews what is known about the use of somatic interventions for the treatment of children and adolescents with major depression, dysthymia, and related conditions. Particular emphasis is placed on interpreting the available scientific data so that they may be rationally applied to current clinical practice.

Tricyclic antidepressants

For decades, tricyclic antidepressants were the benchmarks for pharmacotherapy. Several of these compounds, such as amitriptyline, desipramine, imipramine,

---

This work was supported, in part, by a Clinical Research Center grant from the Stanley Foundation.
* Corresponding author.
E-mail address: robert.findling@uhhs.com (R.L. Findling).

and nortriptyline, were shown to be effective in treating depressed adults. Initial uncontrolled studies in children and adolescents suggested that some tricyclic antidepressants might have beneficial effects when prescribed for depressed youths. Randomized controlled trials, however, have failed to demonstrate that these agents are superior to placebo in ameliorating symptoms of depression in children and adolescents [3–5].

Birmaher and colleagues found that treatment with amitriptyline at an average dose of 173 mg/day was not associated with greater symptom amelioration than placebo in 27 treatment-resistant adolescent patients [6]. The patients treated with amitriptyline experienced more tachycardia and complained more frequently of dry mouth than the patients taking placebo. Another study published within the past few years similarly failed to demonstrate that desipramine at an average daily dose of 214.1 mg/day was superior to placebo in 45 adolescents between the ages of 13 and 18 years who were treated in a double-blind, controlled 6-week study [7].

Most recently, Keller and colleagues treated 182 depressed adolescents from 12 to 18 years of age with imipramine or placebo in a double-blind study over an 8-week period [8]. As discussed later, this study also included a third treatment arm in which 93 teenagers were treated with paroxetine. The patients treated with imipramine received between 200 and 300 mg of medication per day. The authors found no significant differences in changes in depressive symptomatology in the 95 adolescents treated with imipramine at a mean dose of 205.8 mg/day and the 87 teenagers who received placebo. Moreover, the authors found that 31.5% of the patients treated with imipramine but only 9.7% of the patients treated with paroxetine withdrew from the treatment study because of side effects. Perhaps of even greater importance, 14% of the patients treated with imipramine had cardiovascular side effects that led to discontinuation of the study.

There is some evidence that intravenous pulse treatment with the tricyclic antidepressant clomipramine may be superior to placebo when administered to depressed teenagers. In one study, treatment with a single intravenous 200-mg dose of clomipramine was found to be safe and superior to intravenously administered placebo in 16 depressed adolescents, 8 of whom received active treatment [9]. These data may not be applicable to oral treatment with clomipramine. The authors hypothesized that the therapeutic effects of the intravenous clomipramine may have resulted from pharmacodynamic changes that occur specifically with pulse intravenous therapy.

In short, numerous agents from this class of compounds have failed to show superiority to placebo in randomized, clinical trials. Tricyclic antidepressants have the potential for causing significant and potentially life-threatening cardiovascular side effects. Other problematic drug-related side effects (such as anticholinergia and sedation) may also significantly interfere with the use of tricyclic antidepressants in treating pediatric depression [3]. For these reasons, tricyclic antidepressants should generally not be considered as first-line treatments for depressed young people.

Monoamine oxidase inhibitors

Historically, the monoamine oxidase inhibitors (MAOIs) were the second most commonly prescribed class of drugs administered for the treatment of depression in adults. These compounds are effective in the treatment of depressed adults. Older compounds that are nonselective inhibitors of both MAO-A and MAO-B (eg, isocarboxazid, phenelzine, and tranylcypromine) require significant dietary restrictions of tyramine-rich foods to avoid the risk of a hypertensive crisis [10].

In the first randomized, controlled trial to examine the efficacy of antidepressant agents in depressed children, the effects of phenelzine and chlordiazepoxide were compared with those of phenobarbitone plus placebo in a cross-over study [11]. The author noted that most patients treated with phenelzine and chlordiazepoxide for the 2-week study period had some clinical benefit from treatment. The diagnostic heterogeneity of this patient cohort, the small sample size ($n = 32$), the lack of a placebo arm, and the brief duration of treatment significantly impair the definitive interpretation of these results.

A chart review of 23 teenagers between the ages of 11 and 18 years who were unresponsive to tricyclic antidepressant therapy and were subsequently treated with an MAOI suggested that treatment with tranylcypromine or phenelzine alone or adjunctively with the previously prescribed tricyclic antidepressant might be associated with a good or fair response to MAOI treatment in some patients [12]. Approximately 30% percent of the youths, however, failed to comply with the necessary dietary restrictions.

The authors generally do not recommend the routine use of nonselective MAOIs for the treatment of depressed children or teenagers for several reasons. The first relates to the paucity of data from controlled, clinical trials. The second arises from the dietary restrictions that are necessary for these drugs to be administered safely and that may be difficult for most teenagers to comply with. Both phenelzine (Nardil; Parke-Davis Morris, Plains, NJ) and tranylcypromine (Parnate; Glaxo Smith Kline Research, Triangle Park, NC) are still marketed for adults in the United States. Because there is one case report that phenelzine may be useful in treatment-resistant cases of adolescent depression [13], the use of MAOIs that are nonselective inhibitors of MAO-A and MAO-B might be a reasonable consideration for patients with treatment-resistant depression.

Other MAOIs are not associated with the same degree of risk of tyramine-associated hypertensive crises. There is substantial evidence from randomized, clinical trials that moclobemide (a reversible inhibitor of MAO-A) is safe and effective for the treatment of depression in adults [14,15]. Dietary restrictions do not seem to be necessary when adults are treated with moclobemide at the generally recommended doses [14]. Evidence also suggests that open-label treatment with moclobemide might be safe and of benefit to children with attention deficit hyperactivity disorder (ADHD) [16,17]. Whether or not moclobemide may be useful in treating pediatric depression has yet to be adequately considered.

Similarly, some evidence suggests that selegiline (L-deprenyl), a compound that at low doses selectively inhibits MAO-B, might be useful for the treatment of children with ADHD and tic disorders [18,19]. In adults, there is evidence suggesting that selegiline is an effective antidepressant when given at higher oral doses, at which its MAO-B selectivity may be lost. This consideration is important because it is selegiline's MAO-B selectivity at low doses that mediates its modest risk for tyramine-associated hypertensive events. Whether selegiline is an effective antidepressant at the lower doses at which it retains its MAO-B selectivity has yet to be definitively established [20]. At present there are no data regarding the use of selegiline in depressed children or adolescents.

Pirlindole, befloxatone, and toloxatone are other reversible MAO-A inhibitors that are marketed outside the United States or are currently under clinical development in adults [15,20]. Whether these agents can eventually be used to treat depressed young people is not yet known.

Trazodone

Trazodone is a triazolopyridine derivative that was initially marketed in the United States in 1981 for the treatment of depression in adults [21,22]. Its pharmacodynamics seems to result from its action as a serotonin receptor antagonist [23,24]. There is only limited information about the use of this compound in depressed children or adolescents, most probably because of concerns about the possibility of drug-induced priapism [25,26]. Also, sedation seems to be a dose-limiting side effect with this agent.

Some clinicians, however, have taken advantage of trazodone's sedating properties in their treatment of adults with depression. Trazodone, at doses lower than typically given for the treatment of depression, has been reported to be an effective adjunct to antidepressant pharmacotherapy with other agents in adults with depression- or antidepressant-related sleep disturbances [27]. In contrast, a retrospective chart review found that little benefit from the addition of trazodone to fluoxetine pharmacotherapy in adolescent inpatients [28].

Because of the limited data about the use of trazodone in pediatric depression and concerns about priapism and sedation, the authors generally do not prescribe this compound to depressed children or teenagers.

Bupropion

Bupropion is an aminoketone antidepressant that was initially marketed in the United States in 1988. Bupropion seems to act by modulating the reuptake of norepinephrine and dopamine in the CNS [29]. Bupropion has historically been marketed in the United States as Wellbutrin (Glaxo Smith Kline Research, Triangle Park, NC). Recommended daily dosing for Wellbutrin was administration in three divided doses. Of major concern is Wellbutrin's association with a 0.40% seizure rate in adults [30].

A sustained-release formulation, Wellbutrin SR (Glaxo Smith Kline Research, Triangle Park, NC), was approved for use in this country in 1996 and has subsequently been marketed here. Wellbutrin SR is effective in treating adults with depression and allows twice-daily dosing. Of perhaps greater importance, Wellbutrin SR seems to have has a reduced seizure risk than the originally available immediate-release preparation [31–33]. The active ingredient in Zyban (Glaxo Smith Kline Research, Triangle Park, NC), a product marketed as an aid to smoking cessation, is the sustained-release formulation of bupropion [34].

Although evidence from several studies suggests that bupropion may be safe and effective in the treatment of pediatric ADHD [35–38], there is a paucity of data regarding the use of this compound in either formulation in depressed youths. This lack of information probably arises from concerns about the risk of seizures in adults that has been reported with Wellbutrin, particularly at higher doses [30]. In one open-label study, Wellbutrin SR, at doses of approximately 6 mg/kg/day, was found to be safe and associated with amelioration in depressive symptomatology in a cohort of 16 adolescents with ADHD and either major depression or dysthymia [39].

Unfortunately, data about the use of bupropion in depressed children or adolescents are limited. Because Wellbutrin SR seems to have some advantages over Wellbutrin in adults, the safety and efficacy of Wellbutrin SR in children and adolescents with depression should be a topic of future study.

Serotonin-selective reuptake inhibitors

Five serotonin-selective reuptake inhibitors (SSRIs) are currently marketed in the United States. All SSRIs have been shown to be effective in treating depression in adults [40]. Although these agents have different effects on neural transmission, they all seem to act primarily by selectively inhibiting serotonin reuptake [41].

Fluoxetine (Eli Lilly and Company, Indianapolis, IN) was the first SSRI released in the United States. It is currently marketed under the name Prozac for use in adults with depression, obsessive-compulsive disorder, and bulimia nervosa. Fluoxetine is also marketed under the name Sarafem as a treatment for premenstrual dysphoric disorder. At present, fluoxetine is not approved for use in children or adolescents. The second SSRI available in the United States was sertraline (Zoloft; Pfizar Inc., New York, NY). Sertraline is currently approved for use in the treatment of obsessive-compulsive disorder in adults and children and in treating adults with depression, panic disorder, or posttraumatic stress disorder. Paroxetine (Paxil; Glaxo Smith Kline Research, Triangle Park, NC) the next SSRI released in the United States, is indicated for use in adults with depression, obsessive-compulsive disorder, panic disorder, and social anxiety disorder. Presently, paroxetine is not approved for use in children or adolescents. Fluvoxamine (Luvox; Solvey Pharmaceuticals Inc., Maritta, GA) is currently approved for use in the treatment of adults and children with obsessive-

Table 1
Selected studies of fluoxetine in pediatric depressive disorders

Lead author (Year)	Diagnosis	Study design	N	Age (years)	Dosing (mg/d)	Comments
Simeon (1990)	MDD	RPC	40	13–18	60	Two thirds of placebo- and fluoxetine-treated patients had marked or moderate response. No statistically significant differences noted between treatment arms.
Boulos (1992)	MDD	OLP	15	16–24	5–40	Most patients benefited from therapy despite being unresponsive to TCAs. Starting doses of 5–10 mg recommended.
Jain (1992)	MDD, BP-Dep	RCR	31 (27 MDD)	9–18	20–60	Fifty-four percent were much or very much improved; 20% showed minimal improvement.
Gammon (1993)	MDD, DYS, Others	OLP	32 (6 MDD, 25 DYS)	9–17	2.5–20	Adjunctive treatment with fluoxetine at doses at 20 mg/d or lower were found to be effective for patients with ADHD and comorbid depressive disorders who were partially responsive to methylphenidate.
Colle (1994)	MDD	OLP	9	15–18	10–40	Treatment with fluoxetine for up to 1 year was reported to be generally safe and effective.
Ghaziuddin (1995)	MDD	OLP	6	15–18	20–60	Fluoxetine was associated with reductions in depressive symptoms for patients unresponsive to TCA therapy.
Emslie (1997)	MDD	RPC	106	7–17	20	Fluoxetine was found to be safe and superior to placebo in reducing symptoms of depression during an 8-week trial.
Riggs (1997)	MDD, CD, SUD	OLP	8	14–18	20	Fluoxetine was found to be effective in reducing symptoms of depression in depressed teenagers with comorbid CD and histories of SUD while in residential treatment.

Study	Diagnosis	Design	N	Age range	Dose	Comments
Strober (1999)	MDD	OLP	52	13–17	20–40	Fluoxetine was associated with reductions in depressive symptoms in hospitalized teenagers. When compared with 28 historical controls that had been treated with imipramine, fluoxetine seemed to be associated with greater salutary effects over a 6-week trial.
Waslick (1999)	DYS ± MDD	OLP	19	12–18	20	Fluoxetine seemed to be safe and effective for patients with DYS ± MDD who do not respond to psychotherapy.
Dittman (2000)	MDD, Others	RCR	213	11–23	-	Naturalistic use of fluoxetine seems to be generally safe and effective.
Emslie (2000)	MDD	RPC	219	8–17	20	Fluoxetine was found to be safe and superior to placebo in reducing symptoms of depression over an 8-week controlled study.
Emslie (2001)	MDD	RPC	40	8–17	20–60	Patients who responded to 15 weeks of fluoxetine treatment were randomly assigned to receive either continued fluoxetine or placebo. Fluoxetine was found to be superior to placebo in preventing depressive relapses.
Hoog (2001)	MDD	RCT	29	9–17	20–60	Patients unresponsive to 9 weeks of fluoxetine treatment at 20 mg/d were either maintained at their current dose or could have their dose increased to 40–60 mg/d. Clinical response to the increased dose was robust, but statistical between-group significance was not seen, probably because of small sample size.

RPC, randomized, placebo-controlled; MDD, major depressive disorder; BP-Dep, bipolar depression; OLP, open-label prospective; TCA, tricyclic antidepressant; RCR, retrospective clinical review; DYS, dysthymia; ADHD, attention-deficit/hyperactivity disorder; CD, conduct disorder; SUD, substance use disorders; -, data not available; RCT, randomized, controlled trial.

compulsive disorder. Citalopram (Celexa; Forest Pharmaceuticals Inc., St. Louis, MO), the SSRI most recently released in the United States, is approved for the treatment of depression in adults.

Fluoxetine

More is known about fluoxetine than about any of the newer antidepressants (Table 1). Results of open-label studies suggest that fluoxetine is a generally effective treatment in pediatric major depression or dysthymia for patients with and without comorbid psychiatric diagnoses. These reports also suggest that more than 90% of young patients treated with fluoxetine tolerate it well. When considered as a group, these open studies also suggest that fluoxetine is likely to be effective for major depression and dysthymia at doses lower than those typically prescribed for adults [42–50].

The first study that compared the antidepressant efficacy of fluoxetine with placebo failed to demonstrate any difference between the two treatments [51]. The results of this study were difficult to interpret, however, because of the small sample size, high placebo-response rate, and forced titration to 60 mg/day, a higher dose than is generally prescribed.

The two other randomized, double-blind, placebo-controlled studies that have been conducted found that fluoxetine, at a dose of 20 mg/day, was superior to placebo in the acute treatment of depressed children and teenagers [52,53]. There is also evidence that, for patients who do not respond to fluoxetine therapy at the 20-mg/day dose level, increasing the doses of fluoxetine to 40 or 60 mg/day may be of benefit [54]. Finally, evidence suggests that fluoxetine may also be an effective maintenance therapy for the treatment of pediatric depression [55].

In short, more data support the use of fluoxetine in pediatric depressive illnesses than any other compound. In practice, the authors generally initiate treatment at 10 mg/day and increase doses in 10-mg increments every 3 to 4 weeks. Although the data from randomized, controlled studies have shown that higher starting doses and larger dosing increments are generally well tolerated, the open-label literature and the authors' clinical experience suggest the use of smaller dosing increments as a reasonable treatment approach.

Sertraline

Several studies have examined the safety and effectiveness of sertraline in children and adolescents (Table 2). The pharmacokinetics of sertraline was studied in 61 children and adolescents, 44 of whom were depressed [56]. Results of that study found that the pharmacokinetics of sertraline is similar in children, adolescents, and adults. Those findings have clinical relevance because they support the once-daily administration of sertraline.

Although data from double blind studies have demonstrated that sertraline is safe and effective in treating pediatric obsessive-compulsive disorder [57], data from double-blind, placebo-controlled studies in depressed children and teenagers are not available. The data that exist suggest that when a flexible dose strategy is used during open-label treatment, sertraline therapy is generally well tolerated and is associated with high rates of depressive symptom amelioration [56,58–61].

The results of the available studies indicate that sertraline is a promising treatment for children and adolescents with depressive disorders. Data from double-blind, placebo-controlled studies are needed, however.

Paroxetine

Open-label studies of the effectiveness of paroxetine as a treatment for pediatric depressive disorders have reported that this drug may be a safe and well-tolerated agent in a variety of distinct patient cohorts (see Table 2). The results of these open studies also suggest that paroxetine may be an effective antidepressant in children at smaller doses than usually prescribed for adults [62–65]. Although the biotransformation of paroxetine seems to be more rapid in children and adolescents than adults, the available data support once-daily dosing of paroxetine [62].

Published data available from a large, randomized, placebo-controlled clinical trial describe the acute efficacy of paroxetine in adolescents with depression (see Table 2). The authors of that study found that paroxetine was superior to placebo in reducing several measures of depressive symptomatology, whereas imipramine was not [8].

In summary, the evidence suggests that paroxetine is a safe and effective treatment for pediatric depressive-spectrum illnesses. Doses of paroxetine lower than those generally administered to adult patients may be effective for treating depressed children. For this reason the authors initiate treatment with paroxetine at a dose of 10 mg/day and use 10-mg dose increments as needed. More data from randomized, placebo-controlled trials are necessary to confirm or to refute these impressions.

Fluvoxamine

Data from double-blind studies have demonstrated that fluvoxamine is safe and effective in treating pediatric obsessive-compulsive disorder [66]. There are few published data about the use of fluvoxamine in children and adolescents with depressive spectrum disorders (see Table 2). The existing data suggest that fluvoxamine is effective in adolescents with depressive illnesses [67,68,84]. More data about the use of fluvoxamine in this population are needed.

Citalopram

In a recently completed, unpublished study, 178 depressed children and teenagers between the ages of 7 and 17 years were randomly assigned to receive either citalopram at a dose of 20 to 40 mg/day or placebo for 8 weeks. The results

Table 2
Selected studies of antidepressants in pediatric depressive disorders

Lead author (year)	Diagnosis	Study design	N	Age (years)	Dosing (mg/d)	Comments
Sertraline						
Tierney (1995)	MDD	RCR	33	8–18	25–200	Most patients (65%) were much or very much improved. Seven patients developed mania or disinhibition.
McConville (1996)	MDD	OLP	13	12–18	25–200	Eleven of 13 patients had a greater than 50% reduction in their Hamilton Rating Scale for Depression scores.
Alderman (1998)	MDD, OCD	OLP	61	6–17	25–200	Significant improvement in depression severity noted. Pharmacokinetics found to be similar to those seen in adults.
Sallee (1998)	MDD	OLP	18	9–17	200	Seventy-two percent were considered responders.
Ambrosini (1999)	MDD	OLP	53	12–19	50–200	At the end of 10 weeks of treatment, 85% were considered much or very much improved.
Paroxetine						
Masi (1997)	MDD, MR	OLP	7	14–18	20–40	Reductions in depressive symptoms were noted in this cohort of subjects with IQs ranging from 53–68.
Rey-Sánchez (1997)	MDD	OLP	45	Mean = 10.7	Mean = 16.22	With a flexible dose strategy, relatively low doses of paroxetine were found to be safe and effective.

Study	Diagnosis	Design	N	Age	Dose	Comments
Findling (1999)	MDD	OLP	30	6–17	10–20	All patients were considered symptom-free after an average of 8.4 months of treatment.
Nobile (2000)	DYS	OLP	7	11–18	10–40	Paroxetine was found to be safe and well tolerated with most patients responding to the 10–mg/d doses. Pharmacokinetics of paroxetine are also described. Treatment over 3 months was well tolerated with 5/7 subjects being considered responders.
Keller (2001)	MDD	RPC	275	12–18	20–40	Paroxetine, but not imipramine, was found to be superior to placebo on some, but not all, measures of depression. Paroxetine was better tolerated than placebo and was associated with low discontinuation rates from adverse events.
Fluvoxamine						
Apter (1994)	MDD	OLP	6	13–17	100–300	Significant reductions in depressive symptomatology were noted.
Rabe-Joblanska (2000)	DYS	OLP	21	Mean = 15.6	150–200	Treatment with fluvoxamine for up to 26 weeks was associated with symptom amelioration and was generally well tolerated.

RPC, randomized, placebo-controlled; MDD, major depressive disorder; OLP, open-label prospective; RCR, retrospective clinical review; DYS, dysthymia; MR, mental retardation; OCD, obsessive-compulsive disorder.

of this study showed that citalopram was well tolerated and was superior to placebo in ameliorating symptoms of depression when youngsters were assessed with the Children's Depression Rating Scale–Revised (Paul J. Tiseo, PhD, personal communication, 2001).

Doses of citalopram, 70 mg/day, have been reported as being effective in the treatment of a variety of anxiety disorders in children and adolescents [69] including posttraumatic stress disorder [70], obsessive-compulsive disorder [71,72], and panic disorder [73]. The safety and efficacy of citalopram in treating pediatric depression should be a topic of future study.

Venlafaxine

Venlafaxine is a bicyclic phenylethylamine that was initially marketed in the United States as Effexor (Wyeth-Ayerst, Philadelphia, PA). More recently, an extended-release version of this preparation, Effexor XR (Wyeth-Ayerst, Philadelphia, PA) has been marketed. Both preparations are safe and effective in the treatment of adults with depression [74,75]. The extended-release version of the drug seems to have two key advantages: it allows once-daily dosing and seems to be associated with less nausea and dizziness seen with the immediate-release form of the compound [74]. Venlafaxine seems to act by inhibiting the uptake of serotonin and norepinephrine from the synaptic cleft [76,77].

One published study has examined the efficacy of venlafaxine as an adjunct to psychotherapy in pediatric depression. In that trial, venlafaxine was not found to be superior to placebo [78], but the low dose of venlafaxine used and the small sample employed prevent definitive conclusions from being made concerning the efficacy of venlafaxine in treating juvenile depression (Table 3). Because some data suggest that venlafaxine may have salutary effects in ADHD [79,80], it would be of particular interest to clinicians to have data from randomized, clinical trials about the safety, efficacy, and dosing of venlafaxine in depressed youths with and without ADHD.

Nefazodone

Marketed as Serzone (Bristol-Meyers Squibb, Princeton, NJ) in the United States, nefzadone is a phenylpiperazine antidepressant that blocks postsynaptic serotonin 5-HT$_{2a}$ receptors and also inhibits the reuptake of serotonin and norepinephrine. Nefazodone has been shown to be safe and effective in the treatment of depressed adults [81].

There is a modest amount of data pertaining to the use of nefazodone in the young (see Table 3). A pharmacokinetic study of nefazodone found the pharmacokinetics of this drug to be similar in children, adolescents, and adults [82]. Open-label reports suggest that nefazodone is safe and effective in treating depressed young people [82–84]. Adolescents generally seem to respond to doses similar to those used in adults, whereas children seem to benefit from lower doses of medication. Whether nefazodone is truly safe and effective in pediatric depressive illnesses should be a topic of future research.

Mirtazapine

Mirtazapine (Remeron Oregon, Inc., West Orange, NJ) is a 6-aza derivative of the antidepressant mianserin. Mirtazapine potentiates serotonergic and noradrenergic neural transmission and has been shown to be safe and effective in the treatment of depressed adults [85].

Unfortunately, there are no published studies of mirtazapine in depressed children or teenagers. Of clinical interest is a case report of an 8-year-old girl with posttraumatic stress disorder successfully treated with 7.5 mg of mirtazapine at bedtime (half the recommended starting dose of mirtazapine for depressed adults) [86]. More data are needed about the use of mirtazapine in the young.

Lithium

Lithium has been reported to be effective in preventing relapses of depression in adults [87]. Data from adult studies also support the use of lithium as an augmenting agent to antidepressants [88].

There are data from chart reviews and an open clinical trial about the use of lithium as an antidepressant augmentation strategy in youths (see Table 3). What information exists suggests that the addition of lithium may be an effective approach for patients who are not fully responsive to antidepressant pharmacotherapy [89–91]. Whether lithium truly is effective as an antidepressant-augmenting agent remains to be rigorously studied in young patients.

Of particular interest are the results of a randomized, clinical trial in which lithium was compared with placebo in a group of depressed children at risk for developing bipolar disorder. In that study, lithium and placebo were found to have equal efficacy [92].

Light therapy

A growing body of evidence indicates that bright light therapy may be helpful for adult patients who have seasonal patterns to their depressive episodes when they are seen in mental health settings [93]. Despite its potential as a safe, effective treatment for depression, a recent study of bright light therapy in adults did not support its widespread use in a primary care–based population [94]. The optimal light therapy regimen for the treatment of patients with seasonal affective disorder remains to be definitively determined [95,96].

Although a seasonal pattern of depression may have a very early age of onset [97], few studies have carefully looked at the treatment of seasonal depression in

Table 3
Selected studies of other somatic treatments in pediatric depressive disorders

Lead author (year)	Diagnosis	Study design	N	Age (years)	Dosing (mg/d)	Comments
Venlafaxine						
Mandoki (1997)	MDD	RPC	40	8–18	37.5–75	Patients treated with venlafaxine and psychotherapy had outcomes similar to those treated with placebo and psychotherapy.
Nefazodone						
Wilens (1997)	MDD, BP-Dep	RCR	7	9–17	200–600	Clinical improvement was often seen for patients with bipolar depression and unipolar depression.
Findling (2000)	MDD	OLP	28	7–17	200–600	Pharmacokinetics in adolescents and children were found to be similar to those seen in adults. Treatment seemed to be effective and safe.
Goodnick (2000)	MDD	OLP	10	13–17	400	Treatment was generally well tolerated and associated with reduction in depressive symptoms.
Lithium						
Ryan (1988)	MDD	RCR	14	14–19	600–1200	Lithium augmentation to TCA therapy was associated with a good response in 6/14 teenagers who were not responsive to TCAs alone.
Strober (1992)	MDD	OLP	24	Mean = 15.4	Variable	For 10/24 depressed adolescents unresponsive to IMI, 3 weeks of adjunctive lithium was found to be helpful.

Study	Diagnosis	Design	N	Age	Dose	Results
Geller (1998)	MDD	RPC	30	6–12	Variable	Lithium was not found to be superior to placebo in the treatment of depressed children with family history predictors for developing bipolar disorder.
Walter (1998)	MDD	RCR	2	16	500–1250	Lithium was reported to be a useful adjunct to venlafaxine in two adolescents partially responsive to venlafaxine therapy.
Light therapy						
Sonis (1987)	SAD	RCT	19	-	2 hours of bright light therapy	Light therapy was associated with a greater reduction of neuro-vegative symptoms when compared with relaxation therapy.
Swedo (1997)	SAD	RPC	28	7–17	2 hours dawn stimulation and 1 hour of bright light therapy	Light therapy was found to be effective and superior to placebo.
Rosenthal (1986), Giedd (1998)	SAD	RCR	7	13–22	Variable	Patients with SAD who were initially responsive to light therapy were followed up over a 7-year period and were found to have persistent seasonal symptomatology. Light therapy generally continued to ameliorate symptoms in these patients.
Magnusson (1998)	SAD	OLP	18	18–19	40 minutes of bright light therapy	Mild benefit was noted.

RPC, randomized, placebo-controlled; MDD, major depressive disorder; BP-Dep, bipolar depression; OLP, open-label prospective; TCA, tricyclic antidepressant; IMI, imipramine; RCR, retrospective clinical review; SAD, seasonal affective disorder; -, data not available; RCT, randomized clinical trial.

children and adolescents (see Table 3). Most notably, in a randomized, clinical trial, 28 participants between the ages of 7 and 17 years with seasonal affective disorder were found to have greater reductions in depressive symptomatology after bright light therapy than after placebo treatment [98].

At present, light therapy seems to be a promising treatment for patients with seasonal affective disorders. More research into the usefulness of this intervention is needed.

Alternative therapies

Alternative therapies are forms of treatment that are not typically delivered by health care professionals. They consist of interventions such as herbal therapies, folk remedies, biofeedback, acupuncture, and homeopathy [99]. These practices have become commonly used in the United States, and many parents wish to treat their children with these alternative forms of therapy [100,101]. Unfortunately, there are relatively few studies of alternative treatments for adult or pediatric patients with depression.

Electroacupuncture is a form of acupuncture in which electrical stimulation is applied through acupuncture needles. Some evidence to suggests that electro-acupuncture may be an effective form of treatment for depressed adults [102]. There are no studies of acupuncture in children or adolescents with depression.

Probably the best-studied alternative therapy for depression is the extract from St. John's wort (*Hypericum perforatum*). Numerous studies of varying methodologic rigor have suggested that St. John's wort may be a safe and effective treatment of depression in adults [103–106]. A recently published rigorous, placebo-controlled trial has brought the efficacy of St. John's wort for adults with major depression into question, however [107].

Few data are available about the use of St. John's wort in depressed youths. In a case series describing the use of St. John's wort in five adolescents with psychiatric illnesses, Walter and Rey described this naturotherapy as well tolerated and associated with reductions in depressive symptomatology in a single 17-year old girl with major depression and panic attacks [108].

An 8-week, flexible-dose, open-label trial of St. John's wort was recently completed at the University Hospitals of Cleveland/CaseWestern Reserve University. In that study, more than 25 children and adolescents were administered St. John's wort at doses of up to 900 mg/day. Observations from this trial suggest that open-label treatment with St. John's wort may be safe and effective in this population (R.L. Findling, unpublished data, 2002). Because this study was not placebo-controlled, and because the small sample size was relatively small, definitive conclusions about the safety and efficacy of Saint John's wort cannot and should not be made.

Because there are so few data about the use of alternative treatments in children and adolescents, the authors generally recommend that parents eschew these forms of treatment. Parents seem to be quite interested in these forms of therapy, however, so the use of alternative interventions for pediatric depression should be a topic of further study.

Electroconvulsive therapy

Electroconvulsive therapy (ECT) does not seem to be commonly used to treat children or adolescents [109]. Although no controlled studies have examined the use of electroconvulsive therapy in young people, a reasonably extensive body of evidence that suggests that when electroconvulsive therapy is administered to youths, high rates of symptom amelioration generally occur [110–113]. The use of electroconvulsive therapy in young people remains controversial [114,115], mostly because of concerns about the acute- and long-term safety of this intervention. The data that are available about the safety of electroconvulsive therapy in the young suggest that, although it is associated with transient cognitive effects, it is not associated with long-term adverse sequelae [116,117]. The available data suggest that electroconvulsive therapy is a reasonable consideration for the treatment of depressed youths who are not responsive to other forms of therapy.

Repetitive transcranial magnetic stimulation

Data suggest that repetitive transcranial magnetic stimulation may be a safe, effective treatment for adults with major depression [118]. Results of recently published, double-blind studies have provided further evidence that repetitive transcranial magnetic stimulation may be effective in the short-term treatment of major depression [119,120]. The safety and effectiveness of this intervention in the young have yet to be studied.

Vagus nerve stimulation

Evidence from an open clinical trial indicates that vagus nerve stimulation may be useful in the treatment of adults with treatment-resistant depression [121]. What role, if any, vagal nerve stimulation will have in the treatment of pediatric depression has not been determined.

Other clinical considerations with antidepressant medications

A somatic intervention in a young patient with a depressive-spectrum illness should be initiated only after a careful clinical assessment has been made. In addition, such treatments should be administered as part of a treatment plan in which the implementation of other therapeutic modalities has also been considered.

The SSRIs are the antidepressants for which the greatest amount of data is available to support their use, but several other agents seem promising. Unfortunately, when compared with what is known about the treatment of depression in adults, only a modest amount of data is available regarding the safety, efficacy, and optimal dosing of the antidepressants in pediatric depressive disorders.

The adverse event that seems most commonly to interfere significantly with the use of the newer antidepressants in the young is emergence of disruptive behaviors or restlessness during pharmacotherapy. If the patient is not abusing drugs and does not have a general medical condition that could explain these behaviors, this phenomenon can often be explained by (1) the development of mania or hypomania, (2) medication-induced disinhibition, or (3) the unmasking of latent ADHD. When a patient has these difficulties during antidepressant pharmacotherapy, a careful clinical assessment is needed.

A patient who has developed mania, hypomania, or antidepressant-induced disinhibition may well respond to a reduction in antidepressant dose. For some patients the antidepressant must be discontinued. In more severe cases of mania and hypomania in which euthymia does not return after the discontinuation of antidepressant pharmacotherapy, treatment with a mood stabilizer may be indicated. For patients who have latent ADHD that has become more readily manifest as the patient's mood has improved, treatment with an adjunctive psychostimulant may be reasonable [122].

A review of the literature indicates that children may tolerate adult-sized doses of the newer antidepressants, but data also suggest that young people may respond to lower doses of antidepressants than adults. Because some antidepressant side effects seem to be dose related, it is generally reasonable to adhere to the rule, "start low and go slow" when starting medication treatment of pediatric depression.

Future directions

Much remains to be learned about the acute somatic treatment of pediatric depressive disorders. Unfortunately, even fewer data are available regarding the long-term treatment of these conditions. Moreover, for many groups of patients who have historically not been included in research trials, almost no data are available. These groups include youngsters with substance abuse disorders, psychosis, family histories of bipolar disorder, and patients with general medical conditions. There is also little information about how best to combine somatic treatments with psychosocial interventions.

Many avenues need to be considered in future clinical research studies. Only such investigations can generate scientifically sound, empirically based evidence about the treatment of pediatric depressive illnesses.

Acknowledgments

The authors thank Lisa A. Branicky, MA, for her assistance in preparing this article.

References

[1] American Academy of Child and Adolescent Psychiatry. Practice parameters for the assessment and treatment of children and adolescents with depressive disorders. J Am Acad Child Adolesc Psychiatry 1998;37:63S–83S.

[2] American Academy of Child and Adolescent Psychiatry. Practice parameter for the assessment and treatment of children and adolescents with suicidal behavior. J Am Acad Child Adolesc Psychiatry 2001;40(Suppl):24S–51S.

[3] Findling RL, Reed MD, Blumer JL. Pharmacological treatment of depression in children and adolescents. Paediatric Drugs 1999;1:161–82.

[4] Geller B, Reising D, Leonard HL, et al. Critical review of tricyclic antidepressant use in children and adolescents. J Am Acad Child Adolesc Psychiatry 1999;38:513–6.

[5] Hazell P, O'Connell D, Heathcote D, et al. Efficacy of tricyclic drugs in treating child and adolescent depression: a meta-analysis. BMJ 1995;310:897–901.

[6] Birmaher B, Waterman GS, Ryan ND, et al. Randomized, controlled trial of amitriptyline versus placebo for adolescents with "treatment-resistant" major depression. J Am Acad Child Adolesc Psychiatry 1998;37:527–35.

[7] Klein RG, Mannuzza S, Koplewicz HS, et al. Adolescent depression: controlled desipramine treatment and atypical features. Depress Anxiety 1998;7:15–31.

[8] Keller MB, Ryan ND, Strober M, et al. Efficacy of paroxetine in the treatment of adolescent major depression: a randomized, controlled trial. J Am Acad Child Adolesc Psychiatry 2001;40: 762–72.

[9] Sallee FR, Vrindavanam NS, Deas-Nesmith D, et al. Pulse intravenous clomipramine for depressed adolescents: double-blind, controlled trial. Am J Psychiatry 1997;154:668–73.

[10] McGrath PJ, Stewart JW, Quitkin FM. The use of monoamine oxidase inhibitors for treating atypical depression. Psychiatric Annals 2001;31:371–5.

[11] Frommer EA. Treatment of childhood depression with antidepressant drugs. BMJ 1967;1: 729–32.

[12] Ryan ND, Puig-Antich J, Rabinovich H, et al. MAOIs in adolescent major depression unresponsive to tricyclic antidepressants. J Am Acad Child Adolesc Psychiatry 1988b;27:755–8.

[13] Strober M, Pataki C, DeAntonio M. Complete remission of "treatment resistant" severe melancholia in adolescents with phenelzine: two case reports. J Affect Disord 1998a;50:55–8.

[14] Lotufo-Neto F, Trivedi M, Thase ME. Meta-analysis of the reversible inhibitors of monoamine oxidase type A moclobemide and brofaromine for the treatment of depression. Neuropsychopharmacology 1999;20:226–47.

[15] Tanghe A, Geerts S, Van Dorpe J, et al. Double-blind randomized controlled study of the efficacy and tolerability of two reversible monoamine oxidase A inhibitors, pirlindole and moclobemide, in the treatment of depression. Acta Psychiatr Scand 1997;96:134–41.

[16] Antkowiak R, Rajewski A. Administration of moclobemid in children with attention deficit hyperactivity disorder. Psychiatria Polska 1998;32:751–7.

[17] Trott GE, Friese HJ, Menzel M, et al. Use of moclobemide in children with attention deficit hyperactivity disorder. Psychopharmacology (Berl) 1992;106:S134–6.

[18] Feigin A, Kurlan R, McDermott MP, et al. A controlled trial of deprenyl in children with Tourette's syndrome and attention deficit hyperactivity disorder. Neurology 1996;46:965–8.

[19] Jankovic J. Deprenyl in attention deficit associated with Tourette's syndrome. Arch Neurol 1993;50:286–8.

[20] Bodkin JA, Kwon AE. Selegiline and other atypical monoamine oxidase inhibitors in depression. Psychiatric Annals 2001;31:385–91.

[21] Feighner JP, Boyer WF. Overview of USA controlled trials of trazodone in clinical depression. Psychopharmacology (Berl) 1988;95:S50–3.

[22] Schatzberg AF. Trazodone: a 5-year review of antidepressant efficacy. Psychopathology 1987; 20(Suppl 1):48–56.

[23] Marek GJ, McDougle CJ, Price LH, et al. A comparison of trazodone and fluoxetine: impli-

cations for a serotonergic mechanism of antidepressant action. Psychopharmacology (Berl) 1992;109:2–11.

[24] Schatzberg AF, Dessain E, O'Neil P, et al. Recent studies on selective serotonergic antidepressants: trazodone, fluoxetine, and fluvoxamine. J Clin Psychopharmacol 1987;7:44S–9S.

[25] Scher M, Krieger JH, Juergens S. Trazodone and priapism. Am J Psychiatry 1983;140:1362–3.

[26] Warner MD, Peabody CA, Whiteford HA, et al. Trazodone and priapism. J Clin Psychiatry 1987;48:244–5.

[27] Nierenberg AA, Adler LA, Peselow E, et al. Trazodone for antidepressant -associated insomnia. Am J Psychiatry 1994;151:1069–72.

[28] Kallepalli BR, Bhatara VS, Fogas BS, et al. Trazodone is only slightly faster than fluoxetine in relieving insomnia in adolescents with depressive disorders. J Child Adolesc Psychopharmacol 1997;7:97–107.

[29] Horst WD, Preskorn SH. Mechanisms of action and clinical characteristics of three atypical antidepressants: venlafaxine, nefazodone, and bupropion. J Affect Disord 1998;51:237–54.

[30] Johnston JA, Lineberry CG, Ascher JA, et al. A 102-center prospective study of seizure in association with bupropion. J Clin Psychiatry 1991;52:450–6.

[31] Davidson JRT, Connor KM. Bupropion sustained release: a therapeutic overview. J Clin Psychiatry 1998;59(Suppl 4):25–31.

[32] Kavoussi RJ, Segraves RT, Hughes AR, et al. Double-blind comparison of bupropion sustained release and sertraline in depressed outpatients. J Clin Psychiatry 1997;58:532–7.

[33] Settle Jr. EC. Bupropion sustained release: side effect profile. J Clin Psychiatry 1998;59 (Suppl 4):32–6.

[34] Goldstein MG. Bupropion sustained release and smoking cessation. J Clin Psychiatry 1998;59(Suppl 4):66–72.

[35] Barrickman LL, Perry PJ, Allen AJ, et al. Bupropion versus methylphenidate in the treatment of attention-deficit hyperactivity disorder. J Am Acad Child Adolesc Psychiatry 1995;34:649–57.

[36] [-Casat CD, Pleasants DZ, Van Wyck-Fleet J. A double-blind trial of bupropion in children with attention deficit disorder. Psychopharmacol Bull 1987;23:120–2.

[37] Clay TH, Gualtieri CT, Evans RW, et al. Clinical and neuropsychological effects of the novel antidepressant bupropion. Psychopharmacol Bull 1988;24:143–8.

[38] Conners CK, Casat CD, Gualtieri CT, et al. Bupropion hydrochloride in attention deficit disorder with hyperactivity. J Am Acad Child Adolesc Psychiatry 1996;35:1314–21.

[39] Daviss WB, Bentivoglio P, Racusin R, Brown KM, Bostic JQ, Wiley L. Bupropion sustained release for adolescents with comorbid attention-deficit/hyperactivity disorder and depression. J Am Acad Child Adolesc Psychiatry 2001;40:307–14.

[40] Mace S, Taylor D. Selective serotonin reuptake inhibitors: a review of efficacy and tolerability. Expert Opinion on Pharmacotherapy 2000;1:917–33.

[41] Richelson E. Synaptic effects of antidepressants. J Clin Psychopharmacol 1996;6(Suppl 2): 1S–9S.

[42] Boulos C, Kutcher S, Gardner D, et al. An open naturalistic trial of fluoxetine in adolescent and young adults with treatment-resistant major depression. J Child Adolesc Psychopharmacol 1992;2:103–11.

[43] Colle LM, Bélair J-F, DiFeo M, et al. Extended open-label fluoxetine treatment of adolescents with major depression. J Child Adolesc Psychopharmacol 1994;4:225–32.

[44] Dittman RW, Czekalla J, Hundemer HP, et al. Efficacy and safety findings from naturalistic fluoxetine drug treatment in adolescents and young adult patients. J Child Adolesc Psychopharmacol 2000;10:91–102.

[45] Gammon GD, Brown TE. Fluoxetine and methylphenidate in combination for treatment of attention deficit disorder and comorbid depressive disorder. J Child Adolesc Psychopharmacol 1993;3:1–10.

[46] Ghaziuddin N, Naylor MW, King CA. Fluoxetine in tricyclic refractory depression in adolescents. Depression 1995;2:287–91.

[47] Jain U, Birmaher B, Garcia M, et al. Fluoxetine in children and adolescents with mood dis-

orders: a chart review of efficacy and adverse effects. J Child Adolesc Psychopharmacol 1992; 2:259–65.

[48] Riggs PD, Mikulich SK, Coffman LM, et al. Fluoxetine in drug-dependent delinquents with major depression: an open trial. J Child Adolesc Psychopharmacol 1997;7:87–95.

[49] Strober M, DeAntonio M, Schmidt-Lackner S, et al. The pharmacotherapy of depressive illness in adolescents: an open-label comparison of fluoxetine with imipramine-treated historical controls. J Clin Psychiatry 1999;60:164–9.

[50] Waslick BD, Walsh BT, Greenhill LL, et al. Open trial of fluoxetine in children and adolescents with dysthymic disorder or double depression. J Affect Disord 1999;56:227–36.

[51] Simeon JG, Dinicola VF, Ferguson HB, et al. Adolescent depression: a placebo-controlled fluoxetine treatment study and follow-up. Prog Neuropsychopharmacol Biol Psychiatry 1990; 14:791–5.

[52] Emslie GJ, Heiligenstein JH, Hoog SL, et al. Fluoxetine for acute treatment of depression in children and adolescents: a placebo-controlled, randomized clinical trial [poster presentation]. Presented at the Annual Meeting of the American College of Neuropsychopharmacology. San Juan, Puerto Rico; December 10–14, 2000.

[53] Emslie GJ, Rush AJ, Weinberg WA, et al. A double-blind, randomized, placebo-controlled trial of fluoxetine in children and adolescents with depression. Arch Gen Psychiatry 1997;54: 1031–7.

[54] Hoog SL, Heiligenstein JH, Wagner KD, et al. Fluoxetine treatment 20 mg versus 40–60 mg for pediatric fluoxetine 20 mg nonresponders. In: Villani S, editor. American Psychiatric Association Annual Meeting New Research Abstracts. New Orleans: American Academy of Child and Adolescent Psychiatry; 2001. p. 200.

[55] Emslie GJ, Heiligenstein JH, Hoog SL, et al. Fluoxetine for maintenance of recovery from depression in children and adolescents: a placebo-controlled, randomized clinical trial. In: Villani S, editor. American Psychiatric Association Annual Meeting New Research Abstracts. New Orleans: American Academy of Child and Adolescent Psychiatry; 2001. p. 199.

[56] Alderman J, Wolkow R, Chung M, et al. Sertraline treatment of children and adolescents with obsessive-compulsive disorder or depression: pharmacokinetics, tolerability, and efficacy. J Am Acad Child Adolesc Psychiatry 1998;37:386–94.

[57] March JS, Biederman J, Wolkow R, et al. Sertraline in children and adolescents with obsessive-compulsive disorder. A multicenter randomized controlled trial. JAMA 1998;280:1752–6.

[58] Ambrosini PJ, Wagner KD, Biederman J, et al. Multicenter open-label sertraline study in adolescent outpatients with major depression. J Am Acad Child Adolesc Psychiatry 1999;38: 566–72.

[59] McConville BJ, Minnery KL, Sorter MT, et al. An open study of the effects of sertraline on adolescent major depression. J Child Adolesc Psychopharmacol 1996;6:41–51.

[60] Sallee FR, Hilal R, Dougherty D, et al. Platelet serotonin transporter in depressed children and adolescents: ^{3}H-paroxetine platelet binding before and after sertraline. J Am Acad Child Adolesc Psychiatry 1998;37:777–84.

[61] Tierney E, Joshi PT, Llinas JF, et al. Sertraline for major depression in children and adolescents: preliminary clinical experience. J Child Adolesc Psychopharmacol 1995;5:13–27.

[62] Findling RL, Reed MD, Myers C, et al. Paroxetine pharmacokinetics in depressed children and adolescents. J Am Acad Child Adolesc Psychiatry 1999;38:952–9.

[63] Masi G, Marcheschi M, Pfanner P. Paroxetine in depressed adolescents with intellectual disability: an open label study. J Intellect Disabil Res 1997;41:268–72.

[64] Nobile M, Bellotti B, Marino C, et al. An open trial of paroxetine in the treatment of children and adolescents diagnosed with dysthymia. J Child Adolesc Psychopharmacol 2000;10:103–9.

[65] Rey-Sánchez F, Gutiérrez-Casares JR. Paroxetine in children with major depressive disorder: an open trial. J Am Acad Child Adolesc Psychiatry 1997;36:1443–7.

[66] Riddle MA, Reeve EA, Yaryura-Tobias JA, et al. Fluvoxamine for children and adolescents with obsessive-compulsive disorder: a randomized, controlled, multicenter trial. J Am Acad Child Adolesc Psychiatry 2001;40:222–9.

576   R.L. Findling et al / Child Adolesc Psychiatric Clin N Am 11 (2002) 555–578

[67] Apter A, Ratzoni G, King RA, et al. Fluvoxamine open-label treatment of adolescent inpatients with obsessive-compulsive disorder or depresssion. J Am Acad Child Adolesc Psychiatry 1994; 33:342–8.
[68] Rabe-Jablonska J. Therapeutic effects and tolerability of fluvoxamine treatment in adolescents with dysthymia. J Child Adolesc Psychopharmacol 2000;10:9–18.
[69] Lepola U, Leinonen E, Koponen H. Citalopram in anxiety disorder of childhood and adolescence. Eur Child Adolesc Psychiatry 1994;3:277–9.
[70] Seedat S, Lockhat R, Kaminer D, et al. An open trial of citalopram in adolescents with post-traumatic stress disorder. Int Clin Psychopharmacol 2001;16:21–5.
[71] Thomsen PH. Child and adolescent obsessive-compulsive disorder treated with citalopram: findings from an open trial of 23 cases. J Child Adolesc Psychopharmacol 1997;7:157–66.
[72] Thomsen PH, Ebbesen C, Persson C. Long-term experience with citalopram in the treatment of adolescent OCD. J Am Acad Child Adolesc Psychiatry 2001;40:895–902.
[73] Lepola U, Leinonen E, Koponen H. Citalopram in the treatment of early-onset panic disorder and school phobia. Pharmacopsychiatry 1996;29:30–2.
[74] Entsuah R, Chitra R. A benefit-risk analysis of once-daily venlafaxine extended release (XR) and venlafaxine immediate release (IR) in outpatients with major depression. Psychopharmacol Bull 1997;33:671–6.
[75] Rudolph RL, Feiger AD. A double-blind, randomized, placebo-controlled trial of once-daily venlafaxine extended release (XR) and fluoxetine for the treatment of depression. J Affect Disord 1999;56:171–81.
[76] Feighner JP. Mechanism of action of antidepressant medications. J Clin Psychiatry 1999; 60(Suppl 4):4–11.
[77] Harvey AT, Rudolph RL, Preskorn SH. Evidence of the dual mechanism of action of venlafaxine. Arch Gen Psychiatry 2000;57:503–9.
[78] Mandoki MW, Tapia MR, Tapia MA, et al. Venlafaxine in the treatment of children and adolescents with major depression. Psychopharmacol Bull 1997;33:149–54.
[79] Findling RL, Schwartz MA, Flannery DJ, et al. Venlafaxine in adults with attention-deficit/hyperactivity disorder: an open clinical trial. J Clin Psychiatry 1996;57:184–9.
[80] Olvera RL, Pliszka SR, Luh J, et al. An open trial of venlafaxine in the treatment of attention-deficit/hyperactivity disorder in children and adolescents. J Child Adolesc Psychopharmacol 1996;6:241–50.
[81] Davis R, Whittington R, Bryson HM. Nefazodone. A review of its pharmacology and clinical efficacy in the management of major depression. Drugs 1997;53:608–36.
[82] Findling RL, Preskorn SH, Marcus RN, et al. Nefazodone pharmacokinetics in depressed children and adolescents. J Am Acad Child Adolesc Psychiatry 2000;39:1008–16.
[83] Goodnick PJ, Jorge CA, Hunter T, et al. Nefazodone treatment of adolescent depression: an open-label study of response and biochemistry. Ann Clin Psychiatry 2000;12:97–100.
[84] Wilens TE, Spencer TJ, Biederman J, et al. Case study: nefazodone for juvenile mood disorders. J Am Acad Child Adolesc Psychiatry 1997;36:481–5.
[85] Holm KJ, Markham A. Mirtazapine. A review of its use in major depression. Drugs 1999;57: 607–31.
[86] Good C, Petersen C. SSRI and mirtazapine in PTSD. J Am Acad Child Adolesc Psychiatry 2001;40:263–4.
[87] Coppen A. Lithium in unipolar depression and the prevention of suicide. J Clin Psychiatry 2000;61(Suppl 9):52–6.
[88] Nelson JC. Augmentation strategies in depression 2000. J Clin Psychiatry 2000;61(Suppl 2): 13–9.
[89] Strober M, Freeman R, Rigali J, et al. The pharmacotherapy of depressive illness in adolescence: II. effects of lithium augmentation in nonresponders to imipramine. J Am Acad Child Adolesc Psychiatry 1992;31:16–20.
[90] Walter G, Lyndon B, Kubb R. Lithium augmentation of venlafaxine in adolescent major depression. Australia and New Zealand Journal of Psychiatry 1998;32:457–9.

behavioral therapy improved more on these cognitive indices than did those in the other study arms. Three self-rated scales of family-environmental functioning also were administered. The authors did not report, however, whether any changes on these indices occurred during the course of therapy. None of the family-climate measures were associated with treatment outcomes.

An adaptation of group cognitive behavioral therapy for Hispanic adults that focused on dysfunctional cognitions, pleasant activities, social-support systems, and assertiveness was compared with interpersonal psychotherapy targeting the problem areas of grief, interpersonal disputes, role transitions, and interpersonal deficits and with a wait-list control condition. The sample was comprised of 71 13-to 18-year-old depressed youths in Puerto Rico. Both treatments were detailed in manuals and were delivered in 12 weekly individual sessions [26]. Compared with the wait-list control, both treatments resulted in decreased self-rated severity of depression and in fewer youths scoring in the dysfunctional range. On average, 72% of treated youth were functioning better at end of treatment than those wait-listed. Interpersonal psychotherapy and cognitive behavioral therapy were similarly successful in improving self-esteem and social adaptation, and those treated with interpersonal psychotherapy also fared better in these two areas than did control cases. Those receiving interpersonal psychotherapy (but not those receiving cognitive behavioral therapy or the wait-list controls) showed significant changes on measures of social adaptation and school functioning. However, the relationship between improved social adjustment and lessened depression was not reported. Moreover, because interpersonal psychotherapy and cognitive behavioral therapy were equally efficacious in reducing depression, it is not possible to conclude that changes in interpersonal targets were critical to improvement.

Another study compared interpersonal psychotherapy that included weekly telephone contacts during the first 4 weeks of therapy with clinical monitoring in a 12-week trial involving 48 12- to 18-year-old adolescents [27]. The interpersonal psychotherapy resulted in greater reductions in self-rated depressive symptoms and greater recovery in terms of clinician-rated depression scores than did the clinical monitoring. Adolescents who received interpersonal therapy reported more improvement in overall social functioning and in peer and dating relationships than did comparison patients after controlling for baseline scores. Patients treated with interpersonal therapy also fared better in self-reported rational problem solving and in positive problem-solving orientation.

Comments

These studies of clinically diagnosed youths suggest that active, goal-oriented interventions that focus on cognitive behavioral and relationship issues are superior to other interventions and to wait-list conditions for pediatric depression. The success rates for active treatments were suboptimal, however, and, as noted, in some studies a substantial portion of treated participants remained in a depressive episode at the end of the trial. Available follow-up data also suggest that many treated participants continued to experience depressive symptoms and that up to about 45% of the youths had relapses or recurrences during the year following treatment.

One possible explanation for the less than optimal outcomes in these studies is that treatment durations may have been too short. In clinically referred youths, the median time to recovery from an episode of major depression is about 7 to 9 months [28,29]. Other design features of the trials also may have made it difficult to obtain higher rates of response. For example, the inclusion in some studies of youths with major depression, dysthymia, or both [20–23] could have obscured a better response rate possibly associated with one (but not the other) condition [30]. Additionally, as also noted by Harrington et al [31], most studies were not designed to manage comorbid disorders. Comorbid conditions may signal more serious psychopathology or may otherwise interfere with optimal treatment of the depression.

Youths' response to treatment also may have been adversely affected by contextual factors such as parental psychopathology [32–35], parents' marital problems [36], parent-child conflict [37,38], and inadequate overall social support [39,40]. With the exception of the study by Brent et al [7], however, the social context of the youths or the mental health of their parents were neither investigated nor targeted for change [30].

Some studies involving clinically depressed children and adolescents also suggest that cognitive and behaviorally focused interventions can affect conceptually salient and empirically targeted processes. For example, treatments directed at patients' cognitions have been successful in reducing depressogenic cognitions [20] and cognitive distortions [7,22]. There is, however, insufficient evidence to conclude that such outcomes were treatment-modality specific. Namely, in one study, there was no active comparison intervention [20], whereas in another study patients in both the active and the nonspecific treatment arms evidenced more functional cognitions at end of the trial [22]. Do changes in cognitions occur in tandem with reductions in depressive symptomatology? Would cognitive-behavior interventions be similarly successful for two comparably depressed patients who differ in the extent of depressogenic cognitions? No data have been reported in regard to these questions, and thus the relationship between changes in processes salient to cognitive behavioral therapy and overall improvement in depression still remain to be explored.

There are also indications that treatments focusing on interpersonal and social targets do result in improved social functioning. At least some of the evidence, however, suggests that such changes are not intervention-specific. For example, one study that reported improvement in targeted interpersonal processes did not include an active comparison treatment [27]. In another study, social functioning improved in patients receiving both the active and the generic interventions [23]. Only one trial found changes in social adaptation that were specific to the treatment modality [26]. None of the interpersonally focused studies reported whether or how changes in conceptually salient target processes were related to recovery from depression.

Treatment of undiagnosed depressed samples

The authors identified six peer-reviewed intervention studies with undiagnosed but symptomatically depressed children and adolescents. Participants in these studies were accessed in school settings and were primarily selected by cut-off scores on self- or parent-rated scales or teachers' reports. Youth assigned to experimental therapies generally evidenced greater symptomatic improvement than those assigned to control conditions, but there were few differences among the active therapy conditions. Moreover, treatment response rates in these studies seemed to be more favorable, in general, than were the rates in the previously reviewed investigations of clinically diagnosed youths.

The studies

A school-based study examined two target interventions that exemplify components of cognitive behavioral therapy, namely, behavioral role-playing (focusing on recognition of emotions and social and problem-solving skills) and cognitive restructuring (identifying and replacing dysfunctional thoughts, enhancing listening skills, and recognizing the relationship between thoughts and feelings). Participants were 56 symptomatically depressed fifth-and sixth-grade students [41] The two interventions yielded similar reductions in depressive symptoms and increases in self-esteem as compared with attention placebo and no-treatment control conditions. The positive changes also were evident in teachers' reports. Furthermore, both active interventions were successful in reducing cognitive distortions, as quantified by responses to hypothetic problem situations involving family, peers, and school. No information, however, was provided about the relationship between reductions in cognitive distortions and overall treatment response.

Another study compared cognitive-behavioral therapy (self-monitoring, self-evaluation, and self-reinforcement skills) and relaxation (progressive muscle relaxation) techniques with a wait-list control arm in a high-school sample of 30 symptomatically depressed adolescents [42]. Participants in both active interventions fared better than the controls. At end-point, approximately 80% of participants in the active treatments, but none of the wait-list controls, scored below the clinical cut-off for depression on a self-reporting scale. Improvements among the participants receiving active therapy were maintained at 5-week follow up.

A cognitive-behavioral intervention focusing on self-control (self-monitoring and self-reinforcement skills) was compared with behavior problem-solving training (monitoring pleasant events and improving social and problem-solving skills) and a wait-list control in a sample of 28 9- to 12-year-old middle-school students [43]. According to both self-reports and parents' ratings, most participants receiving active treatment improved (78% and 60%, respectively, scored in the nonclinical range in terms of self-reported severity of depression), whereas only 11% of those on the wait list did so. The intervention containing both cognitive and behavioral elements was reportedly as effective in symptom reduction as the more traditional, behaviorally based treatment.

A version of cognitive behavioral therapy based largely on Lewinsohn and colleagues' CWD course was compared with progressive relaxation therapy and self-modeling (feedback from video-taped rehearsal of "nondepressed" behavior) in a sample of 68 10- to 14-year-old middle-school students [44]. The three interventions resulted in similar improvements in self- and clinician-rated severity of depressive symptoms. At 1-month follow-up, gains were maintained among participants who had been assigned to the cognitive behavioral therapy and relaxation therapy arms, whereas 50% of participants in the self-modeling group again scored in the dysfunctional ranges on self-reported scales.

In a school-based study of 7- to 11-year-olds, children received group-based social-competence training involving elements of cognitive behavioral therapy (cognitive restructuring and social and interpersonal problem-solving skills) or were assigned to attention placebo or to a wait-list control [8]. Participants in all three arms (n = 31) evidenced similar declines in the severity of depressive symptoms at the end of treatment. Improvements were maintained at 2-month follow up, with no difference among treatment groups. Even though the social competence training explicitly focused on teaching social skills and interpersonal problem solving, there were no significant end-of-treatment differences on self- or teacher reports of children's social skills or in children's self-reported experiences of social problems.

A cognitive behaviorsl intervention called "Primary and Secondary Control Enhancement Training" (PASCET) was compared with no treatment in a study of 48 children in grades 3 to 6 with mild to moderate depressive symptoms [45]. The 8-session PASCET program targeted primary control (eg, skills and strategies for changing one's situation to maximize reinforcement) and secondary control (eg, altering attributions or using relaxation when objective conditions cannot be modified). The children in the PASCET program showed greater symptomatic improvement and were more likely than untreated children to score in the nonclinical ranges on self- and interviewer ratings of depression. Specifically, at posttreatment assessment, 50% of the treated children and 16% of the controls moved from above the normal range to within the normal range on self-rated measures of severity of depression. These differences also were generally apparent at a 9-month follow up.

Comment

The overall positive response rates in school-based intervention studies involving symptomatically depressed youths are compelling and seem to be higher than the rates in clinically diagnosed samples. It also is notable that several school-based studies included children younger than 10-years of age, whereas studies of youth diagnosed with depression typically were confined to adolescents. In school-based studies, however, outcome assessments by teachers and parents did not uniformly agree with the participants' self-reports [43,44], raising some questions about the cross-situational generalizability of treatment effects. A lack of convergence also has been reported even with identical assessment methods.

The evidence is scant and mixed regarding treatment-specific changes in purported underlying mechanisms. For example, in one study [8], intervention-specific changes in social skills or social problem solving were not detected in comparisons of pretreatment and posttreatment assessments. On the other hand, in another study [41] both role-playing and cognitive restructuring reduced cognitive distortions. The relationship between these changes and improvements in depression were not addressed, however.

Summary and conclusions

There is solid evidence that active and goal-oriented cognitive-behavioral or relationship-focused therapies are generally superior to more generic therapies or to no treatment for clinically diagnosed and for undiagnosed but symptomatic youths. Between 50% to 87% of diagnosed youths who received a targeted treatment had recovered from their depressive episodes, in comparison to 21% to 75% of those who received some other generic therapy and 5% to 48% of wait-listed youths. The cognitive behavioral and relationship-oriented interventions that were tested tended to be even more successful in reducing depressive symptoms in school-based samples, possibly because the participants in the school-based studies may have been less disturbed than the clinically diagnosed cases. Although the targeted treatments generally yielded better results than the comparison conditions, the targeted interventions seem to be similarly successful in ameliorating depression.

Determining which psychosocial therapy works best for a given depressed youngster remains problematic. As noted in recent reviews [30,46,47], little attention has been devoted to which interventions, or parts of an intervention, are likely to be effective with children with various characteristics. This issue acquires added importance because in some diagnosed samples half or more of the treated participants were still in a depressive episode at the end of the trial. Likewise, in intervention studies involving symptomatic, school-based young-sters, not all children improved, and gains were not uniform across domains of functioning (eg, severity of depression, self-esteem, global functioning).

Possibly, for some of the nonresponders, the participant's characteristics and relevant problems and the target interventions were mismatched. For example, a depressed youth with a long history of highly dysfunctional relationships may not respond optimally to a therapy focusing on negative cognitions; alternatively, interpersonal therapy may not be the most effective treatment for a youth dispositionally inclined to negative ruminations about the self and for whom relationship issues are not the most relevant. Empiric information about the relationship between the underlying processes presumed to account for the onset and maintenance of depression and recovery from depression is limited. Few studies of youths provide direct evidence that cognitive-behavioral interventions change depressogenic cognitions, explanatory style, and pleasant events, among others, that relationship-focused approaches predictably alter relevant interpersonal processes, or that improvements in these domains relate to overall depression outcomes.

Admittedly, the designs of extant studies typically preclude conclusions about the relationship between changes in target processes and improvement in depression or about treatment specificity. More compelling evidence linking changes in targeted mechanisms to decreases in depressive symptoms comes from a controlled prevention trial involving 10- to 13-year-olds that used cognitive restructuring, social problem-solving, or a combination intervention [48]. According to the results, changes in explanatory style were related to decreased depression and accounted for a significant portion of the variance in changes in depression even after controlling for treatment assignment. Further research along such lines may help identify which treatment may be most effective for a patient with a given set of characteristics. To improve patients' response rates to specific treatments, it also would be helpful to understand better the impact of other attributes, such as psychiatric comorbidity, and contextual factors, such as parental psychopathology, on the process of recovery. With few exceptions [25], however, such variables have not yet received sufficient attention.

Recent reviews also have noted that researchers typically use multicomponent interventions in treatment trials [46,47]. This design can make it difficult to identify which particular treatment ingredient is instrumental in general or among children with specific characteristics. Thus, empiric initiatives also are needed to determine the active ingredients of experimental therapies for depressed youths. Existing models include component-analysis or dismantling studies of multifaceted treatments for depressed adults [49,50]. Once the important prognostic factors and active ingredients of therapies have been identified, it will be possible to conduct studies in which children are either "matched" or "mismatched" to treatment conditions. To achieve meaningful results and to enroll sufficient numbers of youths, collaborative, multisite efforts may be required.

What treatment should be endorsed for depressed youths from the perspective of health services policy? When the criteria of the Task Force on Promotion and Dissemination of Psychological Procedures [1] are applied broadly, both cognitive behavioral and interpersonally oriented therapies can be deemed efficacious. Both approaches have been tested in different samples by two independent teams and thus may be regarded as well-established treatments for depression in youths. If the criteria are applied more stringently, so that exactly the same intervention is tested independently by two or more research teams, interpersonal therapy and cognitive behavioral therapy would be regarded as "probably efficacious". Namely, the two trials of interpersonal therapy apparently used somewhat different versions because of cultural differences in the samples. The complete CWD course has been tested and the results have been replicated only by its originators [20,21]. Other trials of cognitive behavioral therapy entail various different study-specific approaches and consequently cannot serve as replications

[46,47]. A next step in psychotherapy research might therefore involve further independent replication of standardized, previously studied therapies.

In their landmark meta-analytic study of the efficacy of psychotherapy for adults, Smith et al [51] concluded that all psychotherapies are about equally beneficial and that distinctions among them, although "cherished by those who draw them … make no important differences" (p. 186). Likewise, the various psychotherapies for depressed youths that have been examined seem to produce similar rates of improvement, despite different conceptual bases and somewhat different therapy targets. This evidence of similar rates of improvement (or alternatively, similar limits in efficacy) across the tested therapies and the scant data regarding meaningful prognostic factors might indicate that at present it does not matter what type of brief, goal-oriented nonsomatic therapy is used to treat pediatric depression. Alternatively, one might conclude that patients who fail to respond may have been mismatched to a therapy that was not focused on their primary depression-related deficits.

Thus, clinicians who treat depressed children and adolescents are faced with substantial challenges, and, to date, results of controlled psychotherapy trials with depressed youths offer limited guidance regarding choice of treatment. Nonetheless, some general guidelines can be culled from the available data. For example, interventions or elements of therapies that are structured and directed towards cognitive, behavioral or relationship issues show promise for the treatment of juvenile depression. It also appears that group interventions may be used as profitably as the more traditional individual therapy formats. And although parental participation in empiric treatment trials of pediatric depression has been limited to either separate parent groups as an adjunct [20,21] or family therapy [7], it can be argued that for various practical and clinical reasons [30] direct involvement of parents may be a wise choice. Parents may be critical to the success of interventions with depressed children and should be regarded as potentially important agents of change.

References

[1] Task Force on Promotion and Dissemination of Psychological Procedures. Training in and dissemination of empirically-validated psychological treatments: report and recommendations. The Clinical Psychologist 1995;8:3–24.

[2] Beck AT, Rush AJ, Shaw BF, et al. Cognitive therapy of depression. New York (NY): Guilford Press; 1979.

[3] Beck AT. Thinking and depression: II. theory and therapy. Arch Gen Psychiatry 1964;10: 561–71.

[4] Beck AT. Depression: clinical, experimental, and theoretical aspects. New York (NY): Hoeber; 1967.

[5] Abramson LY, Seligman ME, Teasdale JD. Learned helplessness in humans: critique and reformulation. J Abnorm Psychol 1978;87:49–74.

[6] Rehm LP. A self-control model of depression. Behavior Therapy 1977;8:787–804.

[7] Brent DA, Holder D, Kolko DJ, et al. A clinical psychotherapy trial for adolescent depression comparing cognitive, family, and supportive therapy. Arch Gen Psychiatry 1997;54:877–85.

[8] Liddle B, Spence SH. Cognitive-behavior therapy with depressed primary school children: a cautionary note. Behavioral Psychotherapy 1990;18:85–102.

[9] Wood A, Harrington R, Moore A. Controlled trial of a brief cognitive-behavioral intervention in adolescent patients with depressive disorders. J Child Psychol Psychiatry 1996;37:737–46.

[10] Lewinsohn PM. A behavioral approach to depression. In: Friedman RJ, Katz MM, editors. The psychology of depression: contemporary theory and research. Washington, DC: Winston-Wiley; 1974. p. 157–84.

[11] Clarke GN, Lewinsohn PM, Hops H. Instructor's Manual for the Adolescent Coping with Depression Course. Eugene, OR: Castalia Press, 1990.

[12] Klerman GL, Weissman MM, Rounsaville BJ, et al. Interpersonal psychotherapy of depression. New York (NY): Basic Books; 1984.

[13] Moreau D, Mufson L, Weissman MM, et al. Interpersonal psychotherapy for adolescent depression: description of modification and preliminary application. J Am Acad Child Adolesc Psychiatry 1991;30:642–51.

[14] Mufson LH, Moreau D, Weissman MM, et al. Interpersonal psychotherapy for adolescent depression. In Klerman GL, Weissman MM, editors. New applications of interpersonal psychotherapy. Washington, DC: American Psychiatric Press; 1993. p. 129–66.

[15] Alexander J, Parsons BV. Functional family therapy. Pacific Grove (CA): Brooks/Cole Publishing Co; 1982.

[16] Robin AL, Foster SL. Negotiating parent-adolescent conflict: a behavioral-family systems approach. New York (NY): Guilford Press; 1989.

[17] American Psychiatric Association. Diagnostic and statistical manual of mental disorders. 3rd edition. Washington, DC: American Psychiatric Association; 1980.

[18] American Psychiatric Association. Diagnostic and statistical manual of mental disorders. 3rd edition, revised. Washington, DC: American Psychiatric Association; 1987.

[19] Spitzer RL, Endicott J, Robins E. Research diagnostic criteria: rationale and reliability. Arch Gen Psychiatry 1978;35:773–82.

[20] Lewinsohn PM, Clarke GN, Hops H, et al. Cognitive-behavioral treatment for depressed adolescents. Behavior Therapy 1990;21:385–401.

[21] Clarke GN, Rohde P, Lewinsohn PM, et al. Cognitive-behavioral treatment of adolescent depression: efficacy of acute group treatment and booster sessions. J Am Acad Child Adolesc Psychiatry 1999;38:272–9.

[22] Fine S, Forth A, Gilbert M, et al. Group therapy for adolescent depressive disorder: a comparison of social skills and therapeutic support. J Am Acad Child Adolesc Psychiatry 1991;30:79–85.

[23] Vostanis P, Feehan C, Grattan E, et al. Treatment for children and adolescents with depression: lessons from a controlled trial. Clinical Child Psychology and Psychiatry 1996;1(2):199–212.

[24] Vostanis P, Feehan C, Grattan E, et al. A randomized controlled out-patient trial of cognitive-behavioural treatment for children and adolescents with depression: 9-month follow-up. J Affect Disorders 1996;40(1–2);105–16.

[25] Brent DA, Kolko DJ, Birmaher B, et al. Predictors of treatment efficacy in a clinical trial of three psychosocial treatments for adolescent depression. J Am Acad Child Adolesc Psychiatry 1998;37(9):906–14.

[26] Rosselló J, Bernal G. Treatment of depression in Puerto Rican adolescents: the efficacy of cognitive-behavioral and interpersonal treatments. J Consult Clin Psychol 1999;67:734–45.

[27] Mufson L, Weissmann M, Moreau D, et al. Efficacy of interpersonal psychotherapy for depressed adolescents. Arch Gen Psychiatry 1999;56:573–9.

[28] Kovacs M, Obrosky DS, Gatsonis C, et al. First episode major depressive and dysthymic disorder in childhood: clinical and sociodemographic factors in recovery. J Am Acad Child Adolesc Psychiatry 1997;36:777–84.

[29] McCauley E, Myers K, Mitchell J, et al. Depression in young people: initial presentation and clinical course. J Am Acad Child Adolesc Psychiatry 1993;32:714–22.

[30] Kovacs M, Sherrill JT. The psychotherapeutic management of major depressive and dysthymic disorders in childhood and adolescence: issues and prospects. In: Goodyer I.M. editor. The

depressed child and adolescent: developmental and clinical perspectives. New York (NY): Cambridge University Press; 2001. p 325–52.

[31] Harrington R, Whittaker J, Shoebridge P. Psychological treatment of depression in children. A review of treatment research. Br J Psychiatry 1998;173:291–8.

[32] Kovacs M, Devlin B, Pollock M, et al. A controlled family history study of childhood-onset depressive disorder. Arch Gen Psychiatry 1997;46:776–82.

[33] Mitchell J, McCauley E, Burke P, et al. Psychopathology in parents of depressed children and adolescents. J Am Acad Child Adolesc Psychiatry 1989;28:352–7.

[34] Todd RD, Neuman R, Geller B, et al. Genetic studies of affective disorders: should we be starting with childhood onset probands? J Am Acad Child Adolesc Psychiatry 1993;32:1164–71.

[35] Williamson DE, Ryan ND, Birmaher B, et al. A case-control family history study of depression in adolescents. J Am Acad Child Adolesc Psychiatry 1995;34:1596–607.

[36] Forehand R, Brody G, Slotkin J, et al. Young adolescents and maternal depression: assessment, interrelations, and family predictors. J Consult Clin Psychol 1988;56:422–6.

[37] Puig-Antich J, Kaufman J, Ryan ND, et al. The psychosocial functioning and family environment of depressed adolescents. J Am Acad Child Adolesc Psychiatry 1993;32:244–53.

[38] Puig-Antich J, Lukens E, Davies M, et al. Psychosocial functioning in prepubertal major depressive disorders. I. interpersonal relationships during the depressive episode. Arch Gen Psychiatry 1985;42:500–7.

[39] Armsden GC, McCauley E, Greenberg MT, et al. Parent and peer attachment in early adolescent depression. J Abnorm Child Psychol 1990;18:683–97.

[40] Daniels D, Moos RH. Assessing life stressors and social resources among adolescents: applications to depressed youth. Journal of Adolescent Research 1990;5:268–89.

[41] Butler L, Miezitis S, Friedman R, et al. The effect of two school-based intervention programs on depressive symptoms in pre-adolescents. American Educational Research Journal 1980;17: 111–9.

[42] Reynolds WM, Coats KI. A comparison of cognitive-behavioral therapy and relaxation training for the treatment of depression in adolescents. J Consult Clin Psychol 1986;54:653–60.

[43] Stark KD, Reynolds WM, Kaslow NJ. A comparison of the relative efficacy of self-control therapy and a behavioral problem-solving therapy for depression in children. J Abnorm Child Psychol 1987;15:91–113.

[44] Kahn JS, Kehle TJ, Jenson WR, et al. Comparison of cognitive-behavioral, relaxation, and self-modeling interventions for depression among middle-school students. School Psychology Review 1990;19:196–211.

[45] Weisz J, Thurber C, Sweeney L, et al. Brief treatment of mild to moderate child depression using primary and secondary control enhancement training. J Consult Clin Psychol 1997;65:703–7.

[46] Kaslow NJ, Thompson MP. Applying the criteria for empirically supported treatments to studies of psychosocial interventions for child and adolescent depression. J Clin Child Psychol 1998; 27:146–55.

[47] Kazdin AE, Weisz JR. Identifying and developing empirically supported child and adolescent treatments. J Consult Clin Psychol 1998;66:19–36.

[48] Jaycox LH, Reivich KJ, Gillham J, et al. Prevention of depressive symptoms in school children. Behav Res Ther 1994;32:801–16.

[49] Jacobson NS, Dobson KS, Truax PA, et al. A component analysis of cognitive-behavioral treatment for depression. J Consult Clin Psychol 1996;64:295–304.

[50] Rehm LP, Kaslow NJ, Rabin AS. Cognitive and behavioral targets in a self-control thereapy program for depression. J Consult Clin Psychol 1987;55:60–7.

[51] Smith ML, Glass GV, Miller TL. The benefits of psychotherapy. Baltimore (MD): Johns Hopkins University Press; 1980.

Child Adolesc Psychiatric Clin N Am
11 (2002) 595–617

CHILD AND
ADOLESCENT
PSYCHIATRIC
CLINICS

Somatic treatment of bipolar disorder in children and adolescents

Elizabeth B. Weller, MD[a],*, Arman K. Danielyan, MD[b],
Ronald A. Weller, MD[b]

[a]*Department of Child and Adolescent Psychiatry, Children's Hospital of Philadelphia,
34th and Civic Center Boulevard, Philadelphia, PA 19104, USA*
[b]*Department of Psychiatry, University of Pennsylvania, 3535 Market Street,
Philadelphia, PA 19104, USA*

Despite increasing knowledge about the clinical presentation and phenomenology of juvenile-onset bipolar disorder, pharmacotherapy of this disorder has not been well studied [1]. The use of mood-stabilizing agents such as lithium, carbamazepine, and divalproex sodium in children and adolescents diagnosed with bipolar disorder has sharply increased in recent years. The use of these agents, however, is still based primarily on case reports and studies with small numbers of subjects [2,3]. There are no methodologically sound, controlled studies on which to base treatment decisions for children and adolescents with bipolar disorder [4]. Despite the lack of scientific evidence as to their efficacy and long-term safety, these medications have been widely used in children and adolescents [5]. Often the selection of a particular type of pharmacological treatment in children and adolescents is extrapolated from data from studies of adults with bipolar disorder. In adults, all of the randomized, double-blind, placebo-controlled studies have involved patients hospitalized with acute mania. There are no such studies in children or adolescents. The treatment studies done in children and adolescents have either been discontinuation studies using hospitalized, acutely manic adolescents [6] or outpatients with mania; controlled [7] or open studies of inpatient children [8] or of outpatients with mania, hypomania, bipolar disorder not otherwise specified; or studies in depressed patients with a family history of bipolar disorder [9,10]. Adding to the confusion is increasing tendency for studies not to distinguish between types of bipolar disorder, so that the term "bipolar" can refer to mania or to any other condition within the bipolar spectrum.

Although many classes of psychotropic medications, including mood stabilizers, antidepressants, anticonvulsants and antipsychotics, have been used to treat

---

* Corresponding author.
E-mail address: Weller@email.chap.edu (E.B. Weller).

bipolar disorder in recent years, mood stabilizers seem to be the most efficacious agents for bipolar patients, regardless of age. Although the biopsychosocial approach to treatment is recommended for all patients, this article focuses only on the somatic treatment of bipolar disorder in children and adolescents.

Medication choice and the duration of treatment

The practice parameters of the American Academy of Child and Adolescent Psychiatry [1] state that several factors should be considered in choosing a medication for treatment of juvenile bipolar disorder. These factors include: (1) evidence of efficacy, (2) the phase of illness, (3) the presence of confounding presentations (eg, rapid-cycling mood swings, psychotic symptoms), (4) the agent's side-effect profile, (5) the patient's history of medication response, and (6) the preferences of the family or patient. Lin and colleagues also suggest that the pharmacokinetics of lithium, antidepressants, and other psychotropic agents may vary in different ethnic groups, possibly leading to different side effects, blood levels, and efficacy [11]. Kowatch et al [10] compared the effectiveness of different mood stabilizers in the management of bipolar disorder in children and adolescents. They studied 42 children, aged 8 to 18 years, who were randomly assigned to receive lithium, valproate, or carbamazepine. The response rate in the lithium and carbamazepine groups was 38%, whereas the response rate in the valproate group was 53% [10]. Unfortunately, there are no research-based algorithms to guide clinicians in the choice of medication. One of the key factors in deciding which medication to use in patients with a family history of bipolar disorder is the history of a positive response to a particular medication in a first-degree relative with bipolar disorder.

Preliminary data show that medication in children with early-onset bipolar disorder must be used for an extended and continuous period, often throughout their teenage years. In general when beginning the treatment process, an antimanic agent needs to be given at an adequate dose for at least 4 to 6 weeks before its efficacy can be determined. Evidence to date suggests that the relapse rate is quite high for early-onset bipolar disorder, and one of the main reasons for relapse is noncompliance.

Lithium

Lithium is the oldest and most-studied mood stabilizer for adults with bipolar disorder. In adults, lithium has been found to be effective for the treatment of acute manic and depressive episodes, prevention of recurrent manic and depressive episodes, and reduction of mood instability between episodes [12]. In adults, lithium remains the treatment of choice for acute mania and prophylaxis. The efficacy of lithium in adult mania was established in several placebo-controlled crossover studies with treatment durations of 7 to 14 days [13–16]. A study by Bowden et al, the first to use lithium in a parallel-groups design, reported a response rate of 49% to lithium and 25% to placebo [17]. Lithium has been approved by the Food and Drug Administration (FDA) for treatment of bipolar disorder in adolescents 12 years of age or older but not in prepubertal children.

Lithium has been well studied in adults and is the medication of choice in adults with bipolar disorder, but knowledge of lithium's safety and efficacy for treatment of juvenile-onset bipolar disorder is inadequate [18]. A positive response to lithium in adolescents with bipolar disorder was first reported in 1959 by Van Krevelen and Van Voorst [19]. Currently published treatment studies are limited by small sample size, by lack of placebo control groups [8,20,21], or by the inclusion of subjects of mixed or unclear diagnostic status (eg, subjects with broadly defined psychotic disorders or with combined manic symptoms and disruptive behavior disorders) [7,22,23]. Still, lithium has been reported to have beneficial effects for the treatment of childhood-onset bipolar disorder [8,24], adolescent onset bipolar disorder [25–28], aggressive behaviors in hospitalized children with conduct disorder [29–32], and manic symptoms caused by traumatic brain injury in children [33,34]. Geller et al [35] suggested lithium therapy in "not-yet-bipolar" children (ie, depressed children with family history of bipolar disorder) who may become manic on treatment with antidepressants, especially with tricyclic antidepressants. The authors go on to state that when the depression is unipolar, lithium has a positive effect in only 14% of children under age 14 years [35]. De Long and Aldershof [22] reported positive response to lithium therapy in 82% of depressed children with neurovegetative and other episodic symptoms. Varanka and colleagues [8] also reported improvement in psychotic symptoms of children with bipolar disorder aged 6 to 12 years.

Controlled studies

Of several controlled studies of lithium in youth, only three studied bipolar patients. Two focused on bipolar disorder and one focused on adolescents with bipolar disorder and a secondary substance dependency disorder. McKnew and colleagues [21] studied lithium response in six children with heterogeneous diagnoses who had a lithium-responding parent in a double-blind, multiple crossover study lasting 16 to 18 weeks. Lithium, at serum levels of 0.8 to 1.2 mEq/L, was superior to placebo only in the two children, aged 8 and 12 years, who met adult criteria for bipolar disorder, mixed phase, by modified Research Diagnostic Criteria (RDC). DeLong and Nieman [20] studied lithium response in 11 children, aged 6.3 to 13.5 years, "with symptoms suggesting manic-depressive illness" in a double-blind, placebo-controlled crossover study lasting 3 weeks. For inclusion in the study, a child had to be a known lithium responder with more than two previous episodes in 2 years and with a family history of major affective disorder. Doses of lithium ranged from 600 to 1200 mg/day with resulting blood levels between 0.3 to 1.3 mEq/L (mean, 0.6 mEq/L). The authors reported that subjects tended to improve when taking lithium and to deteriorate when taking placebo. Although both these studies showed a positive response to lithium, their sample sizes were small. In the only published, methodologically sound, double-blind, randomized, controlled prospective study, which used the *Diagnostic and Statistical Manual of Mental Disorders–IV (*DSM-IV*)* criteria for bipolar disorder [9], lithium was administered in a double-blind and placebo-controlled fashion to 25 adolescents with bipolar disorder and a secondary substance dependency disorder (most had alcohol or marijuana dependence). The diagnosis of bipolar disorder preceded the substance abuse by several years. This study included a 2-week, single-blind, placebo washout phase followed by a 10-week, placebo-controlled, double-blind, short-term treatment phase. Those randomly assigned to lithium treatment showed significantly better outcome of both their bipolar disorder and their secondary drug dependency than those randomly assigned to placebo. This study suggests that lithium may be efficacious in the treatment of bipolar adolescents with comorbid substance abuse. The focus of this study, however, was on whether lithium treatment reduced substance use in this population, although effect on mood was also measured.

Open studies

Two large open treatment studies have suggested that lithium is efficacious in bipolar children and adolescents. DeLong and Aldershof [22] studied long-term treatment of bipolar outpatients, most of whom were younger than 14 years. They found 45 (73.7%) of the 59 bipolar children who continued to take lithium for more than 2 months had good response. Strober et al [28] reported the results o a treatment study of 50 hospitalized, acutely manic adolescents, aged 13 to 17 years. Although the main objective was to examine the family history of adolescent bipolar probands, response to lithium treatment was also reported. Psychoactive medications, including carbamazepine and neuroleptics, were administered concurrently with lithium in some patients. Overall, 34 (68%) of the 50 subjects showed a good response after 6 weeks of treatment with lithium, maintained with serum lithium levels between 0.9 and 1.5 mmol/L. The response rate in subjects with juvenile-onset bipolar disorder, however, was only 40%, compared with an 80% response rate in adolescent-onset subjects.

In several other open studies of children and adolescents with bipolar disorder, response to lithium ranged between 50% and 60%, about 20% lower than response rates in adults [12]. Brumback and Weinberg1 [36] reported that two of six children with prepubertal mania or hypomania improved with lithium in dosages of 30 to 40 mg/kg/day. In an open study of 10 children by Varanka and colleagues, lithium alone seemed efficacious in prepubertal children with psychotic bipolar disorder [8]. Campbell et al found only modest, insignificant effects of lithium on aggressiveness, explosive affect, and hyperactivity in 10 children, aged 3 to 6 years, in a study comparing lithium and chlorpromazine [30]. Strober et al examined the efficacy of lithium prophylaxis in 37 bipolar adolescents who were stabilized on lithium. They found that continuation of lithium decreased the 18-month relapse rate from 92.3% to 37.5% [6]. The relapse rate was similar to the 33% failure rate reported in adults [37].

In summary, a few controlled studies, case studies, and individual case reports have found lithium to be effective [6,8,27,28,38–40], especially for patients with adolescent-onset bipolar disorder [41]. The overall response may be less than that for adults, possibly because youth with mania often have mixed manic-depressive syndromes or a predominance of psychotic symptoms, both of which are generally more refractory to treatment.

Dosing

Weller and colleagues [42] devised a lithium dosage guide and based on body weight that is easy to use with outpatient children and adolescents. These guidelines indicate a dosage of 30 mg/kg/day in three divided doses will produce a lithium level of 0.6 to 1.2 mEq/L within 5 days in children between the ages of 6 and 12 years. In lithium treatment, lithium levels as high as 1.2 mEq/L have been reported with minimal side effects. Lithium can be monitored safely in the blood or the saliva [43].

Geller and Fetner [44] proposed a kinetics-based method to determine lithium dose derived from measurements of serum lithium levels in 25 adults 24 hours after a single lithium dose of 600 mg [45] is administered. The investigators tested this nomogram method in six children and state that this method can be used to predict serum lithium levels in children.

Hagino and colleagues [43] compared these two methods during the acute phase of lithium treatment of hospitalized preschool and early school-aged children. Lithium dosages estimated by the two methods were similar, but the investigators suggested that neither the kinetics-based nor the weight-based method of determining lithium dosage is likely to prevent the emergence of adverse effects in the acute treatment of young children. According to the investigators, central nervous system side effects can occur in children aged 6 years and younger during the initiation phase of lithium treatment. Side effects are usually related to higher milligram-per-kilogram doses, higher serum lithium levels, initial phase of treatment, and concurrent medical illness [43]. There seems to be a genetic variation in the rate of elimination of lithium. Slow eliminators can develop unacceptably high serum lithium levels and adverse effects [3].

Duration of treatment

Reports of studies in adults with bipolar disorder suggest that intermittent lithium therapy leads to a worse outcome than continuous, uninterrupted lithium therapy. Furthermore, it may be difficult to restabilize patients after treatment interruptions [46–50]. Because of the chronic course of childhood manic-depressive illness and because of rapid cycling and the occurrence of mixed features that are known to predict poor response in older populations [39,51–53], the decision of how long to maintain treatment in children and adolescents is difficult [54]. The little available data strongly support long-term maintenance treatment with lithium, particularly during the teenage years, because of the significantly higher relapse rate of those who discontinued lithium [6,55].

Side effects

Lithium is administered to children following the same safety precautions as in adults. Renal, thyroid, calcium, and phosphorus indices must be monitored at 6-month intervals [2,56]. Although youth generally tolerate lithium well and may have fewer side effects than adults, younger children tend to be more prone to side effects than older children [57]. Although side effects from lithium have been reported in children as young as 3 years [18], controversy still exists regarding the prevalence of side effects. In 48 children (aged 5–13 years), Campbell et al [57] found more frequent side effects than expected from the research literature and stated that the occurrence of side effects depends greatly on age (the younger the child, the more likely the side effects) and diagnosis (the clearer the clinical picture, the fewer the side effects). In contrast, a large study of lithium by DeLong and Aldershof found only 1of the 196 children had to withdraw from lithium treatment because of side effects and that only 1child developed hypothyroidism [22]. Khandelwal et al [56] also found no side effects 3 to 5 years after they had started lithium treatment in four adolescents aged 13 to 15 years.

Common lithium side effects in children include nausea, diarrhea, tremor, enuresis, fatigue, ataxia, leukocytosis, and malaise [58]; less common side effects are renal, ocular, thyroid, neurologic, dermatologic, and cardiovascular effects. Changes in weight and growth, diabetes, and hair loss are also reported [59]. Growth related side effects are a particular concern in children. Although lithium does not seem to have a negative influence on the growth of bones [60], an indirect influence through an effect on the thyroid might be expected, because lithium has been associated with the development of hypothyroidism, goiter, and thyroid autoantibodies [41].

Lithium treatment may also lead to the common side effects of polyuria and polydipsia. Lithium inhibits the action of antidiuretic hormone on the distal tubules and collecting ducts, and this inhibition may evolve into diabetes insipidus, which is usually reversible if lithium is discontinued [61]. Although the long-term effects of lithium on kidney function are of concern [62], the risk of significant glomerular damage with long-term lithium therapy seems minimal [61,63], as has been demonstrated in adolescents [56]. Khandelwal and colleagues reported renal function was unimpaired in four adolescents who had received lithium for 3 to 5 years.

Adverse effects of lithium on cognitive functioning are of great concern in children and adolescents. A double-blind, placebo-controlled study of lithium in aggressive children has suggested that some children will develop cognitive impairment at low plasma levels [58]. This finding was also noted in a double-blind, placebo-controlled study of lithium treatment of depressed children with risk factors for bipolarity [64]. Carlson et al [7] studied lithium effects in a heterogeneous group of children, most of whom had bipolar disorder and disruptive behavior disorder. They found no evidence of impaired attention, cognitive functioning, or learning.

Although lithium can affect cardiac conduction, including first-degree atrio-ventricular block, irregular sinus rhythms, and increased premature ventricular contractions, serious adverse reactions are rare [61]. Reversible conduction abnormalities have been reported in children [30].

Lithium may also produce a variety of neurologic effects, including muscle weakness, tremor, lethargy, cognitive blunting, and headaches [61,65]. With blood levels above 3.0 mEq/L, patients may develop more devastating neurologic impairments, including seizures, coma, and death [61]. Children younger than 6 years may experience neurologic side effects relatively more frequently than older children [18].

Major drug interactions

Lithium must be used with caution with nonsteroidal anti-inflammatory drugs (NSAIDS), angiotensin-converting enzyme (ACE) inhibitors, xanthines, and calcium-channel blockers.

Predictors of response and resistance to treatment

Several factors may predict response to lithium treatment. For example, previous good response to lithium, a family history of positive response to lithium [22,66], pure but not severe mania, classic bipolar disorder with an episode sequence of mania-depression-euthymia, and therapeutic serum levels are associated with good response to lithium [67,68]. High relapse rates almost certainly correlate with premature discontinuation of lithium maintenance therapy. Strober et al [6] found the relapse rate of 13 adolescents with bipolar I disorder who discontinued prophylactic lithium therapy shortly after hospital discharge was nearly three times greater than the rate in patients who continued lithium without interruption.

Other factors that may be associated with unfavorable responses to lithium treatment include any axis I diagnosis before the age of 12 years [28]. In adults, heavy familial loading of bipolar disorder, multiple previous episodes, presence of prominent psychotic features, rapid cycling, mixed manic states and serum levels below 0.616 are associated with poor response [52,69]. In adolescents, a tendency toward chronic mood instability; significant comorbidity with attention, conduct, and alcohol or substance abuse disorders; and the presence of a personality disorder when euthymic [70] predict poor response. DeLong and Aldershof [22] treated 196 children, adolescents, and young adults (aged 3.1– 20 years) with lithium. Sixty-six percent of these patients, who later developed a bipolar disorder, responded to lithium therapy. This success rate is higher than the 40% response reported in Strober's study of juvenile-onset bipolar disorder [28].

Pharmacokinetics

Pharmacokinetics of lithium clearance in children younger than 9 years has not been systematically studied. Although it has been suggested that renal clearance of lithium in children is high [71], there is not enough published evidence to confirm this hypothesis. One pharmacokinetic study obtained serial blood and saliva lithium samples after administration of a single 300-mg dose of lithium carbonate in nine children aged 9 to 12 years and found that children have a shorter half-life of elimination and higher total clearance of lithium than do adults [72]. In contrast, a study of renal lithium-sodium countertransport in 98 healthy participants aged 5 to 89 years suggested renal clearance of lithium is reduced with advanced age but is not significantly different between children and adults [73].

Anticonvulsants

It has been suggested that anticonvulsants may be more effective than lithium in treating mixed mania and rapid-cycling bipolar disorder [52]. Both open and controlled studies have supported the efficacy of the anticonvulsants carbamazepine and valproate for the acute treatment of bipolar disorder in adults [36]. Only a few studies examined the efficacy of anticonvulsants for early-onset bipolar disorder, and placebo-controlled studies are lacking [65].

Valproate

Divalproex sodium (valproate sodium) is a mood-stabilizing agent that has demonstrated efficacy in adults with bipolar disorder [17,74,75]. In a retrospective comparison with lithium [76], valproate was shown to be as effective as lithium in the treatment of classic mania but more effective than lithium in the treatment of mixed mania. A review of acute treatment studies of divalproex sodium in adults with mania found an average response rate of 56% [77]. Valproate was also effective in the treatment of mania in adolescents [78]. Valproate seems to be relatively well tolerated by children and young adolescents [1] and shows promise as a possible treatment for juvenile-onset bipolar disorder, based on adult studies and limited open trials in adolescents with bipolar disorder. No study, however, has demonstrated the efficacy of valproate in a randomized, controlled trial in children and adolescents. Valproate is approved by the FDA for the treatment of acute mania in adults.

There are several uncontrolled reports, including case reports [79–81] and case series [47,78,82–87], of the use of divalproex sodium in children and adolescents with bipolar disorder. These open studies involved a wide variability of treatment responses, the frequent use of concomitant antipsychotic agents, and extensive occurrence of comorbid psychiatric diagnoses. Whittier et al [81] reported valproate was effective in a 13-year-old girl with dysphoric mania and mild retardation. In an open, naturalistic study of divalproex sodium in 10 adolescents with chronic temper outbursts and mood lability, Donovan et al reported an improvement in all subjects. It also was reported that discontinuation of medication led to relapse with subsequent improvement after restarting valproate in five of six subjects [88].

Kowatch et al [10] reported an increase of bipolar symptoms after 3 weeks of treatment with valproate that typically resolved the following week. A similar phenomenon has not been observed among adult bipolar patients treated with divalproex, suggesting, the investigators believe, a transitory difference between adults and children in their neurochemical response to valproate. They suggest treating physicians should not discontinue the use of valproate if bipolar symptoms worsen after 2 to 3 weeks of treatment but should continue for several more weeks before discontinuing treatment with valproate. A naturalistic study of 20 Swedish adolescent inpatients with bipolar disorder (16 mixed with mania) reported good control of manic and psychotic symptoms and of agitation and aggression with valproate treatment [89]. There were few side effects.

Dosing

Optimum serum levels for adults with bipolar disorder are reported to be 45 to 125 μg/mL [90]. The usual dose for children is 10 to 60 mg/kg/day and for adolescents is 1000 to 3000 mg/day [91]. Optimum serum level for children and adolescents has not been reported.

Side effects

Most youth tolerate valproate well. The most common side effects of valproate include sedation, nausea, vomiting, appetite increase and weight gain, tremor, hepatic toxicity, hyperammonemia, blood dyscrasias, alopecia, decreased serum carnitine, neural tube defects, pancreatitis, hyperglycemia, and menstrual changes [59]. The hepatic toxicity, which may lead to death, seems to occur almost exclusively in relatively young children, especially those younger than 2 years, who are receiving multiple concomitant medications [92,93].

A specific concern has recently been raised that valproate may induce a metabolic syndrome, characterized by obesity, hyperinsulinemia, lipid abnormalities, polycystic ovaries, and hyperandrogenism, particularly in younger women. A report by Isojarvi et al [94] showed that 89% of adolescent girls who started valproate treatment for epilepsy before the age of 20 years developed polycystic ovarian disease, compared with 27% of epileptic women who were not receiving valproate. In a 1996 article, Isojarvi and colleagues [95] reported that valproate was associated with onset of obesity in more than half of 65 women who participated in the study and that polycystic ovarian disease developed in these individuals. On replacing valproate with lamotrigine in 16 women, Isojarvi and colleagues [96] found the severity of this metabolic syndrome to be reduced (suggesting a partial reversibility). It is not known whether these findings can be generalized to psychiatric populations because the reports of this syndrome, so far, are confined to this single cohort with epilepsy [97].

Major drug interactions

Divalproex should be used with caution with carbamazepine, lamotrigine, diazepam, lorazepam, amitriptyline, and nortriptyline.

Carbamazepine

Carbamazepine is an anticonvulsant agent structurally similar to imipramine [98]. The use of carbamazepine to treat bipolar disorder was first described by Japanese investigators [99]. Carbamazepine has demonstrated efficacy in adults with bipolar disorder [100,101], and the combination of lithium and carbamazepine was suggested to be superior to lithium therapy alone [102]. In adults, carbamazepine may be superior to lithium alone in mixed or rapid-cycling mania

[13]. Although carbamazepine has been found to be effective as a second-line treatment of acute mania in adults [77], it has never been studied in a controlled manner with bipolar children and adolescents. Most carbamazepine treatment reports are with children and adolescents with attention deficit hyperactivity disorder (ADHD) or conduct disorder, some of whom also had neurologic disorders [103–105].

Carbamazepine is widely used in the treatment of behavioral disorders in children and adolescents [104], including conduct disorder with a profile of explosiveness and aggression. Although an early pilot study reported promising results [105], a 6-week, double-blind study of 22 children aged 5 to 12 years with conduct disorder, who were hospitalized for aggression, found carbamazepine in doses from 400 to 800 mg with serum levels from 4.98 to 9.1 µg/mL was not superior to placebo in reducing aggressive behavior [103].

There are no controlled studies and few anecdotal data on the use of carbamazepine in children with bipolar disorder. Carbamazepine, however, has been used in the treatment of juvenile bipolar disorder as a monotherapy or as an adjunct to lithium when lithium treatment alone was ineffective. Carbamazepine has been reported to be effective in manic adolescents who have not responded to lithium [106]. Woolston [107] described three adolescents, in whom carbamazepine was a safe and effective treatment for acute mania and long-term maintenance treatment.

Dosing

Treatment with carbamazepine should be started with a low dose (100 mg two times/day for children under 8 years; or 200 mg two times/day for children older than 8 years), and titrated upward based on side effects to achieve a blood level of 6 to 12 µg/mL [108,109]. The dosage for children generally is 10 to 20 mg/kg/day (200 to 600 mg/day). Dosage for adolescents may go as high as 1200 mg/day or more [65,91].

Side effects

Side effects from carbamazepine may be relatively more common than from lithium or placebo [103]. Common side effects include drowsiness, loss of coordination, and vertigo. More serious side effects reported to the manufacturer over an 11-year period during which 4 million patients were treated included 27 cases of aplastic anemia and 10 cases of agranulocytosis [97]. Hematologic, dermatologic, hepatic, and pancreatic effects have been reported. Because side effects can present with sore throat and fever, it is important to perform complete blood cell counts (CBCs) with differential and platelet counts.

There are several adverse cognitive and behavioral side effects with carbamazepine in children [98,110]. In children with seizure disorders, reported cognitive and behavior effects include impaired performance on learning and memory tasks, irritability, agitation, insomnia, and emotional lability [111]. Stores et al [112], however, found no significant cognitive or behavior effects after 1 year of therapy with either carbamazepine or valproate.

Major drug interactions

Carbamazepine must be used with caution with most of the psychotropic medications, because it interacts with most psychiatric medications.

Novel anticonvulsants

It has been suggested that some new anticonvulsants may have mood-stabilizing action in children with bipolar disorder. As with other medications used for the treatment of bipolar disorder, these new compounds have not yet been studied in children and adolescents. Current use is based on the personal experience of physicians and in some cases on the results of open studies and case reports and series.

Lamotrigine

Lamotrigine was recently approved as an adjunctive agent in the treatment of adults with partial seizures. There are several reports of the effectiveness of lamotrigine in adults with bipolar disorder [113–115]. Because of the high incidence (1/1000) of severe skin rashes, some of which progress to Stevens-Johnson syndrome, the FDA issued a "black-box" warning against using lamotrigine in patients younger than 16 years of age [116–118].

Calabrese et al [119] examined lamotrigine as maintenance monotherapy in a prospective placebo-controlled study of adults with rapid-cycling bipolar disorder. Three hundred twenty-four patients with rapid-cycling bipolar disorder (DSM-IV criteria) received open-label lamotrigine, and 182 patients were randomly assigned to a double-blind maintenance phase. Forty-one percent of lamotrigine patients versus 26% of placebo patients ($P = 0.03$) were stable without relapse during 6 months of monotherapy. Lamotrigine was well tolerated. There were no treatment-related changes in laboratory parameters, vital signs, or body weight. No serious rashes occurred.

Although lamotrigine is becoming increasingly popular in the treatment of childhood bipolar disorder, its usefulness as an antimanic (as well as an anticonvulsant) agent for children and adolescents is limited by its age-related association with the potentially life-threatening Stevens-Johnson syndrome [82,117,120].

Gabapentin

Gabapentin received FDA approval in the United States in 1994 for treatment of adults with partial seizures, either alone or with secondarily generalized seizures. Gabapentin is structurally similar to the inhibitory neurotransmitter Gamma amino butyric acid (GABA). Its mechanism of action in humans is unknown [121]. Gabapentin has been used as an adjunct to treat adult bipolar disorder with good results, and clinical trials are underway with gabapentin as monotherapy for adults with bipolar disorder [122–124].

A potential adverse effect of gabapentin is behavioral disinhibition, which has been reported in several children treated with gabapentin for seizure disorders [125,126].

Combinations of anticonvulsants.

There are several studies on combinations of anticonvulsants in the treatment of bipolar disorder in children and adolescents.

Garfinkel et al [127] reported on 19 treatment-resistant bipolar adolescents (11 with acute mania and 8 with mixed mania) who all had an excellent response to the combination of lithium and carbamazepine. Valproic acid has been used in open studies of hospitalized manic adolescents in combination with other psychoactive medications [78,83]. Finally, a recently published 6-week open, randomized trial of valproate, lithium, and carbamazepine in 42 children and adolescents with bipolar I and II disorder demonstrated a 40% to 50% response rate as assessed by a drop in the Young Mania Rating Scale 168 scores [10]. In this study, lithium dosage was determined using the weight algorithms devised by Weller and colleagues [42], with a starting dose of approximately 30 mg/kg/ day in three divided doses. The initial dose of carbamazepine was 15 mg/kg/day in three divided doses. The initial dose of valproate was 20 mg/kg/day in three divided doses. Dosages were then titrated until the following serum levels were reached: lithium, 0.8 to 1.2 mEq/L; carbamazepine, 7 to 10 μg/L; valproate, 85 to 110 μg/L. By the end of the trial, the following effect sizes were found: divalproex sodium, 1.63; lithium, 1.06; and carbamazepine, 1.00, with no serious side effects.

Soutullo et al [128] report a favorable response to gabapentin plus carbamazepine in a 13-year-old boy with bipolar disorder. The pediatric neurology literature, however, suggests that gabapentin has potential for inducing disruptive and aggressive behavior in children treated for seizure control [125,126,129]. Investigation into its efficacy in pediatric bipolar disorder is clearly needed.

Antipsychotics

It has been suggested that adolescents with mania may have more psychotic and schizophreniform symptoms than do adults [130–132]. There is, however, no definitive proof that the addition of neuroleptics is necessary to treat psychotic symptoms associated with mania in children and adolescents. A small preliminary study reported resolution of mood-congruent delusions and hallucinations within a mean of 11 days in an open trial of lithium alone in 10 psychotic manic children, aged 6 to 12 years [8]. Horowitz [27] reported on lithium treatment in eight manic-depressive adolescents, aged 15 to 18 years. All had delusions, and five hallucinated. All symptoms responded to lithium alone within 5 to 14 days. Goodnick and Meltzer reported that psychotic symptoms in adult mania and schizoaffective mania respond to lithium alone [133]. They found that achieving "comparable remission" could take significantly longer for schizoaffective patients than for manic patients (4 weeks or more, compared with 2 weeks).

In the literature on manic adults, neuroleptics have been shown to be effective for the treatment of acute mania [12], to be superior to placebo, but less effective than lithium [134]. It is not clear whether the effects of neuroleptics are truly antimanic or a result of sedation [12].

Clozapine

In studies of clozapine in treating adult patients with bipolar disorder who did not respond to lithium, anticonvulsants, and neuroleptics, response has ranged between 72% and 87% [135]. A similar response was reported in a series of five children and adolescents with mixed mania, who had not improved with other neuroleptics [136]. Clozapine has also been reported to be effective in an adolescent with bipolar disorder [137]. Side effects of treatment with clozapine include agranulocytosis, sedation, weight gain, and salivation. A recent report [138] highlights a small but potentially fatal risk of myocarditis.

Quetiapine

Quetiapine fumarate is an antipsychotic agent belonging to a new chemical class, the dibenzothiazepine derivatives. Quetiapine is an antagonist at multiple neurotransmitter receptors in the brain, including the serotonin 5HT1A and 5HT2; dopamine D1 and D2; histamine H1, and adrenergic α1 and α2 receptors. The efficacy of quetiapine in the management of psychotic disorders in adults was established in four short-term, controlled trials involving adult psychotic inpatients who met DSM–III-R criteria for schizophrenia [139–142]. To date there has been one case report that quetiapine was helpful in a child with bipolar disorder.

Schaller and Behar [143] reported that a 9-year-old girl with severe mania receiving valproic acid with a blood level of 72 ng/mL was treated with quetiapine, starting with a dosage of 25 mg two times per day and increasing to 150 mg three times per day over 6 days. She tolerated the increase, with only 1 to 2 days of mild sedation. After 3 days of receiving 450 mg/day, she had a complete remission of her manic symptoms. No occurrence of psychiatric symptoms was observed for 4 months except for mild symptoms of major depression, which were successfully treated with 37.5 mg of sertraline.

Risperidone

Risperidone has been associated with improved mood stabilization in adult bipolar patients with incomplete response to mood stabilizers [144–148].

Frazier et al [149] retrospectively reviewed the charts of 28 outpatients with bipolar disorder (mean age, 10.4 ± 3.8 years) who were treated with risperidone. They found risperidone treatment for 6 months (mean dose, 1.7 mg) was associated with an 82% reduction in manic, psychotic, and aggressive symptoms in most of the children. The most common adverse effects were weight gain and sedation, each observed in 18% of cases. Wozniak et al [150] have suggested risperidone may be effective in treating dysphoric aggression in manic children.

Olanzapine

The atypical antipsychotic olanzapine has a pharmacologic and receptor affinity profile similar to that of clozapine [151,152]. Preliminary data suggest that olanzapine, like clozapine, may have mood-stabilizing properties in adults with schizoaffective disorder, bipolar type I [153,154] and treatment-resistant bipolar disorder [155]. Olanzapine is approved by the FDA for the treatment of acute mania in adults.

Soutullo et al [156] reported on six consecutively hospitalized patients and one outpatient with bipolar I disorder, treated with olanzapine (mean age, 15 ± 1 years, range, 12–17 years). All seven patients (three young men and four young women) met *DSM-IV* criteria for a manic episode. Five (71%) displayed moderate or marked improvement with open-label olanzapine treatment.

Chang and Ketter reported marked improvement within 3 to 5 days in three acutely manic prepubertal children treated with olanzapine in addition to their existing mood stabilizer regimen. Adverse side effects were sedation and weight gain [157]. The same side effects were described by Krishnamoorthy and King, who reported that olanzapine treatment was discontinued in all five children within the first 6 weeks of treatment because of adverse effects, including sedation ($n = 3$), weight gain of up to 16 pounds ($n = 3$), akathisia ($n = 2$), or lack of clinically significant therapeutic response [158].

Electroconvulsive therapy

In adults, electroconvulsive therapy (ECT) has been reported to be as effective as lithium for the treatment of mania [159,160]. A randomized, double-blind controlled study by Small et al [161] also showed ECT to be effective in mania.

Electroconvulsive therapy has been considered a treatment of choice for adults with bipolar disorder in the following clinical situations: (1) pregnancy; (2) catatonia; (3) neuroleptic malignant syndrome, and (4) any other medical condition for which more standard medication regimens are contraindicated.

Although research on the use of ECT in children is limited, several case reports indicate that ECT was beneficial for children and adolescents with bipolar disorder, including those in manic, rapid cycling, and depressed phases [162]. Ketcher and Robertson retrospectively studied 22 adolescents. Treatment was successful for eight of nine patients (aged 5 to 15 years), treated for mania, for two rapid-cycling adolescents (aged 15 and 18 years), and for all 11 depressed adolescents, (aged 12 to 18 years). The authors suggested that ECT may be an acutely well tolerated, efficacious, and cost-effective treatment in adolescents with bipolar disorder (in either manic or depressed phases), who had not responded to optimized psychopharmacologic interventions [163]. In adolescents, response rates to ECT of up to 80% have been reported by Walter et al [157]. Potential side effects include short-term cognitive impairment, anxiety reactions, disinhibition, and altered seizure threshold [162].

The renewed interest in ECT to treat adult mania [161] may encourage new systematic research on the safety and efficacy of ECT, particularly for the acute treatment of severe mania, in children and adolescents.

Calcium-channel blockers

Calcium-channel blockers are another group of medications that have many clinical applications, including their possible use in the treatment of bipolar disorder. The efficacy of these compounds as mood stabilizers has not been studied sufficiently, however, and there are few data on their potential efficacy as mood stabilizers in children or adolescents [85].

There is a single case report of an open trial of the calcium-channel blocker nimodipine (Nimotop), a dihydropyridine-type calcium antagonist, in the treatment of a 13-year-old boy with refractory, ultradian rapid cycling, bipolar disorder type I [164]. Prior clinical trials with calcium-channel blockers in adults with ultrarapid cycling affective disorder supported an empirical trial of nimodipine for treatment of ultradian rapid cycling in this adolescent. Authors reported a marked decrease in rapid, repeated, and significant mood changes after 9 days of treatment with nimodipine, 180 mg/day. No adverse effects were noticed. Remission persisted with continued treatment at 36-month follow-up. The response was partially attributed to adjunctive therapy with levothyroxine.

Omega-3 fatty acids

Omega-3 fatty acids are also compounds described as having beneficial effect in patients with bipolar disorder. Omega-3 fatty acids are obtained from marine or plant sources [165], and their mechanism of action is associated with a general dampening of signal transduction pathways associated with phosphatidylinositol, arachidonic acid, and other systems [166,167].

The information on the use of omega-3 fatty acids in children is lacking. In the only controlled trial in adults, Stoll et al studied 30 patients (aged 18 to 65 years) with bipolar disorder in a 4-month, double-blind, placebo-controlled study, comparing omega-3 fatty acids (9.6 g/day) with placebo (olive oil), in addition to usual treatment. Based on the results of the study, the authors concluded that use of the omega 3 fatty acids resulted in significant symptom reduction and a better outcome when compared with placebo in this pilot study. Improvement on almost every assessment measure was significantly greater in the omega-3 fatty acid group than in the control group receiving olive oil.

Further studies in children and adolescents are needed.

Summary

The currently available data from randomized, controlled trials and a considerable amount of open clinical data suggest that adolescent-onset bipolar disorder probably responds to the same agents as adult-onset bipolar disorder. Research examining psychopharmacologic treatment approaches in the early-onset bipolar disorder is limited, however. Methodologic problems include small sample sizes, lack of comparison groups, retrospective designs, and lack of standardized measures. In addition, sometimes no clear differentiation is made between mania and bipolar disorder, the latter term being used broadly in the literature. Often the studies show that symptoms improve because of treatment, but the functioning of the patients does not improve significantly. More research is clearly needed in all aspects of this disorder but especially in examining the efficacy of various types of treatment, its longitudinal course, and diagnostic issues. The indications for, and the overall duration of, long-term maintenance therapy need further study.

Many adolescents and children with bipolar disorder do not respond to any of the first-line pharmacologic treatments; therefore, studies with novel agents should be extended to patients in this age range. Furthermore, physicians will probably continue to use combination therapies when confronted by either lack of efficacy or delayed onset of efficacy with a single agent. Thus, such resultant drug-drug interactions also should also be systematically studied [97].

References

[1] American Academy of Child and Adolescent Psychiatry. Practice parameters for the assessment and treatment of children and adolescents with bipolar disorder. J Am Acad Child Adolesc Psychiatry 1997;36:138–57.

[2] Fetner HH, Geller B. Lithium and tricyclic antidepressants. Psychiatr Clin North Am 1992;15: 223–4.

[3] Youngerman J, Canino IA. Lithium carbonate use in children and adolescents: a survey of the literature. Arch Gen Psychiatry 1978;35:216–24.

[4] Kafantaris V. Treatment of bipolar disorder in children and adolescents. J Am Acad Child Adolesc Psychiatry 1995;34:732–41.

[5] Weller E. Bipolar children and adolescents: controversies in diagnosis and treatment. Proceedings of the American Psychiatric Association 153rd Annual Meeting. Chicago (IL); 2000.

[6] Strober M, Morrell W, Lampert C, et al. Relapse following discontinuation of lithium maintenance therapy in adolescents with bipolar I illness: a naturalistic study. Am J Psychiatry 1990; 147:457–61.

[7] Carlson GA, Rapport MD, Pataki CS, et al. Lithium in hospitalized children at 4 and 8 weeks: mood, behavior and cognitive effects. J Child Psychol Psychiatry 1992;33:411–25.

[8] Varanka TM, Weller RA, Weller EB, et al. Lithium treatment of manic episodes with psychotic features in prepubertal children. Am J Psychiatry 1988;145:1557–9.

[9] Geller B, Cooper TB, Sun K, et al. Double-blind and placebo-controlled study of lithium for adolescent bipolar disorders with secondary substance dependency [see comments]. J Am Acad Child Adolesc Psychiatry 1998;37:171–8.

[10] Kowatch RA, Suppes T, Carmody TJ, et al. Effect size of lithium, divalproex sodium, and carbamazepine in children and adolescents with bipolar disorder. J Am Acad Child Adolesc Psychiatry 2000;39:713–20.

[11] Lin KM, Anderson D, Poland RE. Ethnicity and psychopharmacology. Bridging the gap. Psychiatr Clin North Am 1995;18:635–47.

[12] Goodwin F, Jamison K. Manic-depressive illness. New York (NY): Oxford University Press; 1990.

[13] Goodwin FK, Murphy DL, Bunney WE. Lithium-carbonate treatment in depression and mania. A longitudinal double-blind study. Arch Gen Psychiatry 1969;21:486–96.

[14] Maggs R. Treatment of manic illness with lithium carbonate. Br J Psychiatry 1963;109:56–65.

[15] Schou M, Juel-Nielsen N, Stromgren E, et al. The treatment of manic psychoses by the administration of lithium salts. J Neurol Neurosurg Psychiatry 1954;17:250–60.

[16] Bowden CL, Janicak PG, Orsulak P, et al. Relation of serum valproate concentration to response in mania. Am J Psychiatry 1996;153:765–70.

[17] Bowden CL, Brugger AM, Swann AC, et al. Efficacy of divalproex vs lithium and placebo in the treatment of mania. The Depakote Mania Study Group. [published erratum appears in JAMA 1994;271(23):1830] [see comments] JAMA 1994;271:918–24.

[18] Hagino OR, Weller EB, Weller RA, et al. Untoward effects of lithium treatment in children aged four through six years. J Am Acad Child Adolesc Psychiatry 1995;34:1584–90.

[19] Van Krevelen DA, Van Voorst JA. Lithium in the treatment of a cryptogenetic psychosis in a juvenile. Zeitschrift Fuer Kinderpsychiatrie 1959;26:148–52.

[20] DeLong GR, Nieman GW. Lithium-induced behavior changes in children with symptoms suggesting manic-depressive illness. Psychopharmacol Bull 1983;19:258–65.

[21] McKnew DH, Cytryn L, Buchsbaum MS, et al. Lithium in children of lithium-responding parents. Psychiatry Res 1981;4:171–80.

[22] DeLong GR, Aldershof AL. Long-term experience with lithium treatment in childhood: correlation with clinical diagnosis. J Am Acad Child Adolesc Psychiatry 1987;26:389–94.

[23] Gram LF, Overo KF, Andersen J, et al. Check to see if these outside brackets are right [Lu 5–003 in antidepressive therapy. A controlled clinical trial with simultaneous measurement of pharmacokinetic parameters. [review]. Nord Psykiatr Tidsskr 1972;26:361 [in Norwegian].

[24] Brumback RA, Weinberg WA. Mania in childhood. II. therapeutic trial of lithium carbonate and further description of manic-depressive illness in children. Am J Dis Child 1977;131:1122–6.

[25] Carlson G, Strober M. Manic-depressive illness in early adolescence. A study of clinical and diagnostic characteristics in six cases. J Am Acad Child Adolesc Psychiatry 1978;17:138–53.

[26] Hassanyeh F, Davison K. Bipolar affectiv psychosis with onset before age 16 years: report of 10 cases. Br J Psychiatry 1980;137:530–9.

[27] Horowitz HA. Lithium and the treatment of adolescent manic depressive illness. Dis Nerv Syst 1977;38:480–3.

[28] Strober M, Morrell W, Burroughs J, et al. A family study of bipolar I disorder in adolescence. Early onset of symptoms linked to increased familial loading and lithium resistance. J Affect Disord 1988;15:255–68.

[29] Campbell M, Adams PB, Small AM, et al. Lithium in hospitalized aggressive children with conduct disorder: a double-blind and placebo-controlled study. [published erratum appears in J Am Acad Child Adolesc Psychiatry 1995;34(5):694] J Am Acad Child Adolesc Psychiatry 1995;34:445–53.

[30] Campbell M, Fish B, Korein J, et al. Lithium and chlorpromazine: a controlled crossover study of hyperactive severely disturbed young children. J Autism Child Schizophr 1972;2:234–63.

[31] Campbell M, Small AM, Green WH, et al. Behavioral efficacy of haloperidol and lithium carbonate. A comparison in hospitalized aggressive children with conduct disorder. Arch Gen Psychiatry 1984;41:650–6.

[32] Siassi I. Lithium treatment of impulsive behavior in children. J Clin Psychiatry 1982;43:482–4.

[33] Cohn CK. Lithium. Texas Medicine 1977;73:73–5.

[34] Joshi P, Capozzoli JA, Coyle JT. Effective management with lithium of a persistent, post-traumatic hypomania in a 10-year-old child. J Dev Behav Pediatr 1985;6:352–4.

[35] Geller B, Fox LW, Fletcher M. Effect of tricyclic antidepressants on switching to mania and on

the onset of bipolarity in depressed 6-to 12-year-olds. J Am Acad Child Adolesc Psychiatry 1993;32:43–50.

[36] American Psychiatric Association. Practice guideline for the treatment of patients with bipolar disorder. American Psychiatric Association. Am J Psychiatry 1994;151:1–36.

[37] Prien RF, Potter WZ. NIMH workshop report on treatment of bipolar disorder. Psychopharmacol Bull 1990;26:409–27.

[38] Geller B, Cooper TB, Sun K, et al. Double-blind and placebo-controlled study of lithium for adolescent bipolar disorders with secondary substance dependency. J Am Acad Child Adolesc Psychiatry 1998;37:171–8.

[39] Hsu LK, Starzynski JM. Mania in adolescence. J Clin Psychiatry 1986;47:596–9.

[40] Young RC, Biggs JT, Ziegler VE, et al. A rating scale for mania: reliability, validity and sensitivity. Br J Psychiatry 1978;133:429–35.

[41] Alessi N, Naylor MW, Ghaziuddin M, et al. Update on lithium carbonate therapy in children and adolescents [see comments]. J Am Acad Child Adolesc Psychiatry 1994;33:291–304.

[42] Weller EB, Weller RA, Fristad MA. Lithium dosage guide for prepubertal children: a preliminary report. J Am Acad Child Psychiatry 1986;25:92–5.

[43] Hagino OR, Weller EB, Weller RA, et al. Comparison of lithium dosage methods for preschool-and early school-age children. J Am Acad Child Adolesc Psychiatry 1998;37:60–5.

[44] Geller B, Fetner HH. Children's 24-hour serum lithium level after a single dose predicts initial dose and steady-state plasma level. J Clin Psychopharmacol 1989;9:155.

[45] Cooper TB, Bergner PE, Simpson GM. The 24-hour serum lithium level as a prognosticator of dosage requirements. Am J Psychiatry 1973;130:601–3.

[46] Ahrens B, Grof P, Moller HJ, et al. Extended survival of patients on long-term lithium treatment. Can J Psychiatry 1995;40:241–6.

[47] Muller-Oerlinghausen B, Ahrens B, Grof E, et al. The effect of long-term lithium treatment on the mortality of patients with manic-depressive and schizoaffective illness. Acta Psychiatr Scand 1992;86:218–22.

[48] Muller-Oerlinghausen B, Wolf T, Ahrens B, et al. Mortality during initial and during later lithium treatment. A collaborative study by the International Group for the Study of Lithium-treated Patients. Acta Psychiatr Scand 1994;90:295–7.

[49] Schou M. Prophylactic lithium treatment of unipolar and bipolar manic-depressive illness. Psychopathology 1995;28:81–5.

[50] Schou M, Hansen HE, Thomsen K, et al. Lithium treatment in Aarhus. 2. Risk of renal failure and of intoxication. Pharmacopsychiatry 1989;22:101–3.

[51] Geller B, Sun K, Zimerman B, et al. Complex and rapid-cycling in bipolar children and adolescents: a preliminary study. J Affect Disord 1995;34:259–68.

[52] Himmelhoch JM, Garfinkel ME. Mixed mania: diagnosis and treatment. Psychopharmacol Bull 1986;22:613.

[53] Keller MB, Lavori PW, Coryell W, et al. Bipolar I: a five-year prospective follow-up. J Nerv Ment Dis 1993;181:238–45.

[54] Geller B, Luby J. Child and adolescent bipolar disorder: a review of the past 10 years. J Am Acad Child Adolesc Psychiatry 1997;36:1168–76.

[55] Strober M, Schmidt-Lackner S, Freeman R, et al. Recovery and relapse in adolescents with bipolar affective illness: a five-year naturalistic, prospective follow-up. J Am Acad Child Adolesc Psychiatry 1995;34:724–31.

[56] Campbell M, Silva RR, Kafantaris V, et al. Predictors of side effects associated with lithium administration in children. Psychopharmacol Bull 1991;27:373–80.

[57] Khandelwal SK, Varma VK, Srinivasa Murthy R. Renal function in children receiving long-term lithium prophylaxis. Am J Psychiatry 1984;141:278–9.

[58] Silva RR, Campbell M, Golden RR, et al. Side effects associated with lithium and placebo administration in aggressive children. Psychopharmacol Bull 1992;28:319–26.

[59] Rosenberg DR, Holttum J, Gershon S. Textbook of pharmacotherapy for child and adolescent psychiatric disorders. New York (NY): Brunner/Mazel; 1994.

[60] Birch NJ, Horsman A, Hullin RP. Lithium, bone and body weight studies in long-term lithium-treated patients and in the rat. Neuropsychobiology 1982;8:86–92.

[61] Gelenberg AJ, Schoonover SC. Bipolar disorder. In: Bassuk EL, Schoonover SC, Gelenberg AJ, editors. The practitioner's guide to psychoactive drugs. 3rd edition. New York (NY): Plenum; 1991. p. 91–124.

[62] Reisberg B, Gershon S. Side effects associated with lithium therapy. Arch Gen Psychiatry 1979; 36:879–87.

[63] Hetmar O, Povlsen UJ, Ladefoged J, et al. Lithium: long-term effects on the kidney. A prospective follow-up study ten years after kidney biopsy. Br J Psychiatry 1991;158:53–8.

[64] Geller B, Fox LW, Clark KA. Rate and predictors of prepubertal bipolarity during follow-up of 6- to 12-year-old depressed children [see comments]. J Am Acad Child Adolesc Psychiatry 1994;33:461–8.

[65] Viesselman JO, Yaylayan S, Weller EB, et al. Antidysthymic drugs (antidepressants and antimanics). In: Werry JS, Aman MG, editior. Practitioner's guide to psychoactive drugs for children and adolescents. New York, NY: Plenum; 1993. p. 239–68.

[66] Fristad MA, Weller EB, Weller RA. The Mania Rating Scale: can it be used in children? A preliminary report. J Am Acad Child Alolesc Psychiatry 1992;31:252–7.

[67] Faedda GL, Baldessarini RJ, Tohen M, et al. Episode sequence in bipolar disorder and response to lithium treatment. Am J Psychiatry 1991;148:1237–9.

[68] Gelenberg AJ, Kane JM, Keller MB, et al. Comparison of standard and low serum levels of lithium for maintenance treatment of bipolar disorder. N Engl J Med 1989;321:1489–93.

[69] Post RM, Rubinow DR, Uhde TW, et al. Dysphoric mania. Clinical and biological correlates. Arch Gen Psychiatry 1989;46:353–8.

[70] Lena B. Lithium in child and adolescent psychiatry. Arch Gen Psychiatry 1979;36:854–5.

[71] Kutcher SP, Marton P, Korenblum M. Adolescent bipolar illness and personality disorder. J Am Acad Child Adolesc Psychiatry 1990;29:355–8.

[72] Vitiello B, Behar D, Malone R, et al. Pharmacokinetics of lithium carbonate in children. J Clin Psychopharmacol 1988;8:355–9.

[73] De Santo NG, Coppola S, Coscarella G, et al. Tubular function by lithium clearance, plasma amino acids and hormones following a meat meal in childhood. Ren Physiol Biochem 1991;14: 63–70.

[74] McElroy SL, Keck Jr. PE, Pope Jr HG, et al. Valproate in the treatment of bipolar disorder: literature review and clinical guidelines. J Clin Psychopharmacol 1992;12:42S–52S.

[75] Pope HG, McElroy SL, Keck PE, et al. Valproate in the treatment of acute mania. A placebo-controlled study. Arch Gen Psychiatry 1991;48:62–8.

[76] Strober M. The naturalistic prospective course of juvenile bipolar illness. Pittsburgh (PA); 1977.

[77] Janicak PG. The relevance of clinical pharmacokinetics and therapeutic drug monitoring: anticonvulsant mood stabilizers and antipsychotics. J Clin Psychiatry 1993;54:35–41.

[78] West SA, Keck PE, McElroy SL, et al. Open trial of valproate in the treatment of adolescent mania. J Child Adolesc Psychopharmacol 1994;4:263–7.

[79] Kastner T, Friedman DL. Verapamil and valproic acid treatment of prolonged mania. J Am Acad Child Adolesc Psychiatry 1992;31:271–5.

[80] Kastner T, Friedman DL, Plummer AT, et al. Valproic acid for the treatment of children with mental retardation and mood symptomatology. Pediatrics 1990;86:467–72.

[81] Whittier MC, West SA, Galli VB, et al. Valproic acid for dysphoric mania in a mentally retarded adolescent [letter]. J Clin Psychiatry 1995;56:590–1.

[82] Messenheimer J, Mullens EL, Giorgi L, et al. Safety review of adult clinical trial experience with lamotrigine. Drug Saf 1998;18:281–96.

[83] Papatheodorou G, Kutcher SP. Divalproex sodium treatment in late adolescent and young adult acute mania. Psychopharmacol Bull 1993;29:213–9.

[84] Papatheodorou G, Kutcher SP, Katic M, et al. The efficacy and safety of divalproex sodium in the treatment of acute mania in adolescents and young adults: an open clinical trial. J Clin Psychopharmacol 1995;15:110–6.

[85] Wagner JG, Rocchini AP, Vasiliades J. Prediction of steady-state verapamil plasma concentrations in children and adults. Clin Pharmacol Ther 1982;32:172–81.

[86] Walter G, Rey JM, Mitchell PB. Practitioner review: electroconvulsive therapy in adolescents. J Child Psychol Psychiatry 1999;40:325–34.

[87] West SA, McElroy SL, Strakowski SM, et al. Attention deficit hyperactivity disorder in adolescent mania. Am J Psychiatry 1995;152:271–3.

[88] Donovan SJ, Susser ES, Nunes EV, et al. Divalproex treatment of disruptive adolescents: a report of 10 cases. J Clin Psychiatry 1997;58:12–5.

[89] Deltito JA, Levitan J, Damore J, et al. Naturalistic experience with the use of divalproex sodium on an in-patient unit for adolescent psychiatric patients. Acta Psychiatr Scand 1998;97: 236–40.

[90] Calabrese JR, Fatemi SH, Kujawa M, et al. Predictors of response to mood stabilizers. J Clin Psychopharmacol 1996;16:24S–31S.

[91] Pedley TA, Scheuer ML, Walczak TS. Epilepsy. In: Rowland LP, editor. Merrits textbook of neurology. 9th edition. Baltimore, Md: Williams & Wilkins; 1995. p. 845–69.

[92] Bryant AE. 3, Dreifuss FE: Valproic acid hepatic fatalities. III. U.S. experience since 1986. Neurology 1996;46:465–9.

[93] Silberstein SD, Wilmore LJ. Divalproex sodium: migraine treatment and monitoring. Headache 1996;36:239–42.

[94] Isojarvi JI, Laatikainen TJ, Pakarinen AJ, et al. Polycystic ovaries and hyperandrogenism in women taking valproate for epilepsy. N Engl J Med 1993;329:1383–8.

[95] Isojarvi JI, Laatikainen TJ, Knip M, et al. Obesity and endocrine disorders in women taking valproate for epilepsy [see comments]. Ann Neurol 1996;39:579–84.

[96] Isojarvi JI, Rattya J, Myllyla VV, et al. Valproate, lamotrigine, and insulin-mediated risks in women with epilepsy. Ann Neurol 1998;43:446–51.

[97] Ryan ND, Bhatara VS, Perel JM. Mood stabilizers in children and adolescents. J Am Acad Child Adolesc Psychiatry 1999;38:529–36.

[98] Pleak RR, Birmaher B, Gavrilescu A, et al. Mania and neuropsychiatric excitation following carbamazepine. J Am Acad Child Adolesc Psychiatry 1988;27:500–3.

[99] Okuma T, Kishimoto A, Inoue K, et al. Anti-manic and prophylactic effects of carbamazepine (Tegretol) on manic depressive psychosis. A preliminary report. Folia Psychiatr Neurol Jpn 1973;27:283–97.

[100] Post RM, Ketter TA, Denicoff K, et al. The place of anticonvulsant therapy in bipolar illness. Psychopharmacology (Berl) 1996;128:115–29.

[101] Stuppaeck C, Barnas C, Miller C, et al. Carbamazepine in the prophylaxis of mood disorders. J Clin Psychopharmacol 1990;10:39–42.

[102] Solomon DA, Keitner GI, Ryan CE, et al. Polypharmacy in bipolar I disorder. Psychopharmacol Bull 1996;32:579–87.

[103] Cueva JE, Overall JE, Small AM, et al. Carbamazepine in aggressive children with conduct disorder: a double-blind and placebo-controlled study. J Am Acad Child Adolesc Psychiatry 1996;35:480–90.

[104] Evans RW, Clay TH, Gualtieri CT. Carbamazepine in pediatric psychiatry. J Am Acad Child Adolesc Psychiatry 1987;26:2–8.

[105] Kafantaris V, Campbell M, Padron-Gayol MV, et al. Carbamazepine in hospitalized aggressive conduct disorder children: an open pilot study [published erratum appears in Psychopharmacol Bull 1992;28(3):220]. Psychopharmacol Bull 1992;28:193–9.

[106] Hsu LK. Lithium-resistant adolescent mania. J Am Acad Child Psychiatry 1986;25:280–3.

[107] Woolston JL. Case study: carbamazepine treatment of juvenile-onset bipolar disorder. J Am Acad Child Adolesc Psychiatry 1999;38:335–8.

[108] Ballenger JC. The use of anticonvulsants in manic-depressive illness. J Clin Psychiatry 1988; 49:21–5.

[109] Post RM, Uhde TW, Roy-Byrne PP, et al. Correlates of antimanic response to carbamazepine. Psychiatry Res 1987;21:71–83.

[110] Bhatara VS, Carrera J. Medications for aggressiveness. J Am Acad Child Adolesc Psychiatry 1994;33:282–3.

[111] Carpenter RO, Vining EPG. Antiepileptics (anticonvulsants). In: Werry JS, Aman MG, editors. Practitioner's guide to psychoactive drugs for children and adolescents. New York (NY): Plenum; 1993. p. 321–46.

[112] Stores G, Williams PL, Styles E, et al. Psychological effects of sodium valproate and carbamazepine in epilepsy. Arch Dis Child 1992;67:1330–7.

[113] Calabrese JR, Fatemi SH, Woyshville MJ. Antidepressant effects of lamotrigine in rapid cycling bipolar disorder [letter] [see comments]. Am J Psychiatry 1996;153:1236.

[114] Fatemi SH, Rapport DJ, Calabrese JR, et al. Lamotrigine in rapid-cycling bipolar disorder. J Clin Psychiatry 1997;58:522–7.

[115] Fogelson DL, Sternbach H. Lamotrigine treatment of refractory bipolar disorder. J Clin Psychiatry 1997;58:271–3.

[116] Chaffin JJ, Davis SM. Suspected lamotrigine-induced toxic epidermal necrolysis. Ann Pharmacother 1997;31:720–3.

[117] Dooley J, Camfield P, Gordon K, et al. Lamotrigine-induced rash in children. Neurology 1996; 46:240–2.

[118] Fogh K, Mai J. Toxic epidermal necrolysis after treatment with lamotrigine (Lamictal). Seizure 1997;6:63–5.

[119] Calabrese JR, Suppes T, Bowden CL, et al. A double-blind, placebo-controlled, prophylaxis study of lamotrigine in rapid-cycling bipolar disorder. Lamictal 614 Study Group. J Clin Psychiatry 2000;61:841–50.

[120] Mackay FJ, Wilton LV, Pearce GL, et al. Safety of long-term lamotrigine in epilepsy. Epilepsia 1997;38:881–6.

[121] Dichter MA, Brodie MJ. New antiepileptic drugs. N Engl J Med 1996;334:1583–90.

[122] Ryback RS, Brodsky L, Munasifi F. Gabapentin in bipolar disorder [letter]. J Neuropsychiatry Clin Neurosci 1997;9:301.

[123] Schaffer CB, Schaffer LC. Gabapentin in the treatment of bipolar disorder. Am J Psychiatry 1997;154:291–2.

[124] Young LT, Robb JC, Patelis-Siotis I, et al. Acute treatment of bipolar depression with gabapentin. Biol Psychiatry 1997;42:851–3.

[125] Tallian KB, Nahata MC, Lo W, et al. Gabapentin associated with aggressive behavior in pediatric patients with seizures. Epilepsia 1996;37:501–2.

[126] Lee DO, Steingard RJ, Cesena M, et al. Behavioral side effects of gabapentin in children. Epilepsia 1996;37:87–90.

[127] Garfinkel M, Garfinkel L, Himmelhoch J, et al. Lithium carbonate and carbamazepine: an effective treatment for adolescent manic or mixed bipolar patients. Proceedings of the Annual Meeting of the American Academy of Child and Adolescent Psychiatry, 1985. p. 41–2.

[128] Soutullo CA, Casuto LS, Keck Jr PE. Gabapentin in the treatment of adolescent mania: a case report. J Child Adolesc Psychopharmacol 1998;8:81–5.

[129] Wolf SM, Shinnar S, Kang H, et al. Gabapentin toxicity in children manifesting as behavioral changes. Epilepsia 1995;36:1203–5.

[130] Ballenger JC, Reus VI, Post RM. The "atypical" clinical picture of adolescent mania. Am J Psychiatry 1982;139:602–6.

[131] Joyce PR. Age of onset in bipolar affective disorder and misdiagnosis as schizophrenia. Psychol Med 1984;14:145–9.

[132] Rosen LN, Rosenthal NE, Van Dusen PH, et al. Age at onset and number of psychotic symptoms in bipolar I and schizoaffective disorder. Am J Psychiatry 1983;140:1523–4.

[133] Goodnick PJ, Meltzer HY. Treatment of schizoaffective disorders. Schizophr Bull 1984;10: 30–48.

[134] Janicak PG, Newman RH, Davis JM. Advances in the treatment of mania and related disorders. Annals of Psychiatry 1992;22:92–103.

[135] Calabrese JR, Kimmel SE, Woyshville MJ, et al. Clozapine for treatment-refractory mania. Am J Psychiatry 1996;153:759–64.

[136] Kowatch RA, Suppes T, Gilfillan SK, et al. Clozapine treatment of children and adolescents with bipolar disorder and schizophrenia: a clinical case series. J Child Adolesc Psychopharmacol 1995;5:241–53.

[137] Fuchs DC. Clozapine treatment of bipolar disorder in a young adolescent. J Am Acad Child Adolesc Psychiatry 1994;33:1299–302.

[138] Killian JG, Kerr K, Lawrence C, et al. Myocarditis and cardiomyopathy associated with clozapine. Lancet 1999;354:1841–5.

[139] Arvanitis LA, Miller BG. Multiple fixed doses of "Seroquel" (quetiapine) in patients with acute exacerbation of schizophrenia: a comparison with haloperidol and placebo. The Seroquel Trial 13 Study Group. Biol Psychiatry 1997;42:233–46.

[140] Copolov DL, Link CG, Kowalcyk B. A multicentre, double-blind, randomized comparison of quetiapine (ICI 204,636, 'Seroquel') and haloperidol in schizophrenia. Psychol Med 2000;30:95–105.

[141] Peuskens J, Link CG. A comparison of quetiapine and chlorpromazine in the treatment of schizophrenia. Acta Psychiatr Scand 1997;96:265–73.

[142] Small JG, Hirsch SR, Arvanitis LA, et al. Quetiapine in patients with schizophrenia. A high-and low-dose double-blind comparison with placebo. Seroquel Study Group. Arch Gen Psychiatry 1997;54:549–57.

[143] Schaller JL, Behar D. Quetiapine for refractory mania in a child. J Am Acad Child Adolesc Psychiatry 1999;38:498–9.

[144] Vieta E, Gasto C, Colom F, et al. Treatment of refractory rapid cycling bipolar disorder with risperidone [letter]. J Clin Psychopharmacol 1998;18:172–4.

[145] Ghaemi SN, Sachs GS, Baldassano CF, et al. Acute treatment of bipolar disorder with adjunctive risperidone in outpatients. Can J Psychiatry 1997;42:196–9.

[146] Goodnick PJ. Risperidone treatment of refractory acute mania [letter]. J Clin Psychiatry 1995;56:431–2.

[147] McIntyre R, Young LT, Hasey G, et al. Risperidone treatment of bipolar disorder [letter]. Can J Psychiatry 1997;42:88–90.

[148] Tohen M, Zarate Jr. CA, Centorrino F, et al. Risperidone in the treatment of mania. J Clin Psychiatry 1996;57:249–53.

[149] Frazier JA, Meyer MC, Biederman J, et al. Risperidone treatment for juvenile bipolar disorder: a retrospective chart review. J Am Acad Child Adolesc Psychiatry 1999;38:960–5.

[150] Wozniak J, Biederman J, Kiely K, et al. Mania-like symptoms suggestive of childhood-onset bipolar disorder in clinically referred children [see comments]. J Am Acad Child Adolesc Psychiatry 1995;34:867–76.

[151] Frye MA, Ketter TA, Altshuler LL, et al. Clozapine in bipolar disorder: treatment implications for other atypical antipsychotics. J Affect Disord 1998;48:91–104.

[152] Keck Jr. PE, McElroy SL. The new antipsychotics and their therapeutic potential. Psychiatr Ann 1997;27:320–31.

[153] Friedman L, Findling RL, Kenny JT, et al. An MRI study of adolescent patients with either schizophrenia or bipolar disorder as compared to healthy control subjects [published erratum appears in Biol Psychiatry 1999;46(4):following 584]. Biol Psychiatry 1999;46:78–88.

[154] Tollefson GD, Beasley Jr. CM, Tran PV, et al. Olanzapine versus haloperidol in the treatment of schizophrenia and schizoaffective and schizophreniform disorders: results of an international collaborative trial. Am J Psychiatry 1997;154:457–65.

[155] McElroy SL, Frye M, Denicoff K, et al. Olanzapine in treatment-resistant bipolar disorder. J Affect Disord 1998;49:119–22.

[156] Soutullo CA, Sorter MT, Foster KD, et al. Olanzapine in the treatment of adolescent acute mania: a report of seven cases. J Affect Disord 1999;53:279–83.

[157] Chang KD, Ketter TA. Mood stabilizer augmentation with olanzapine in acutely manic children. J Child Adolesc Psychopharmacol 2000;10:45–9.

[158] Krishnamoorthy J, King BH. Open-label olanzapine treatment in five preadolescent children. J Child Adolesc Psychopharmacol 1998;8:107–13.

[159] Black DW, Winokur G, Nasrallah A. Treatment of mania: a naturalistic study of electrocon-vulsive therapy versus lithium in 438 patients. J Clin Psychiatry 1987;48:132–9.

[160] Welch CA. Electroconvulsive therapy. In: Treatment of psychiatric disorders: a task force report of the American Psychiatric Association. Washington, DC: The American Psychiatric Associ-ation; 1989. p. 1803–13.

[161] Small JG, Klapper MH, Kellams JJ, et al. Electroconvulsive treatment compared with lithium in the management of manic states. Arch Gen Psychiatry 1988;45:727–32.

[162] Bertagnoli MW, Borchardt CM. A review of ECT for children and adolescents. J Am Acad Child Adolesc Psychiatry 1990;29:302–7.

[163] Kutcher S, Robertson HA. Electroconvulsive therapy in treatment-resistant bipolar youth. J Child Adolesc Psychopharmacol 1995;5:167–75.

[164] Davanzo PA, Krah N, Kleiner J, et al. Nimodipine treatment of an adolescent with ultradian cycling bipolar affective illness. J Child Adolesc Psychopharmacol 1999;9:51–61.

[165] Stensby ME. Nutritional properties of fish oils. World Rev Nutr Diet 1969;11:46–105.

[166] Sperling RI, Benincaso AI, Knoell CT, et al. Dietary omega-3 polyunsaturated fatty acids inhibit phosphoinositide formation and chemotaxis in neutrophils. J Clin Invest 1993;91: 651–60.

[167] Tappia PS, Ladha S, Clark DC, et al. The influence of membrane fluidity, TNF receptor bind-ing, cAMP production and GTPase activity on macrophage cytokine production in rats fed a variety of fat diets. Mol Cell Biochem 1997;166:135–43.

Child Adolesc Psychiatric Clin N Am
11 (2002) 619–637

CHILD AND
ADOLESCENT
PSYCHIATRIC
CLINICS

Course and outcome of child and adolescent major depressive disorder

Boris Birmaher, MD[a],*, Clara Arbelaez, MD[b],
David Brent, MD[c]

[a]Department of Psychiatry, University of Pittsburgh School of Medicine,
Western Psychiatric Institute and Clinic, Pittsburgh, Pennsylvania, 3811 O'Hara Street,
Pittsburgh, PA 15213–3811, USA
[b]Colombian School of Medicine, Bogotá, Colombia
[c]Departments of Psychiatry, Pediatrics, and Epidemiology,
University of Pittsburgh School of Medicine, Western Psychiatric Institute and Clinic,
Pittsburgh, PA 15213–3811, USA

Major depressive disorder is a familial recurrent illness that significantly interferes with a child's normal emotional and cognitive development. Major depressive disorder is associated with increased risk for suicidal behavior and suicide attempts, development of other psychiatric disorders (eg, substance abuse) and behavior problems, increased nicotine use, and poor psychosocial, academic, and work functioning. Childhood- and adolescence-onset major depressive disorder increases the risk for recurrences of depression recurrences and for psychosocial difficulties during adulthood [1–9].

The prevalence of major depressive disorder is approximately 2% in children and 6% in adolescents [10–13]. The lifetime prevalence rate of major depressive disorder in adolescents has been estimated to be 20%, which is comparable to lifetime prevalence rates of major depressive disorder in adult populations [13]. Birth-cohort studies in adults and children have found that individuals born more recently are at a greater risk for developing mood disorders and that these disorders are manifesting at a younger age [14–17]. Thus, early identification and understanding the natural course and factors associated with increased risk for major depressive disorder are critical for developing effective acute and preventative strategies to help youth with this condition.

This work was supported in part by grants from the Course and Outcome for Adolescents with Bipolar Illness (MH 59929) and the Child and Adolescent Developmental Psychopathology Research Center for Early-Onset Affective and Anxiety Disorders (MH 55123)
    * Corresponding author.
    E-mail address: birmaherb@msx.upmc.edu (B. Birmaher).

This article reviews the existing longitudinal studies of children and adolescents with major depressive disorder, describes the limitations of the extant literature, and addresses the following questions:

- Do children with major depressive disorder become depressed adolescents?
- Do children with major depressive disorder become depressed adults?
- Are depressed adolescents at risk for further episodes of major depressive disorder during their later adolescent years?
- Do depressed adolescents become depressed adults?
- What psychosocial and biologic correlates are associated with the relapse and recurrences of major depressive disorder?
- Are children and adolescents with major depressive disorder at increased risk of developing bipolar disorder?

This article reviews only naturalistic longitudinal studies that include children and adolescents with major depressive disorder and excludes studies that evaluate only depressive symptoms and not the disorder. Throughout this article the authors use the extant definitions of outcome (eg, response, recurrence) as shown in the box [18–23].

Definitions of outcome

Absence of major depressive disorder: ≤ 1 symptom of major depressive disorder

Response: No major depressive disease or a significant reduction in the symptoms of major depressive disorder (eg, a 50% reduction in symptomatology from baseline, a Children's Depression Rating Scale (CDRS) score ≤ 28, a Beck Depression Inventory score ≤ 9) for at least 2 weeks

Remission: Absence of major depressive disorder for a period of at least 2 weeks but less than 2 months

Relapse: An episode of depression during the period of remission

Recurrence: The emergence of symptoms of major depressive disorder during the period of recovery (ie, a new episode of major depressive disorder)

Because several of the studies reviewed did not use uniform definitions of outcome, the terms remission/recovery and relapse/recurrence are used interchangeably unless otherwise specified.

Do children with major depressive disorder become depressed adolescents?

Longitudinal studies of clinically referred depressed children [3,19,22–26] and one community study of depressed children [27] have shown that childhood-onset major depressive disorder increases the risk for adolescent depression (Table 1). The average duration of a depressive episode in clinically referred children is between 8 and 13 months [3,22,23]. At follow up (12 to 78 months), 50% to 90% of children with major depressive disorder had recovered from their depressions. Thirty percent to 70% of these children, however, will experience a relapse or recurrence, 24 to 70 months after recovery from the index episode. In general, at intake, the presence of comorbid non–mood disorders and dysthymic disorder predicts the persistence of these disorders at follow up. Although at 5-years follow up, approximately 70% of children with dysthymia have developed major depressive disorder, this interval provides a window of opportunity to treat the symptoms of dysthymia actively before the appearance of major depressive disorder [28]. All studies showed that childhood-onset major depressive disorder is associated with greater risk for suicide, behavioral problems, substance abuse, and academic, social, and familial problems than seen in nondisordered controls. Nondepressed controls with other psychiatric conditions also showed increased psychiatric morbidity and psychosocial difficulties at follow up, but depressed children had higher risk for suicidal behaviors and depressive recurrences.

Do children with major depressive disorder become depressed adults?

As many as 50% of adults with major depressive disorder have reported that their depressions began while they were children (Table 2) [29]. Although these studies are subject to problems of recall bias, they suggest that depressed children are at high risk for recurrence of depression during their adult years.

Three clinical, retrospective, catch-up longitudinal studies have evaluated adults who were depressed during their childhoods [2,30,31]. Harrington and colleagues [30] compared 52 adults (mean age, 30.7 years) who were depressed during their childhoods ($n = 22$) and adolescence ($n = 30$) with a matched sample of 52 adults that had psychiatric non–mood disorders during their youth. The risk of any depressive disorder (major depressive disorder or minor depression) by adulthood was significantly higher in the groups with childhood- and adolescence-onset depression (60%) than in those with psychiatric non–mood disorders (25%). When adult Research Diagnostic Criteria (RDC) for major depressive disorder were used as the criterion of outcome, however, the adults with adolescence-onset major depressive disorder ($n = 24$), but not those with childhood-onset major depressive disorder ($n = 13$) differed from the psychiatric controls. Study participants with major depressive disorder and conduct disorder were less likely to have recurrences than those with major depressive disorder alone. Weissman et al [31] assessed the psychiatric and psychosocial outcomes of a group of adults who had been diagnosed with major depressive disorder ($n = 83$), psychiatric non–mood disorders (mainly separation anxiety) ($n = 91$), and no psychiatric disorders ($n = 91$) during their childhoods. There were no significant differences in the risk of developing major depressive

Table 1
Depressed children become adolescents

Author	Depressed group	Comparison Groups	Total duration of follow up (months)	Duration of index episode (mean in months)	Recovery (mean in months)[a]	Relapse/recurrence (months)[a]	Retention
Clinical samples							
Poznanski et al, 1976	10	-	78	-	50%, (78)	50%, (78)	100%
Kovacs et al, 1984a,b	65[b]	49[c]	72	MDD (8), ADDM (6), DD (48)	MDD = 92% (18)[d] DD = 89% (72)[d] DDM = 90% (42)[d]	MDD = 40% (24) DD = 72% (60)	100%
Asarnow et al, 1988	28	18[e]	72	-	-	DD = 40% (24) MDD = 49% (24)	100%
McCauley et al, 1993	65	25[c]	36	9	80% (12).	54% (36)	100%
Goodyer et al, 1997	68	17[c]	9	10, 8[c]	25% (9).	27% (9)	87%
Emslie et al, 1997	70[f]	-	80	-	98% (12)	69.4% (24)	84%
Community samples							
McGee and Williams, 1988	40[g]	81[c]	48	-	50%(48)	50%(48)	90%

-, data not available.
[a] Months when maximum percentage of recovery or recurrence was attained.
[b] Major depressive disorder (MDD) = 42, Dysthymic disorder (DD) = 28, Adjustment disorder with depressive mood (ADDM) = 11. The total number exceeds the cohort size because of overlaps between MDD and DD.
[c] Nondepressed psychiatric controls.
[d] median (8 male, 4 female).
[e] Schizophrenia spectrum disorders.
[f] Inpatients.
[g] 17 current depression: 6 with MDD, 11 with minor depression; 23 past depression: 5 MDD, 18 with minor depression.

Table 2
Depressed children become adults

Author	Depressed group	Comparison groups	Total duration of follow up (mean in months)	Relapse / recurrence (months)[a]	Retention
Harrington et al, 1990[b]	80[c]	80[d]	216	60%(216)[c] 27% (216)[d]	82%
Weissman et al, 1999a[b]	83	135[e]	141	32.5% (12)[f] 45.4% (12)[g] 35.2% (12)[h]	70%
Fombonne et al, 2001	149[i]	-	240	53.6%[j] 64.9%[k]	61%

-, data not available.
[a] Months when maximum percentage of recovery or recurrence was attained.
[b] Clinical samples.
[c] 21 children and 31 adolescents had major depressive disorder (MDD). Only 13 children had MDD.
[d] Nondepressed psychiatric controls.
[e] 44 subjects with anxiety disorder and no major depressive disorder (MDD); 91 with no evidence of past or current psychiatric disorder.
[f] Major depressive disorder (MDD).
[g] Anxiety disorders.
[h] Normal controls.
[i] 96 with MDD; 53 with MDD + conduct disorder, inpatients and outpatients, 28 prepubertal.
[j] Prepubertal.
[k] Pubescent + postpubertal.

disorder during adulthood among the three groups (32.5%, 45.4%, and 32%, respectively), but children who had first-degree relatives with recurrent depressions were at higher risk for major depressive disorder during adulthood. Fombonne et al [2] evaluated a 149 adults who had had major depressive disorder ($n = 96$) or major depressive disorder and conduct disorder during childhood ($n = 28$) or adolescence. The overall rate of recurrence of major depressive disorder was 64%, without significant differences between childhood- and adolescence-onset major depressive disorder (53.6% and 64.9%, respectively) (Eric Fombonne, personal communication, 2001). As in other follow-up studies, the presence of comorbid disorders in childhood or adolescence increased the likelihood of these disorders during adulthood. For example, Fombone [32] reported that patients with comorbid conduct disorder had significantly more behavioral difficulties and antisocial behaviors at follow up than those with only major depressive disorder.

At follow up, adults with a history of major depressive disorder during childhood had increased psychiatric morbidity (eg, substance abuse), psychosocial difficulties, poor work history, increased risk for suicidal behaviors and suicide, and increased use of psychiatric services (eg, hospitalization).

As discussed later in this article, these three studies, although informative, have limitations. Further investigations are needed that follow larger clinical and community samples of depressed children into adulthood.

Are depressed adolescents at risk for further episodes of major depressive disorder during their later adolescent years?

Clinical [25,33–37] and community studies have consistently shown that young adolescents with major depressive disorder are at risk of developing further episodes of major depressive disorder during their late adolescent years (Table 3) [7,13,38–41]. The duration of the index episode in clinical and community samples of depressed adolescents ranged between 4 and 9 months and 3 and 6.5 months, respectively. In clinical studies, 12- to 72-month follow-up studies have shown that 50% to 90% of depressed youth recovered from their index episode of major depressive disorder. Twelve to 72 months after recovery, however, 20% to 54% had one or more recurrences.

Major depressive disorder in adolescents was associated with increased psychiatric (eg, substance abuse, personality disorders) and psychosocial morbidity (eg, poor academic and work performance) and suicidal attempts. Moreover, adolescents who had experienced two or more episodes of major depressive disorder showed significantly more psychosocial morbidity and increased risks for further recurrences, for suicide, and for developing other psychiatric problems such as substance abuse than did controls without psychiatric disorders or with non–mood psychiatric disorders [13,40].

These studies also showed that comorbid disorders at intake were associated with increased non–mood disorders at follow up. In general, however, there were no differences in the rates of non–mood disorders between the depressed adolescents and the non–mood-disordered psychiatric controls.

Do depressed adolescents become depressed adults?

Clinical [2,8,30,31,42–46] and community [6,9,47] studies have also consistently found that adolescence-onset major depressive disorder caries a strong risk for adult major depressive disorder and is associated with high rates of psychiatric morbidity, personality difficulties, work problems, poor academic performance, and potential mortality from suicide in the young-adult years. Table 4 depicts all the extant longitudinal studies with the exception of investigations that used self-reports assessing only depressive symptoms or not reporting rates of relapse/recurrence [8,44,46]. These studies, however, also found continuity between depressive symptomatology during adolescence and adult depression.

As shown in Table 4, the average length of the depressive episode was 7 months in a clinical sample [45] and 2.5 months in a community sample [9]. Follow up (at 74–216 months) of clinical cases showed a higher rate of recurrence of major depressive episodes in persons with major depressive disorder alone than in controls with non–mood psychiatric disorders and those without psychiatric disorders (approximately 65% versus 11–27%, respectively) [30,45,48,49]. Follow up of community samples (at 48–72 months) also showed

Table 3
Late-adolescent outcome of young depressed adolescents

Author	Depressed group	Comparison Group(s)	Total duration of follow-up (months)	Duration of Index Episode (mean - months)	Recovery (mean-months)[a]	Relapse /Recurrence (months)[a]	Retention
Clinical samples							
King and Pitman, 1970	26	25[b]	72	-	50% (72)	50% depressed, 20% bipolar	86%
Strober and Carlson, 1982	60[c]	-	42	5	66% (42)	21% MDD, 20% bipolar	100%
Hammen et al, 1990	22[d]	70[e]	36	4	90% (24)	23%	80%
McCauley et al, 1993	100[f]	38[b]	36	9	80% (12)	54% (36)	65%
Strober et al, 1993	58[c]	-	24	5	90% (24)	-	100%
Sanford et al, 1995	67[g]	-	12	-	66% (12)	33% (12)	100%
Community samples							
Keller et al, 1988	38	-	24	4[h]	90% (24)	-	100%
Warner et al, 1992	174[i]	29[j]	24	3	87% (24)	16.1% (24)	93%
Fleming et al, 1993	45	607[k]	48	-	80% (12)	25% (42)	84%
Lewinsohn et al, 1994	362	1146[L]	48	6.5	75% (6)	33% (48)	88%

-, data not available.
[a] Months when maximum percentage of recovery or recurrence was attained.
[b] Other non–mood psychiatric diagnoses.
[c] Inpatients.
[d] Offspring of unipolar women.
[e] Offspring of women with chronic medical illness and normal controls.
[f] Current or past episode of major depressive disorder (MDD).
[g] 50 outpatients, 17 inpatients.
[h] Median.
[i] Offspring of one or more depressed parents.
[j] Offspring of nondepressed parents.
[k] Conduct disorder (N = 34) and normal controls.
[L] Normal or non–mood psychiatric disorders.

Table 4
Depressed adolescents become adults

Author	Depressed groups	Comparison group	Total duration of follow up (in months)	Mean duration of index episode (in months)[a]	Recovery (mean, in months)	Relapse /recurrence (months)	Retention
Clinical samples							
Garber et al, 1988	11[b]	9[c]	96	-	-	64% (96)[b] 11% (96)[c]	100%
Harrington et al, 1990	80[d]	80[c]	216	-	-	60% (48) 27% (48)	82%
Rao et al, 1995	28	35[e]	74	7	-	69% (84)[f] 18% (84)[c]	94%
Weissman et al, 1999b	73	135[c]	150	-	37% (180)	-	82%
Fombonne et al, 2001	149[g]	-	240	-	-	62.4%[h] 75.2%[i]	61%
Community samples							
Bardone et al, 1996	27[j]	378[k]	72	-	-	54% (72)[j] 20.8% (72)[e] 25% (72)[L]	94%

Lewinsohn et, al 1999	261	73[m] 133[c] 272[e]	48	-	45% (60)[f] 34.2%[m] 28.2%[c] 18.5%[c]	93%
Rao et al, 1999	70[n]	-	60	2.5	47% (48)	86%

-, data not available.

[a] Months when maximum percentage of recovery or recurrence was attained;

[b] Inpatients.

[c] Non–depressed psychiatric controls.

[d] 31 adolescents and 21 children with major depressive disorder (MDD) and minor depression.

[e] Normal controls.

[f] MDD.

[g] MDD 96; MDD + CD = 53; inpatients and outpatients, 28 prepubertal.

[h] MDD.

[i] MDD + minor depression + dysthymia.

[j] Females with MDD and Dysthymic Disorder (DD).

[k] Females with conduct disorder (n = 37) and normal controls.

[L] Conduct disorder.

[m] Adjustment disorders.

[n] Females with MDD.

a 45% to 54% rate of recurrence in persons with major depressive disorder alone, in comparison with rates of recurrent episodes of major depressive disorder of 20% to 34% in controls with non–mood psychiatric disorders or without psychiatric disorders [6,7,9,47].

Adolescents who experience two or more depressive episodes have more recurrences [13,40,45], and those with only one episode of major depressive disorder seem to have clinical outcomes similar to those of normal controls [45]. These results need to be replicated with larger samples, however.

Early-onset depression has also been associated with personality disorders in both retrospective and prospective studies [7].

Correlates of duration and relapse/recurrence

Table 5 depicts a preliminary list of the risk factors associated with protracted depression and with relapses and recurrences of major depressive disorder. Although the topic is beyond the scope of this article, Table 5 also includes, for comparison, the correlates associated with the onset of major depressive disorder [1,4,7,28,30,50].

Several demographic factors (eg, age, gender), psychiatric factors (eg, anxiety disorders, dysthymia), cognitive factors (eg, negative cognitions), psychosocial stressors (eg, conflicts, sexual or physical abuse), biologic factors (eg, hyperticortisolemia), and psychiatric family history (eg, a parent with recurrent major depressive disorder) have been associated with longer duration and relapse or recurrence of major depressive disorder [1,3,4,8,9,17,18,24,30, 31,33,39,41,45,46,48–73].

Although there is overlap among the risk factors for onset, duration, and recurrence (see Table 5), some factors seem to influence the length of the episode or the number and timing of the recurrences or new onsets differentially [3,13,41]. For example, anxiety disorders are associated with the onset and longer episodes of depression but seem not to affect the risk for recurrence [3,8,25,35,45,54,64, 74–77]. Family conflicts may trigger the onset of a depressive episode, increase the length of the episode, and increase the risk for recurrences [7,18,51]. Female gender has been associated with an increased risk for onset but not with an increased likelihood for long and more recurrent episodes [7,22,25,39,45,78].

These risk factors usually affect the natural course of depression through complex interactions, but few studies have addressed this issue [7,29,37,45,46,55, 56,63,72,79]. For example, exposure to stressful life events seems to interact with other factors such as subsyndromal depressive and anxiety symptoms, cognitive style, history of loss, family history of depression, and other prior psycho-pathology to create a predisposition for depression [1,7,21,46,48,55,56, 61,62,79–82]. A higher cortisol/dehydroepiandrosterone (DHEA) ratio, together with one or more disappointing life events, was associated with persistent major depressive disorder at 9-months follow up [55,56]. In addition, the onset of major depressive disorder in never-depressed adolescents was predicted by the additive

Table 5
Factors associated with the onset, duration, and relapse or recurrence of major depressive disorder

	Demographic factors	Clinical picture	Comorbid psychiatric disorders	Cognitive factors	Stressors	Biologic factors	Psychiatric family history
Onset	Female, Low SES	Subsyndromal symptoms of depression Suicide attempts	Anxiety, disruptive, dysthymic, eating, substance abuse disorders	Negative cognitions	High- EE; conflicts; Exposure to negative event (eg, abuse)	High REM density High cortisol and DHEA Rapid increase of nocturnal GH secretion following sleep onset	Parental MDD (specially early onset or recurrent) and anxiety disorders; increased family loading for mood and anxiety
Longer duration	Early age of onset older	Severe depressions Suicide ideation or attempts	Anxiety, disruptive, dysthymic disorders	-	Family conflicts	High cortisol/DHEA	-
Relapse or recurrence	Low SES Non-caucasian Older age	Prior depressive episodes Severe depressions Subsyndromal depression Psychosis Prior suicidal attempts Borderline or antisocial personality traits	Dysthymic Disorder Disruptive disorder (?)	Negative attributional style	Exposure to stress (eg, abuse) EE, conflict with parents	High cortisol levels High cortisol/DHEA Sleep EEG abnormalities[a]	Mood disorders, in particular recurrent MDD in first degree relatives

-, data not available.
DHEA, dehydroepiandrosterone; EEG, electroencephalogram; EE, expressed emotion; GH, growth hormone; MDD, major depressive disorder; REM, rapid eye movement; SES, socioeconomic status.
[a] Sleep latency (initial insomnia), sleep period time (hypersomnia), REM latency, and slow-wave sleep.

effects of high saliva cortisol and DHEA levels (measured two times/day for 4 days), higher depressive symptoms at intake, and personal disappointments and losses experienced within the month before onset [55]. These studies emphasize the importance of simultaneously assessing the psychopathologic, psychologic, environmental, and biologic factors (and their interactions) associated with the onset and course of major depressive disorder in children and adolescents.

Familial factors that influence the course of major depressive disorder may be genetic or nongenetic. Twin and adoption studies show clear evidence that genetic factors influence age of onset and recurrence [83,84]. On the other hand, factors in the family environment such as exposure to parental depression (eg, a parent's modeling of poor ways of coping with stress, poor parenting skills, or inability to perform parental duties, living with a parent who is frequently irritable, economic difficulties caused by a parent's inability to work) may increase the risk for depression [17,41,60,67,69]. Also, factors such as exposure to negative events (eg, losses, sexual abuse, ongoing conflict) may trigger and perpetuate the depression in susceptible individuals [1,18,48,85]. Although controversial, these stressors seem not to be specific for major depressive disorder. It is also not clear whether some risk factors precede, appear during, or are a consequence of the depression. In any case, the identification, evaluation, and management of these factors are important for the successful acute, continuation, and maintenance treatment of the child's mood disorder [48]. For example, ongoing family conflict is associated with more protracted episodes of depression [18,51], and treatment of the conflicts may help ameliorate, decrease the duration, or prevent recurrence of depression during this critical developmental stage. Comorbid attention deficit hyperactivity disorder and conduct problems may create stressful situations and perpetuate the depressive symptomatology. Poor socioeconomic status may increase the likelihood of exposure to stressful situations.

Variables that have consistently shown strong predictive power for onset and recurrence are a family history of major depressive disorder (particularly recurrent or early-onset), a child's history of prior major depressive episodes, and dysthymic disorder. On the other hand, several of the risk factors shown in Table 5 have either not been replicated or have yielded inconsistent results. For example, some studies have found that early age of onset is associated with the greatest hazard of recurrence [22], whereas others have found that adolescence-onset disorder has a greater risk of recurrence [6,30]. Comorbid disruptive disorders have predicted less frequent [4], similar [32], or more frequent rates of recurrence [35]. These inconsistencies may result from methodologic differences, which are discussed in detail later.

Are children and adolescents with major depressive disorder at increased risk of developing bipolar disorder?

Longitudinal studies in depressed children [22,31,86] and depressed adolescents [25,30,31,34,36,37,45,87–89] have reported that at follow up, 5% to 30%

of depressed youth will have developed mania or hypomania. (The rates depend on whether the sample was clinical or epidemiologic.) Although it is difficult to predict who will develop bipolar disorder, the presence of psychosis, psychomotor retardation, pharmacologically induced hypomania or mania, and a family history of bipolar disorder have been associated with increased risk of a manic episode [36,37,86,87]. Thus, caution must be used in prescribing antidepressants for youth whose major depressive disorder has these clinical characteristics.

Summary: limitations of the extant longitudinal studies

There is compelling evidence that for most children and adolescents, the index episode of major depressive disorder is the beginning of a chronic, recurrent, lifelong disorder. Approximately 5% to 10% will develop chronic depression, and others will experience only partial remissions and will continue to have subsyndromal symptoms of depression [3,6,7,18,22,23,30,37,43,90,91]. These ongoing mild depressive symptoms increase the likelihood for future recurrences [7,13,90,92], indicating the need for intensive and ongoing treatment to achieve full recovery.

Although not included in the tables, follow-up studies of depressed children and adolescents after an acute treatment trial with antidepressants or cognitive behavior therapy have found rates of recurrence and poor psychosocial outcome similar to those in the previously described longitudinal studies [5,18,91,93,94]. Continued treatment is needed to prevent further relapses or recurrences.

The extant follow-up studies have shown that there is considerable continuity of major depressive disorder across a person's life span. More specifically, childhood-onset major depressive disorder increases the risk for adolescent major depressive disorder, and adolescent major depressive disorder increases the risk for further depressive recurrences during later adolescence and adulthood. It is logical that if childhood-onset major depressive disorder increases the risk for adolescent major depressive disorder, and adolescence-onset major depressive disorder increases the risk for adult major depressive disorder, childhood-onset major depressive disorder should be associated with adult major depressive disorder. The few studies so far published, however, have shown controversial results, with one study [2] showing continuity, another showing continuity only in children of parents with recurrent major depressive disorder [31], and a third showing no increased risk for adult major depressive disorder [30]. Consistent evidence for the continuity of major depressive disorder across the life span is also given by family studies of children of depressed parents and relatives of depressed children [1,17,33,60,69].

Major depressive disorder is usually accompanied by other comorbid disorders [1,45,77]. Once present, these comorbid conditions are likely to persist [7,13,22, 23,30,32,41,47,49,90].

Both childhood- and adolescence-onset major depressive disorder increase the risks for suicide and suicidal behavior, for behavior problems, and for bipolar, anxiety, substance abuse, and personality disorders and are associated with academic, work-related, and other psychosocial difficulties. Thus, there is an urgent need for early recognition and treatment and for preventative strategies for this chronic and disabling condition that affects youth at a crucial stage of their development.

A family history of mood disorder, particularly recurrent types in first-degree relatives, and a child's prior history of mood disorder are risk factors for the onset, duration, and recurrence of major depressive disease. Factors such as dysthymia, other comorbid psychiatric conditions, negative cognitive style, and exposure to negative life events (eg, abuse and ongoing family conflicts) seem to increase the risk for protracted and difficult-to-treat depressions and further depressive recurrences. Further studies on the effects of these factors on the outcome of depression are needed. Some of these risk factors seem to be nonspecific for major depressive disorder [7,48,77]. The successful treatment of new-onset major depressive disorder and prevention of recurrence [5,50,92,95] may depend, at least in part, on earlier and accurate identification of these risk factors and their appropriate management (eg, diminishing ongoing family conflicts, cognitive restructuring) [48].

Because major depressive disorder is a condition that is prone to relapse and recurrence, it is important that treatment be of sufficient duration to avoid relapse. Studies of short-term treatment have documented the high risk of relapse after discontinuation of psychotherapy or antidepressant treatment [85,91,93]. Both naturalistic and controlled studies have shown that continuation treatment is more likely than acute treatment alone to prevent relapse [91,93].

The prevention of suicide and suicidal behavior in mood-disordered youth rests in part on effective acute and continuation treatment of mood disorders [81,93,96]. It may also be necessary to address concomitant contributors to suicidal behavior, such as comorbid externalizing or substance abuse disorders, family discord, sexual abuse, interpersonal skill deficits, hopelessness, and impulsive aggression.

The differences and inconsistencies among the studies presented here may result from several design issues, such as the use of small samples, variations in participants' ages and gender, lack of uniform definitions for outcome measures (eg, time of onset and offset of the disorder), and differences in duration of follow-up periods, in settings, and in assessment methods. These studies also had one or more of the following limitations:

Initial diagnoses made retrospectively and reconstructed from clinical data summaries.
Failure to evaluate pubertal status (Evaluation of the stage of puberty is important because puberty has been shown to be more sensitive than chronologic age as a risk factor for the onset of major depressive disorder) [80,97].
Infrequent follow-up assessments accompanied by long retrospective recall intervals.

Lack of evaluation for the presence of symptoms of bipolar disorder (This evaluation is important because even subsyndromal bipolar symptomatology is accompanied by poor psychosocial outcome) [98].
No control for the effects of treatment, comorbid disorders, ongoing or past negative events, and inclusion of siblings in the sample.
Lack of control for the effects of family psychiatric history, in particular the effects of parental current and lifetime psychiatric mood and non–mood disorders.
Lack of psychiatric or normal controls.

Future studies should address these limitations.

Acknowledgments

The authors thank Mary Kay Gill, MSN, and Guiomar Arbelaez, PhD, for editorial assistance and Carol Kostek for manuscript preparation.

References

[1] Birmaher B, Ryan ND, Williamson DE, et al. Childhood and adolescent depression: a review of the past ten years. Part I. J Am Acad Child Adolesc Psychiatry 1996;35:1427–39.
[2] Fombonne E, Wostear G, Cooper V, et al. The Maudsley long term follow up of child and adolescent depression. Psychiatric outcomes in adulthood. Br J Psychiatry 2001;179:210–7.
[3] Goodyer IM, Herbert J, Secher SM, et al. Short term outcome of major depression. I: comorbidity and severity at presentation as predictors of persistent disorder. J Am Acad Child Adolesc Psychiatry 1997;36:179–87.
[4] Harrington R, Fudge H, Rutter M, et al. Adult outcomes of childhood and adolescent depression: II. links with antisocial disorders. J Am Acad Child Adolesc Psychiatry 1991; 30(3):434–9.
[5] Harrington R, Whittaker J, Shoebridge P. Psychological treatment of depression in children and adolescents. A review of treatment research. Br J Psych 1998;173:291–8.
[6] Lewinsohn PM, Allen NB, Seeley JR, et al. First onset versus recurrence of depression: differential processes of psychosocial risk. J Abnorm Psychol 1999;108:483–9.
[7] Lewinsohn PM, Rohde P, Seeley JR, et al. Natural course of adolescent major depressive disorder in a community sample: predictors of recurrence in young adults. Am J Psychiatry 2000;157:1584–91.
[8] Pine DS, Cohen P, Gurley D. The risk for early-adulthood anxiety and depressive disorders in adolescents with anxiety and depressive disorders. Arch Gen Psychiatry 1988;55:56–64.
[9] Rao U, Hammen C, Daley SE, et al. Continuity of depression during the transition to adulthood: a 5-year longitudinal study of young women. J Am Acad Child Adolesc Psychiatry 1999;38: 908–15.
[10] Fleming JE, Offord DR. Epidemiology of childhood depressive disorders: a critical review. J Am Acad Child Adolesc Psychiatry 1990;29:571–80.
[11] Kashani JH, Beck NC, Hoeper EW, et al. Psychiatric disorders in community sample of adolescents. Am J Psychiatry 1987;144:584–9.
[12] Lewinsohn PM, Duncan EM, Stanton AK, et al. Age at onset for first unipolar depression. J Abnorm Psychol 1986;95:378–83.

[13] Lewinsohn PM, Clarke GN, Seeley JR. Major depression in community adolescents: age at onset, episode duration, and time to recurrence. J Am Acad Child Adolesc Psychiatry 1994; 33:809–18.

[14] Kovacs M, Gatsonis C. Secular trends in age at onset of major depressive disorder in a clinical sample of children. J Psychiatr Res 1994;28:319–29.

[15] Lewinsohn PM, Rohde P, Seeley JR, et al. Age-cohort changes in the lifetime occurrence of depression and other mental disorders. J Abnorm Psychol 1993;102:110–20.

[16] Ryan ND, Williamson DE, Iyengar S, et al. A secular increase in child and adolescent onset affective disorder. J Am Acad Child Adolesc Psychiatry 1992;31:600–5.

[17] Wickramaratne PJ, Weissman MM. Onset of psychopathology in offspring by developmental phase and parental depression. J Am Acad Child Adolesc Psychiatry 1998;37:933–42.

[18] Birmaher B, Brent DA, Kolko D, et al. Clinical outcome after short-term psychotherapy for adolescents with major depressive disorder. Arch Gen Psychiatry 2000;57:29–36.

[19] Emslie GJ, Rush AJ, Weinberg WA, et al. Recurrence of major depressive disorder in hospitalized children and adolescents. J Am Acad Child Adolesc Psychiatry 1997;36:785–92.

[20] Frank E, Prien RF, Jarrett RB, et al. Conceptualization and rationale for consensus definitions of terms in major depressive disorder: remission, recovery, relapse, and recurrence. Arch Gen Psychiatry 1991;48:851–5.

[21] Goodyer IM, Herbert J, Secher S, et al. Short-term outcome of major depression: I. Comorbidity and severity at presentation predictors of persistent disorder. J Am Acad Child Adolesc Psychiatry 1997;36:179–87.

[22] Kovacs M, Feinberg TL, Crouse-Novak MA, et al. Depressive disorders in childhood: I. a longitudinal prospective study of characteristics and recovery. Arch Gen Psychiatry 1984;41: 229–37.

[23] Kovacs M, Feinberg TL, Crouse-Novak MA, et al. Depressive disorders in childhood: II: a longitudinal study of the risk for a subsequent major depression. Arch Gen Psychiatry 1984; 41:643–9.

[24] Asarnow JR, Goldstein MJ, Carlson GA. Childhood-onset depressive disorders: a follow-up study of rates of rehospitalization and out-of-home placement among child psychiatric patients. J Affect Disord 1988;15:245–53.

[25] McCauley E, Myers K, Mitchell J, et al. Depression in young people: initial presentation and clinical course. J Am Acad Child Adolesc Psychiatry 1993;32:714–22.

[26] Poznanski EO, Krahenbuhl V, Zrull JP. Childhood depression. A longitudinal perspective. J Am Acad Child Adolesc Psychiatry 1976;15:491–501.

[27] McGee R, Williams S. A longitudinal study of depression in nine-year-old children. J Am Acad Child Adolesc Psychiatry 1988;27:342–8.

[28] Kovacs M, Obrosky DS, Gatsonis C, et al. First episode major depressive and dysthymic disorder in childhood: clinical and sociodemographic factors in recovery. J Am Acad Child Adolesc Psychiatry 1997;36:777–84.

[29] Newman DL, Moffit TE, Caspi A, et al. Psychiatric disorder in a birth cohort of young adults: prevalence, comorbidity, clinical significance, and new case incidence from ages 11 to 21. J Consult Clin Psychol 1996;64:552–62.

[30] Harrington R, Fudge H, Rutter M, et al. Adult outcomes of child and adolescent depression: I psychiatric status. Arch Gen Psychiatry 1990;47:465–73.

[31] Weissman MM, Wolk S, Wickramaratne P, et al. Children with prepubertal onset major depressive disorder and anxiety grown up. Arch General Psychiatry 1999;56:794–801.

[32] Fombonne E, Wostear G, Cooper V, et al. The Maudsley long term follow-up of child and adolescent depression. Suicidality, criminality and social dysfunction in adulthood. Br J Psychiatry 2001;179:218–23.

[33] Hammen C, Burge D, Burney E, et al. Longitudinal study of diagnoses in children of women with unipolar and bipolar affective disorder. Arch Gen Psychiatry 1990;47:1112–7.

[34] King L, Pittman G. A six-year follow-up study of 65 adolescent patients. Arch Gen Psychiatry 1970;22:230–6.

[35] Sanford M, Szatmari P, Spinner M, et al. Predicting the one year course of adolescent major depression. J Am Acad Child Adolesc Psychiatry 1995;34:1618–28.

[36] Strober M, Carlson G. Bipolar illness in adolescents with major depression. Arch Gen Psychiatry 1982;39:549–55.

[37] Strober M, Lampert C, Schmidt S, et al. The course of major depressive disorder in adolescents: I: recovery and risk of manic switching in a follow-up of psychotic and nonpsychotic subtypes. J Am Acad Child Adolesc Psychiatry 1993;32:34–42.

[38] Fleming JE, Boyle MH, Offord DR. The outcome of adolescent depression in the Ontario Child Health Study follow-up. J Am Acad Child Adolesc Psychiatry 1993;32:28–33.

[39] Hankin BL, Abramson LY, Moffitt TE, et al. Development of depression from preadolescence to young adulthood: emerging gender differences in a 10-year longitudinal study. J Abnorm Psychol 1988;107:128–40.

[40] Keller MB, Beardslee W, Lavori PW. Course of major depression in non-referred adolescents: a retrospective study. J Affect Disord 1988;15:235–43.

[41] Warner V, Weissman M, Fendrich M, et al. The course of major depression in the offspring of depressed parents. Arch Gen Psychiatry 1992;49:795–801.

[42] Daley SE, Hammen C, Burge D. Depression and axis II symptomatology in an adolescent community sample: concurrent and longitudinal associations. J Personal Disord 1999;13: 47–59.

[43] Garber J, Kriss MR, Hoch M, et al. Recurrent depression in adolescents: a follow-up study. J Am Acad Child Adolesc Psychiatry 1988;27:49–54.

[44] Kandel D, Davies M. Adult sequelae of adolescent depressive symptoms. Arch General Psychiatry 1986;43:255–43.

[45] Rao U, Dahl RE, Ryan ND, et al. Unipolar depression in adolescents: clinical outcome in adulthood. J Am Acad Child Adolesc Psychiatry 1995;34:566–78.

[46] Rueter MA, Scaramella L, Wallace LE, et al. First onset of depressive symptoms or anxiety disorder predicted by the longitudinal course of internalizing symptoms and parent-adolescent disagreements. Arch Gen Psychiatry 1999;56:726–32.

[47] Bardone AM, Moffitt TE, Caspi A, et al. Adult mental health and social outcomes of adolescent girls with depression and conduct disorder. Dev Psychopathol 1996;8:811–29.

[48] Garber J, Hilsman R. Cognition, stress, and depression in children and adolescents. Child Adolesc Psychiatric Clin North Am 1992;1:129–67.

[49] Weissman MM, Wolk S, Goldstein RB, et al. Depressed adolescents grown up. JAMA 1999;281:1707–13.

[50] Beardslee WR, Versage EM, Gladstone TR. Children of affectively ill parents: a review of the past ten years. J Am Acad Child Adolesc Psychiatry 1998;37:1134–41.

[51] Asarnow JR, Tompson M, Hamilton EB, et al. Expressed emotion, childhood-onset depression, and childhood-onset schizophrenia spectrum disorders: is expressed emotion a nonspecific correlate of child psychopathology or a specific risk factor for depression? J Abnorm Child Psychol 1994;22:129–46.

[52] Coplan JD, Wolk SI, Goetz RR. Nocturnal growth hormone secretion studies in adolescents with and without major depression re-examined: integration of adult and clinical data. Biol Psychiatry 2000;47:594–604.

[53] Goetz RR, Wolk SI, Coplan JD, et al. Premorbid polysomnographic signs in depressed adolescents: a reanalysis of EEG sleep after longitudinal follow up in adulthood. Biol Psychiatry 2001;49:930–42.

[54] Goodyer IM, Herbert J, Tamplin A, et al. Recent life events, cortisol, dehydroepiandrosterone, and the onset of major depression in high-risk adolescents. Br J Psychiatry 2001;177: 499–504.

[55] Goodyer IM, Herbert J, Altham PME. Adrenal steroid secretion and major depression in 8- to 16-year-olds. III: influence of cortisol/DHEA ratio at presentation and subsequent rates of disappointing life events and persistent major depression. Psychol Med 1998;28:265–73.

[56] Goodyer IM, Herbert J, Tamplin A, et al. Short term outcome of major depression. II: life

events, family dysfunction and friendship difficulties as predictors of persistent disorder. J Am Acad Child Adolesc Psychiatry 1997;36:474–80.

[57] Hammen C, Adrian C, Hiroto D. A longitudinal test of the attributional vulnerability model in children at risk for depression. Br J Clin Psychol 1988;27:37–46.

[58] Hammen C, Burge D, Stransbury K. Relationship of mother and child variables to child out-comes in a high-risk sample: a casual modeling analysis. Dev Psychol 1990;26:24–30.

[59] Kashani J, Burback D, Rosenberg T. Perceptions of family conflict resolution and depressive symptomatology in adolescents. J Am Acad Child Adolesc Psychiatry 1988;27:42–8.

[60] Klein DN, Lewinsohn PM, Seeley JR, et al. A family study of major depressive disorder in a community sample of adolescents. Arch Gen Psychiatry 2001;58:13–20.

[61] Metalsky GI, Halberstadt LJ, Abramson LY. Vulnerability to depressive mood reactions: toward a more powerful test of the diathesis-stress and causal mediation components of the reformu-lated theory of depression. J Pers Soc Psychol 1987;52:386–93.

[62] Nolen-Hoeksema S, Girgus JS, Seligman MEP. Predictors and consequences of childhood depressive symptoms: a 5-year longitudinal study. J Abnorm Psychol 1992;101:405–22.

[63] Rao U, Dahl RE, Ryan ND, et al. The relationship between longitudinal clinical course and sleep and cortisol changes in adolescent depression. Biol Psychiatry 1996;40:474–84.

[64] Reinherz HZ, Giaconia RM, Pakis B, et al. Psychosocial risks for major depression in late adolescence: a longitudinal community study. J Am Acad Child Adolesc Psychiatry 1993;32:1155–63.

[65] Rhode P, Lewinsohn PM, Seeley JR. Are adolescents changed by an episode of major depres-sion? J Am Acad Child Adolesc Psychiatry 1994;33(9):1289–98.

[66] Stein D, Williamson DE, Birmaher B, et al. Parent-child bonding and family functioning in depressed children and children at high-risk and low risk for future depression. J Am Acad Child Adolesc Psychiatry 2000;39:1220–6.

[67] Weissman MM, Wickramaratne P, Adams PB, et al. The relationship between panic disorder and major depression. A new family study. Arch Gen Psychiatry 1993;50:767–80.

[68] Wickramaratne PJ, Weissman MM, Leaf PJ, et al. Age, period, and cohort effects on the risk of major depression: results from five United States communities. J Clin Epidemiol 1989;42:333–43.

[69] Wickramaratne PJ, Greenwald S, Weissman MM. Psychiatric disorders in the relatives of probands with prepubertal-onset or adolescent-onset major depression. J Am Acad Child Ado-lesc Psychiatry 2000;39:1396–405.

[70] Williamson DE, Birmaher B, Anderson BP, et al. Stressful life events in depressed adolescents: the role of dependent events during the depressive episode. J Am Acad Child Adolesc Psy-chiatry 1995;34:591–8.

[71] Williamson DE, Birmaher B, Dahl RE, et al. Stressful life events influence nocturnal growth hormone secretion in depressed children. Biol Psychiatry 1996;40:1176–80.

[72] Williamson DE, Dahl RE, Birmaher B, et al. Stressful life events and EEG sleep in depressed and normal control adolescents. Biol Psychiatry 1995;37:859–65.

[73] Williamson DE, Birmaher B, Frank E. Nature of life events and difficulties in depressed adolescents. J Am Acad Child Adolesc Psychiatry 1998;37:1049–57.

[74] Alpert JE, Maddocks A, Rosenbaum JF. Childhood psychopathology retrospectively assessed among adults with early onset major depression. J Affect Disord 1994;31:165–71.

[75] Breslau N, Schultz L, Peterson E. Sex differences in depression: a role for preexisting anxiety. Psychiatric Res 1995;58:1–12.

[76] Kovacs M, Gatsonis C. Stability and change in childhood-onset depressive disorders in chil-dren: IV. a longitudinal study of comorbidity with and risk for anxiety disorders. Arch Gen Psychiatry 1989;46:776–82.

[77] Lewinsohn PM, Rohde P, Seeley JR. Adolescent psychopathology: III: the clinical consequen-ces of comorbidity. J Am Acad Child Adolesc Psychiatry 1995;34:510–9.

[78] Kovacs M. Gender and the course of major depressive disorder through adolescence in clin-ically referred youngsters. J Am Acad Child Adolesc Psychiatry 2001;40:1079–85.

[79] Kaufman J, Birmaher B, Perel J, et al. Serotonergic functioning in depressed abused children: clinical and familial correlates. Biol Psychiatry 1998;44:973–81.

[80] Angold A, Costello EJ, Worthman CM. Puberty and depression: the roles of age, pubertal status and pubertal timing. Psychol Med 1998;28:51–61.

[81] Brent DA, Perper JA, Moritz G, et al. Psychiatric risk factors for adolescent suicide: a case-controlled study. J Am Acad Child Adolesc Psychiatry 1993;32:521–9.

[82] Woodward LJ, Fergusson DM. Life course outcomes of young people with anxiety disorders in adolescence. J Am Acad Child Adolesc Psychiatry 2001;40:1086–93.

[83] Kendler KS, Walters EE, Truett KR, et al. Sources of individual differences in depressive symptoms: analysis of two samples of twins and their families. Am J Psychiatry 1994;151: 1605–14.

[84] McGuffin P, Murray R. The new genetics of mental illness. Oxford: Butterworth-Heinemann; 1991.

[85] Brent DA, Holder D, Kolko D, et al. A clinical psychotherapy trial for adolescent depression comparing cognitive, family, and supportive therapy. Arch Gen Psychiatry 1997;54:877–85.

[86] Geller B, Fox LW, Clark KA. Rate and predictors of prepubertal bipolarity during follow-up of 6- to 12-year-old depressed children. J Am Acad Child Adolesc Psychiatry 1994;33:461–8.

[87] Akiskal HS, Walker P, Puzantian VR, et al. Bipolar outcome in the course of depressive illness. J Am Acad Child Psychiatry 1983;5:115–28.

[88] Garber J, Kriss MR, Hoch M, et al. Recurrent depression in adolescents: a follow-up study. J Am Acad Child Adolesc Psychiatry 1988;27:49–54.

[89] Lewinsohn PM, Klein DN, Seeley JR. Bipolar disorders in a community sample of older patients: prevalence, phenomenology, comorbidity, and course. J Am Acad Child Adolesc Psychiatry 1995;34:453–4.

[90] Brent DA, Birmaher B, Kolko D, et al. Subsyndromal depression in adolescents after a brief psychotherapy trial: course and outcome. J Affect Disord 2001;63:51–8.

[91] Emslie GJ, Rush AJ, Weinberg WA, et al. Fluoxetine in child and adolescent depression: acute and maintenance treatment. Depress Anxiety 1998;7:32–9.

[92] Clarke GN, Hawkins W, Murphy M, et al. Targeted prevention of unipolar depressive disorder in an at-risk sample of high school adolescents: a randomized trial of a group cognitive intervention. J Am Acad Child Adolesc Psychiatry 1995;34:312–21.

[93] Birmaher B, Ryan ND, Brent DA, et al. Childhood and adolescent depression: a review of the past ten years. Part II. J Am Acad Child Adolesc Psychiatry 1996;35:1575–83.

[94] Geller B, Zimerman B, Williams M, et al. Adult psychosocial outcome of prepubertal major depressive disorder. J Am Acad Child Adolesc Psychiatry 2001;40:673–7.

[95] Jaycox LH, Reivich KJ, Gillham J, et al. The prevention of depressive symptoms in school children. Behav Res Ther 1994;32:801–16.

[96] Shaffer D, Garland A, Gould M, et al. Preventing teenage suicide: a critical review. J Am Acad Child Adolesc Psychiatry 1988;27:675–87.

[97] Angold A, Rutter M. Effects of age and status of depression in a large clinical sample. Dev Psychopathol 1992;4:5–28.

[98] Lewinsohn PM, Klein DN, Seeley JR: Bipolar disorder during adolescence and young adulthood in a community sample. Bipolar Disorders 2000;2(3Pt 2):281–93.

Child Adolesc Psychiatric Clin N Am
11 (2002) 639–647

CHILD AND
ADOLESCENT
PSYCHIATRIC
CLINICS

Suicide in mood disordered children and adolescents

Cynthia R. Pfeffer, MD

Department of Psychiatry, Weill Medical College of Cornell University,
New York Presbyterian Hospital, 21 Bloomingdale Road, White Plains, NY 10605, USA

Suicide among youth is a national mental health problem in the United States. It is the third leading cause of death in the United States among adolescents and young adults 15 to 24 years of age. According to the Surgeon General's "call to action" report [1], identifying youth at risk is an important means of preventing suicide. The recognition of significant risk factors is among the most important endeavors in reducing the risk of suicide and preventing suicidal behavior among young people. Mood disorders are among the most significant risk factors for suicidal behavior in youth. This article describes the relationships between mood disorders and suicide and between mood disorders and nonfatal suicidal behavior.

Epidemiology of suicidal behavior in youth

Since the early 1980s, community recognition of the high incidence of suicide among adolescents has stimulated national efforts to prevent this tragic phenomenon. It was hoped that by the end of the twentieth century the rates of suicide in youth would be significantly decreased. Although rates of suicide in youth did decrease by the year 2000, these rates are still high. Preliminary data for year 2000 in the United States indicate that suicide continues to be the third leading cause of death among youth aged 15 to 24 years and that 3877 youths committed suicide during that year. The age-adjusted suicide rate was 10.1 per 100,000 [2], a decrease in age-adjusted suicide rate for this age group from 1999, when the suicide rate was 10.3 per 100,000. Suicide by firearms in 1999 accounted for 975 deaths of persons between the ages of 15 and 19 years and 1340 deaths of persons

Support for this research was provided by Nanette Laitman and the William and Mildred Lasdon Foundation.

E-mail address: cpfeffer@med.cornell.edu (C.R. Pfeffer).

between the ages of 20 and 24 years [3]. Among children and young adolescents aged 5 to 14 years, suicide was the fifth leading cause of death, and 297 children died as a result of suicide in 2000. This age-adjusted suicide rate of 0.7 per 100,000 people [2] increased from 0.6 per 100,000 people in 1999. Suicide by firearms in 1999 accounted for 103 deaths of persons aged 10 to 14 years [3]. For comparison, in 2000 suicide was the 11th leading cause of death for all ages, and 28,332 people committed suicide during that year [2]. The age-adjusted suicide rate of 10.3 per 100,000 population represents an overall decrease of 3.7% from 1999, when the age-adjusted suicide rate was 10.7 per 100,000.

There are persistent developmental and demographic differences in suicide rates. Children and young adolescents have the lowest suicide rates of all age groups. White males have the highest suicide rates in all age categories. The difference in rates of suicide between whites and blacks is decreasing [4]. The rate of suicide among black youths has risen since 1987, and the rate of suicide among whites has decreased during that period. Although the rates of suicide in both white and black youths have been decreasing, the gap in suicide rates between these two groups has lessened. The reasons for this phenomenon have not been identified. Loss of social support resulting from a decrease in religious practices and from changes in family life may have affected the risk for suicide among blacks [4]. For all ages, firearms are the method most commonly used to commit suicide. Preventing access to firearms is an important strategy for preventing suicide among youth.

The Youth Risk Behavior Surveillance survey reported a high prevalence of suicidal behavior among high school students [5]. Specifically, 19.3% of respondents reported suicidal ideation and 2.6% reported a medically lethal suicide attempt in the year of this survey.

Psychologic autopsy studies

Studies using psychologic autopsy methods gather data about suicide victims by interviewing individuals who knew the suicide victim. Such methods have been shown to be reliable and valid in identifying psychopathology and social factors influencing youthful suicide victims [6]. Most such studies have consistently found that approximately 90% of youth who commit suicide suffer from psychiatric disorders at the time of their deaths [7]. This rate may be an underestimate. Psychologic autopsy studies of adolescent suicide victims report that mood disorders, especially major depressive disorder, is the most prevalent psychiatric disorder among the youthful suicide victims [8–10]. In addition, major depressive disorder increases the risk for suicide associated with other psychiatric disorders. The relative risks (RR) for youth suicide imparted by psychopathology was reported in a case-control study of 67 adolescent suicide victims who were compared with 67 age- and demographically matched community-based controls [8]. The relative risks associated with psychiatric disorders were major depression, 27.0 (95% confidence interval [CI], 1.6–199.8); bipolar mixed state, 9.0 (95% CI, 1.1–71.0); substance abuse, 8.5 (95% CI, 2.0–36.8); and conduct disorder 6.0 (95% CI, 1.8–20.4). Substance abuse was a more significant risk factor when comorbid with mood disorder (RR, 17.0; 95% CI, 1.0–294.0) than when alone (RR, 3.3; 95% CI, 0.9–11.9). Prior suicidal ideation with a plan, previous suicide attempts, and violent behavior were significantly associated with suicide. Specifically, the relative risk for suicide if there was a history of a suicide attempt was 17.0 (95% CI, 2.3–127.7), and for a young person with a history of suicidal ideation with a plan the relative risk was 21.0 (95% CI, 2.8–156.3).

To understand the predictors of suicide among adolescents with mood disorders, 63 adolescent suicide victims with a history of a mood disorder were compared with 23 adolescents in the community with a lifetime history of a mood disorder [11]. The results indicated higher rates of major depressive disorder comorbid with substance abuse, past suicide attempts, family history of major depressive disorder, history of legal problems, a handgun available in the home, and treatment with a tricyclic antidepressant among the suicide victims than among the adolescents in the community. These data indicate that an important means of reducing suicide rates in youth is to identify and treat children and adolescents who suffer from mood disorders, especially major depressive disorder.

Studies of nonfatal youth suicidal behavior

The effects of psychopathology on increasing the risks for childhood and adolescent suicidal ideation and suicide attempts have been consistently reported in empiric studies of community-based and psychiatric samples. A community-based sample of 1709 adolescents showed a lifetime prevalence of 1% for bipolar disorders, primarily bipolar II disorders [12]. An additional 5.7% of adolescents had suffered at least one distinct episode of abnormally and persistently elevated, expansive, or irritable mood [12]. The adolescents with bipolar disorders and expansive mood states had significantly higher rates of comorbid anxiety and disruptive disorders, more functional impairment, and higher prevalence of suicide attempts than did the 316 adolescents with a history of major depressive disorder or the 845 adolescents who never had experienced a psychiatric disorder. Specifically, 44.4% of adolescents with bipolar disorder, 22.2% of adolescents with major depressive disorder, and 1.2% of adolescents without psychopathology reported a suicide attempt. Furthermore, adolescents with hypomanic personality traits, as measured with the Hypomanic Personality Scale, and a history of major depressive disorder had significantly higher rates of suicide attempts [13].

Comparative studies of adolescent psychiatric inpatients attempting suicide and adolescent suicide victims suggest that similar psychiatric disorders are associated with the risks for nonfatal and fatal suicidal acts [14]. The most significant among these disorders is major depressive disorder. Bipolar disorder I and bipolar disorder II were more common among the suicide victims (22.2%; RR, 13.7; 95% CI, 2.1–89.9) than among the suicidal inpatients (5.4%). The adolescent suicide victims were more likely than suicidal adolescent psychiatric inpatients to have a mood disorder comorbid with non–mood disorders (RR, 2.0; 95% CI, 1.1–3.8). Suicide victims were more likely (RR, 2.7; 95% CI, 1.1–6.4) than suicidal psychiatric patients to have firearms in the home. This study indicates that removing firearms from the home might be a suicide-preventive strategy.

The influence of mood disorders on the risk for suicide attempts in adolescents was suggested in a study of 73 high school students [15]. Seventy-four percent of the sample had at least one psychiatric disorder. The most prevalent psychiatric disorders were major depressive disorder (40%) and oppositional defiant disorder (29%). Fifty-six percent of the adolescents reported suicidal ideation. Severity of suicidal ideation was measured by a self-reporting questionnaire, the Modified Scale for Suicidal Ideation. The results indicated a significant relationship between the presence of psychiatric disorders and suicidal ideation. Although the severity of symptoms of other psychiatric disorders, such as generalized anxiety, oppositional defiant disorder, attention deficit hyperactivity disorder, and substance abuse was significantly associated with suicidal ideation, these associations were intensified by the presence of either major depressive disorder or dysthymic disorder. This study revealed that major depressive disorder and dysthymic disorder alone are associated with suicidal ideation; the other disorders are not independently associated with suicidal ideation when analyses are adjusted for the presence of major depressive or dysthymic disorders. This study suggested that identification of adolescents suffering from mood disorders is an important aspect of suicide prevention.

Most studies have not highlighted the risk imparted by bipolar disorder among youth, probably because of the low rate of such disorders or inadequate identification of these disorders in children and adolescents. Controversy continues about the appropriate diagnostic criteria for bipolar disorder in children and adolescents. Nevertheless, when samples of children and adolescents with bipolar disorder are described, suicidal risk is elevated for youth with bipolar disorder. A characteristic of bipolar disorder in youth is the rapid cycling that is prevalent in such samples. This changing psychiatric state may be an important aspect that elevates risk for suicidal behavior. A preventive strategy is to identify children and adolescents with rapidly cycling mood states.

Longitudinal studies

Prospective studies offer distinct advantages in understanding risk for suicidal behavior because they are able to identify risk factors, that is, the factors present before the suicidal ideation, suicide attempt, or suicide. Because longitudinal studies require large samples, however, they are generally not feasible for the study of suicide.

Prospective studies have consistently identified mood disorders as significant risk factors for suicidal behavior in youth. For example, among the rare prospective studies of a large, representative community sample of adolescents, the incidence of a suicide attempt within the year after an initial assessment was 1.7% in the total sample of 1508 adolescents [16]. The results indicated that, after controlling for the presence of depressive symptoms, the psychosocial factors that predict a future suicide attempt are a past suicide attempt (RR, 5.8; 95% CI, 2.5–13.6), a recent suicide attempt by a friend (RR, 3.2; 95% CI, 1.4–7.3), and poor self esteem (RR, 1.8; 95% CI, 1.0–3.1).

Most prospective studies have used psychiatric patient populations. For example, among prepubertal psychiatric inpatients the relative risk for suicidal ideation was found to be 3.7 (95% CI, 1.0–13.0) times greater, and for suicide attempts the risk was 6.2 (95% CI, 1.9–20.6) times greater in adolescents than in prepubertal children without psychopathology and those who do not report suicidal behavior [15]. Prepubertal psychiatric inpatients who suffer from major depressive disorder have a 5.3 (95% CI, 1.8–15.8) times greater risk for suicide attempts in adolescence than do prepubertal children without psychopathology [17]. Such results have been supported by other studies of prepubertal children with major depressive disorder. For example, 60 prepubertal children with major depressive disorder, 32 prepubertal children with major depressive and comorbid dysthymic disorders, 23 prepubertal children with dysthymic disorder, 19 prepubertal children with adjustment disorder with depressed mood, and a psychiatric comparison group of 49 prepubertal children with non–mood psychiatric disorders were followed for as long as 12 years [18]. At the initial assessment, 58% children reported a history of suicidal ideation, and 9% reported a history of a suicide attempt. There were no differences at the initial assessment in rates of suicidal ideation or suicide attempts among children with major depression, those with comorbid major depression and dysthymia, and those with dysthymia. At initial assessment, however, children with mood disorder involving major depression or dysthymia had significantly higher rates of suicidal ideation or suicide attempts than children with non–mood disorders or adjustment disorder with depressed mood. Specifically, children with mood disorder had a 2.6-fold (95% CI, 1.39–4.76) greater likelihood for suicidal ideation and a 10.83-fold (95% CI, 1.40–83.64) greater likelihood for a suicide attempt than children without a mood disorder. Over the 7-year follow-up period, the rates of suicidal ideation were comparable to those at initial assessment, but the rates of suicide attempts doubled during the follow-up period. Rates of suicidal ideation and suicide attempts in the follow-up period were significantly greater among children with a mood disorder than among those without a mood disorder. The increasing rates of suicidal acts as the children grow older and in those suffering from a mood disorder parallel the trends among youth who committed suicide.

Prospective studies of prepubertal children with major depressive disorder suggest the long-term continuity of mood disorders and the poor outcome with regard to emergence of other disorders in adulthood. In a study of 83 prepubertal children with major depressive disorder, 44 prepubertal children with anxiety disorder, and 91 prepubertal children without these disorders, all of whom were followed into adulthood, the lifetime relative risk for suicide attempts was 4.4 times higher (95% CI, 1.7–11.6) in children with major depressive disorder and

2.8 tiems higher (95% CI, 1.0–7.5) in children with anxiety disorders than in children without psychopathology [19]. The lifetime relative risk for a suicide attempt was 3.0 (95% CI, 1.0–8.7) times higher in prepubertal children with a major depressive disorder than in prepubertal children with anxiety disorders [19]. Compared with children without psychopathology, children with prepubertal-onset major depressive disorder had a significantly higher rate of bipolar I disorder, a 2.3 relative risk (95% CI, 1.2–4.5) for any substance abuse or dependence disorder, a 3.0 relative risk (95% CI, 1.3–6.6) for alcohol abuse or alcohol dependence disorder, and a 3.9 relative risk (95% CI 1.0–15.0) for conduct disorder [19]. Compared with children without psychopathology, children with anxiety disorders had a 2.1 relative risk (95% CI, 1.0–4.3) for any substance abuse or dependence disorder, a 2.3 relative risk (95% CI, 1.0–5.6) for alcohol abuse or dependence disorder, and a 4.7 relative risk (95% CI, 1.2–18.8) for conduct disorder [19]. Another prospective study of 73 adolescents with major depressive disorder and of 37 adolescents without psychiatric disorders who were followed up 10 to 15 years later reported a suicide rate of 7.7% and a 5.6-fold increased risk (95% CI, 1.2–25.2) for a suicide attempt during the follow-up years among those with adolescent onset major depressive disorder [20]. This study is one of many that point out the significant risk for suicidal behavior imparted by history of a mood disorder.

Family studies

Family studies of adolescent suicide victims and of children and adolescents who attempt suicide suggest that there is a significantly higher rate of suicidal behavior among parents and siblings of youth who commit or attempt suicide [11,21]. Brent et al [7] have suggested that the relationships between youthful suicide and family suicidal behavior are independent of the prevalence of mood disorders within the family. The results of psychologic studies also suggest that the presence of specific psychiatric disorders in adolescent suicide victims is significantly related to the increased rate of that psychiatric disorder among the suicide victims' first-degree relatives [6]. The data of a study of prepubertal suicidal children [21] support Brent and colleagues' [22] assertion that although there are significant relationships between child and adolescent suicide attempts and family histories of suicidal behavior, there are no significant relationships between a family history of mood disorders and suicidal behavior in children and adolescents. It has not been conclusively determined, however, if suicidal behavior is independent of family transmission of mood disorders. A comparative study of 192 children and adolescents of emotionally healthy and depressed mothers suggests children of depressed mothers are significantly more likely than children of emotionally healthy mothers to exhibit suicidal ideation or suicide attempts [23]. There is also a significant relationship between children's suicidal behavior and parental suicidal behavior. These researchers noted that it is not possible to differentiate the effects of parental depression from those of parental suicidal behavior. It is important to identify a family history of mood disorder, because such a history may indicate a risk for major depressive disorder in children and thereby suggest a higher risk for suicidal behavior. Specifically, the rate of any mood disorder in first-degree relatives of prepubertal children with recurrent major depressive disorder is significantly higher (59.7%) than among first-degree relatives of children with only one episode of major depressive disorder (34.1%) [19].

Features of mood disorders associated with suicidal behavior

Cognitive aspects of mood disorders have been studied as important components of suicidal risk. Recent research with 200 incarcerated juvenile delinquents using a self-reporting questionnaire, the Children's Depression Inventory (CDI), that measures severity of depressive symptoms suggests that hopelessness and poor self esteem are significantly associated with suicidal ideation [24]. This report suggests that specific factors within criteria for depressive disorders should be foci for identification of suicide risk. Another study also indicates that attributional style, hopelessness, and poor self-esteem are associated with suicidal ideation among psychiatrically hospitalized children and adolescents [25]. Among a sample of 68 adolescent who have attempted suicide, self-criticism has been strongly associated with hopelessness [26]. This study suggests that interventions focusing on cognitive features of self-criticism may be helpful in preventing suicidal acts among adolescents. Notably, hopelessness has been identified as a significant risk factor for suicide in adults and youth [27].

Recent efforts to understand predictors of lethality of a suicidal act suggest that cognitive components and impulsivity may be important factors. Sixty adolescent psychiatric inpatients who attempted suicide while suffering from major depressive disorder were grouped according to the levels of severity of their suicide attempts [28]. The level of lethality of the suicide attempt did not correlate with the patient's severity of hopelessness, depressive symptoms, lack of self-esteem, substance abuse, or bipolar disorder. Those whose suicide attempts were more lethal had comorbid major depressive and attention deficit hyperactivity disorders and expressed the strongest desire to kill themselves. This study suggests that evaluation of suicidal intent and degree of impulsivity may indicate those who are at greater risk for highly lethal suicide attempts. Support for the significance of impulsivity in raising the risk for suicidal acts was provided in a study of 33 adolescents who attempted suicide by overdosing, 30 adolescents with psychopathology but no suicidal behavior, and 30 adolescents without psychopathology [29]. The results suggested that when severity of depressive symptoms was controlled, all the variables studied, except impulsivity, were similar among the three groups of adolescents. Adolescents who attempted suicide had significantly higher levels of impulsivity. Depression was the most significant correlate of suicidal behavior, but impulsivity was associated with suicidal behavior independent of depression.

Prevention of suicidal behavior in youth

A significant means of reducing the incidence of suicidal behavior is practicing preventive approaches. One of the most important approaches is to identify children and adolescents who may be at risk before the manifestation of suicidal behavior. Use of screening techniques involving self-reporting question- naires and subsequent diagnostic interviews may be a sequenced method to identify children and adolescents at risk for suicidal behavior [30]. Identification of children and adolescents at risk for mood disorders and interventions to prevent the onset of such disorders may be the best primary preventive method. For example, children whose parents have mood disorders are at significant risk for developing mood disorders. Preventive intervention offered to such families has limited the onset of mood disorders in children [31]. Recognition and treatment of children and adolescents who manifest symptoms of mood disor- ders or who have a history of suicidal behavior is another important preven- tive approach.

Future research is needed to evaluate the effectiveness of interventions to treat children and adolescents with mood disorders. By using effective interventions in conjunction with early identification of those at risk for suicidal behavior, suicide among children and adolescents may be prevented.

References

[1] US Public Health Service. The surgeon general's call to action to prevent suicide. Washington, DC: US Public Health Service; 1999.

[2] Minino AM, Smith BL. Deaths: preliminary data for 2000. National vital statistics reports, vol 49, no 12. Hyattsville (MD): National Center for Health Statistics; 2001.

[3] Hoyert DL, Arias E, Smith BL, et al. Deaths: final data for 1999. National vital statistics reports, vol 49, no 8. Hyattsville (MD): National Center for Health Statistics; 2001.

[4] Shaffer D, Gould M, Hicks RC. Worsening suicide rate in black teenagers. Am J Psychiatry 1994;151:1810–2.

[5] Kann L, Kinchen SA, Williams BI, et al. Youth risk behavior surveillance–United States, 1999. J Sch Health 2000;70:271–85.

[6] Brent DA, Perper JA, Moritz G, et al. The validity of diagnoses obtained through the psycho- logical autopsy procedure in adolescent suicide victims: use of family history. Acta Psychiatr Scand 1993;87:118–22.

[7] Shaffer D, Gould MS, Fisher P, et al. Psychiatric diagnosis in child and adolescent suicide. Arch Gen Psychiatry 1996;53:339–48.

[8] Brent DA, Perper JA, Moritz G, et al. Psychiatric risk factors for adolescent suicide: a case- control study. J Am Acad Child Adolesc Psychiatry 1993;32:521–9.

[9] Shaffer D, Garland A, Gould M, et al. Preventing teenage suicide: a critical review. J Am Acad Child Adolesc Psychiatry 1988;27:675–87.

[10] Shafii M, Carrigen S, Whittinghill JR, et al. Psychological autopsy of completed suicide in children and adolescents. Am J Psychiatry 1985;142:1061–4.

[11] Brent DA, Perper JA, Moritz G, et al. Suicide in affectively ill adolescents. A case-control study. J Affect Disord 1994;31:193–202.

[12] Lewinsohn PM, Klein DN, Seeley JR. Bipolar disorders in a community sample of older adolescents: prevalence, phenomenology, comorbidity, and course. J Am Acad Child Adolesc Psychiatry 1995;34:454–63.

[13] Klein DN, Lewinsohn PM, Seeley JR. Hypomanic personality traits in a community sample of adolescents. J Affect Disord 1996;38:135–43.

[14] Brent DA, Perper JA, Goldstein CE, et al. Risk factors for adolescent suicide: a comparison of adolescent suicide victims with suicidal inpatients. Arch Gen Psychiatry 1988;45:561–88.

[15] Esposito CL, Clum GA. Psychiatric symptoms and their relationship to suicidal ideation in a high-risk adolescent community sample. J Am Acad Child Adolesc Psychiatry 2002;41:44–51.

[16] Lewinsohn PM, Rohde P, Seeley JR. Psychosocial risk factors for future adolescent suicide attempts. J Consult Clin Psychol 1994;62:297–305.

[17] Pfeffer CR, Klerman GL, Hurt SW, et al. Suicidal children grow up: rates and psychosocial risk factors for suicide attempts during follow-up. J Am Acad Child Adolesc Psychiatry 1993;32: 106–13.

[18] Kovacs M, Goldston D, Gatsonis C. Suicidal behaviors and childhood-onset depressive disorders: a longitudinal investigation. J Am Acad Child Adolesc Psychiatry 1993;32:8–20.

[19] Weissman MM, Wolk S, Wickramaratne P, et al. Children with prepubertal-onset major depressive disorder and anxiety grown up. Arch Gen Psychiatry 1999;56:794–801.

[20] Weissman MM, Wolk S, Goldstein RB, et al. Depressed adolescents grown up. JAMA 1999; 281:1707–13.

[21]. Pfeffer CR, Normandin L, Kakuma T. Suicidal children grow up: suicidal behavior and psychiatric disorders among relatives. J Am Acad Child Adolesc Psychiatry 1994;33:1087–97.

[22] Brent DA, Perper JA, Moritz G, et al. Familial risk factors for adolescent suicide: a case-control study. Acta Psychiatr Scand 1994;89:52–8.

[23] Klimes-Dougan B, Free K, Ronsaville D, et al. Suicidal ideation and attempts: a longitudinal investigation of children of depressed and well mothers. J Am Acad Child Adolesc Psychiatry 1999;38:651–9.

[24] Esposito CL, Clum GA. Specificity of depressive symptoms and suicidality in a juvenile delinquent population. J Psychopath Behav Assess 1999;21:171–82.

[25] Wagner KD, Rouleau M, Joiner T. Cognitive factors related to suicidal ideation and resolution in psychiatrically hospitalized children and adolescents. Am J Psychiatry 2000;157:2017–21.

[26] Donaldson D, Spirito A, Farnett E. The role of perfectionism and depressive cognitions in understanding the hopelessness experienced by adolescent suicide attempters. Child Psychiatry Hum Dev 2000;31:99–111.

[27] Beck AT, Steer RA, Kovacs M, et al. Hopelessness and eventual suicide: a 10-year prospective study of patients hospitalized with suicidal ideation. Am J Psychiatry 1985;142:559–63.

[28] Nasser EH, Overholser JC. Assessing varying degrees of lethality in depressed adolescent suicide attempters. Acta Psychiatr Scand 1999;99:423–31.

[29] Kingsbury S, Hawton K, Steinhardt K, et al. Do adolescents who take overdoses have specific psychological characteristics? A comparative study with psychiatric and community controls. J Am Acad Child Adolesc Psychiatry 1999;38:1125–31.

[30] Pfeffer CR, Jiang H, Kakuma T. Child-Adolescent Suicidal Potential Index (CASPI): a screen for risk for early onset suicidal behavior. Psychol Assess 2000;12:304–18.

[31] Beardslee WR, Gladstone TRG. Prevention of childhood depression: recent findings and future prospects. Biol Psychiatry 2001;49:1101–10.

CHILD AND
ADOLESCENT
PSYCHIATRIC
CLINICS

Child Adolesc Psychiatric Clin N Am
11 (2002) 649–671

Aggression and violence in mood disorders

Deborah M. Weisbrot, MD[a],*, Alan B. Ettinger, MD[b]

[a]*Division of Child and Adolescent Psychiatry, Department of Psychiatry and Behavioral Sciences, Putnam Hall-South Campus, State University of New York at Stony Brook, NY 11790-8794, USA*
[b]*Long Island Jewish Comprehensive Epilepsy Center, Department of Neurology, Albert Einstein College of Medicine, New Hyde Park, NY 11040, USA*

Severe aggression in childhood is one of the earliest and most intractable psychiatric problems, placing some children on a maladjusted trajectory and at risk for the development of mood disorders [1,2]. Aggression is currently the most common reason that children and adolescents are referred for psychiatric evaluation and is associated with potentially severe psychosocial, behavioral, and academic impairments. Aggression presents in a diverse array of psychiatric conditions, including mood disorders. Aggressive behavior may be a manifestation of irritability, a core symptom of both mania and depression. Aggression may also be a symptom of conditions frequently comorbid with mood disorder, such as oppositional defiant disorder, conduct disorder, attention deficit disorder, and substance use disorders. Identifying a comorbid mood disorder can be challenging when the clinician's attention is drawn primarily toward severe aggressive behavior. Symptoms of aggression and mood disturbances also occur as adverse effects of psychotropic therapies for other psychiatric conditions [3]. To understand the relationships between aggression and mood, the clinician must thoughtfully consider associated conditions and situations that give a context to the aggressive behavior.

This article summarizes the current understanding of the multidimensional relationships between aggression and mood disorder. It addresses the neurophysiologic, neuroanatomic, and genetic underpinnings of aggression and cognitive, dynamic family, and environmental influences. It also examines psychiatric disorders with affective components in which aggression is particularly common. Finally, it highlights the treatment of aggression in the context of a mood disorder and how responses to treatment lend further insight into the interrelationships between aggression and mood.

---

* Corresponding author.
E-mail address: Deborah.Weisbrot@StonyBrook.edu (D.M. Weisbrot)

1056-4993/02/$ – see front matter © 2002, Elsevier Science (USA). All rights reserved.
PII: S 1 0 5 6 - 4 9 9 3 (0 2) 0 0 0 1 6 - 0

Definitions and subtypes of aggression

In the psychiatric literature and in clinical practice there are numerous definitions of anger and aggression. For the purposes of this article the authors define aggression as "behaviors by one person intended to cause pain, damage or destruction to another" [4]. Hostility is the motive or desire to hurt someone. Anger is aroused when a person feels thwarted or treated unfairly [5]. Irritability is defined as a readiness to explode with negative affect at the slightest provocation and includes a display of quick temper and exasperation [5–8].

Aggression may be classified as either instrumental or reactive. Instrumental aggression is purposeful and is unaccompanied by strong emotion. Reactive aggression occurs in response to a perceived provocation. Because reactive aggression is accompanied by strong emotion (usually anger) and is not premeditated, it is also called "impulsive" or "emotional" aggression. In interpersonal contexts, aggression is typically reactive. Although many studies argue for a clear delineation between these two types of aggression, patients in clinical practice often exhibit a mixture of both forms.

Vitiello and Stoff [9], in their critical review of childhood aggression, categorize aggression according to phenomenologic constructs, dividing aggression into emotive and predatory types. They emphasize early- and late-onset variants and the overt or covert nature of aggression. They argued for a dichotomy in childhood aggression between an impulsive-reactive-hostile-affective subtype and a controlled-proactive-instrumental-predatory subtype. The impulsive subtype is more common in mood disorders. It is a response to a perceived threat or provocation, and its retaliatory nature connects it to affective types of aggression. This dichotomy is yet to be validated, however. Impulsive aggression (alternatively termed reactive aggression) is characterized by disinhibition and affective instability but not necessarily by antisocial tendencies [9]. Reactive aggression is explosive, uncontrolled, is accompanied by anger or fear, is characterized by high levels of arousal, and at times is self-directed.

Proactive, or predatory, aggression is initiated to obtain specific rewards and can be expressed by behaviors such as coercion, attacks with the purpose to steal, and bullying of weaker children. A rating scale has been developed for teachers' use in differentiating proactive and reactive forms of aggression [10].

A meta-analysis of childhood antisocial behavior [11] found empiric support for categorizing aggression as overt or covert. Highly overt aggression is more likely to be impulsive, accompanied by strong affect (fear, anger), and poorly controlled, in contrast with the instrumental and overcontrolled character of covert aggression.

Pathophysiology and treatments of each type vary widely. Boys with reactive aggression misinterpret peers' behavior as hostile and overreact with aggression when faced with peers' rejection. Reactively aggressive boys are perceived to be angry and unhappy, whereas boys with proactive aggression are viewed less negatively by their peers [9,10]. These investigators found that boys with purely predatory aggression are unlikely to receive appropriate psychiatric treatment. In this series, patients with affective aggression had lower verbal IQs, higher rates of psychotic disorders, higher rates of prior treatments with neuroleptics or lithium, and higher rates of substance abuse than did children with a predatory aggression. These findings support the dichotomy of aggressive subtypes.

The lack of uniformity among different studies in the classification of aggression subtypes and in the specific definitions of aggression and its subtypes compromises makes it difficult to synthesize the diverse literature on this subject. Some studies fail to distinguish verbal from physical aggression or to distinguish aggression from oppositional, hyperactive, or other disruptive and troublesome behaviors or comorbid disorders. The lack of a longitudinal perspective on the development of behavior problems is also a failing of many studies.

Causes

This section briefly summarizes a number of different theoretic perspectives on the complex causative relationships between aggression and mood disorders.

Genetic perspectives

It is generally believed that no individual is genetically programmed to develop violent behavior in later life. A confluence of genetic and environmental influences may ultimately lead to aggressive tendencies, however. Temperament, which can be conceptualized as a style of behavior, is significantly influenced by constitutional factors and by gene-environment interactions. Studies [12] suggest that there are significant associations between difficult temperaments (ie, negative emotionality) and later behavior problems or psychiatric disturbances, including mood disorders [12–14]. Difficult temperament in a child could also directly influence a parent's response by eliciting negative responses. These negative responses from the parents could lead to difficulties in parent-child interaction and reduce the child's social skills, including the ability to handle stressful situations without becoming aggressive. In summary, a difficult temperament (eg, irritability, poor emotional regulation, and temper tantrums) may be a precursor of both aggressive behavior and childhood-onset mood disorders.

Parent-child dynamics

The family has been described as the cradle of violence [15]. Mood disturbance in immediate family members can powerfully affect the development of aggressive behavior or mood disorder in the child [5]. Depressed parents are often irritable, angry, and disconnected from their children [16]. Interactions with an angry parent can be frightening for a child, can model angry and aggressive behavior, and can contribute to the child's problems in emotional regulation. Studies suggest that complex associations exist between childhood depressive symptoms and aggression in children and also between maternal depressive symptoms and behavior problems in children [5,17]. Cicchetti [2] has speculated that early childhood aggression may be associated with an insecure attachment between mother and child. An insecure mother-child bond may also be a significant factor in the development of later mood disorders.

Abusive experiences in childhood provide lifelong models of violent behavior. The longer and earlier the abuse, the more severe is the long-term impact. Multiple studies [2,18–20] have demonstrated that an abused child is more likely to be impulsive and emotionally labile and to have learning difficulties and cognitive impairments. In a study of reactive aggression among maltreated children, a history of abuse predicted emotional dysregulation, affective lability and negativity, and socially inappropriate emotional expressions [21].

Commonalities in biologic mechanisms of aggression and mood disorders

Many studies in animals and humans have identified serotonin and norepinephrine deficiencies in depression [22–25]. As in depression, reduced cerebrospinal fluid (CSF) 5-HIAA levels are seen in aggressive or violent psychiatric patients [26–29], so it has been suggested that serotonin may have an inhibitory effect on impulsive aggression.

Norepinephrine is involved in arousal and reactivity to the environment [27]. Heightened reactivity may lead to affective instability, irritability, and a predisposition toward aggression [30]. Humans with aggressive or impulsive behavior show higher levels of the norepinephrine metabolite 5-hydroxy-3 methyoxypheneleneglycol (5-MHPG) [31]. Violent suicide victims have increased β-adrenergic receptor binding in prefrontal and temporal cortex. The normal release of growth hormone in response to administration of an α-adrenergic agonist is blunted in patients with irritability [32].

How does one reconcile the reduction of norepinephrine in depression and the increase in norepinephrine seen in aggression? One possibility is that the decreased norepinephrine activity in depression reflects withdrawal from the environment. Serotonin deficiency may be associated with either self-directed or outwardly directed impulsive aggression. Low serotonin levels accompanied by high norepinephrine activity may predispose outwardly directed impulsive aggression directed, whereas, low serotonin levels accompanied by low norepinephrine activity may generate inwardly directed aggression leading to depression and sometimes violent and aggressive suicide attempts [29]. Further study is needed to confirm these relationships.

Psychodynamic perspectives on depression and aggression

Freud's, and later Abraham's [15], basic formulation was that depression represents aggression turned against the self after the loss of an ambivalently loved object. Contemporary psychoanalytic writings have emphasized interpersonal causes of depression and dysregulation of self-esteem. The role of aggression in the development of depressive symptoms has been downplayed [33,34].

From a psychodynamic perspective, violent behavior occurs because the individual's defenses fail in channeling or controlling this reaction. For example, when an adolescent is depressed, he or she may be attempting to manage a sense of overwhelming helplessness [35]. The adolescent needs to try to master this experience of being overwhelmed by whatever means are in his or her control. In this context, violence can become a method of dissipating anger. Subsequent feelings of guilt are relieved through remorse for the violent act or, more usually, through externally imposed punishment [35]. Some adolescents make suicide attempts, engage in criminal acts, die "accidentally," or sustain "accidental" injuries, especially in automobile accidents.

Object-relations theorists such as Klein et al [36] suggest that early or repeated object loss may lead to self-criticism and related depressive symptoms as well as to hostility over abandonment. These reactions may lead to aggressive behavior toward other objects or people. In this model, a pattern of ongoing hostility, described as frequent anger, suspicion, resentment, or the belief that one is being mistreated, is predictive of depression and aggressive acting-out behaviors.

Cognitive influences on aggression in mood disorders

The original cognitive perspective on aggression and mood relationships was developed by Dollard in 1939 [37] and was termed the frustration-aggression hypothesis. Dollard claimed that frustration could create aggressive inclinations even when the frustration is not arbitrary or personally aimed at the subject. A revision of the original model [38] holds that frustrating experiences produce aggressive tendencies when they evoke negative affect. Accordingly, the presence of a mood disorder greatly heightens the possibility of aggressive tendencies, because an individual with mood disorder is much more likely to have symptoms of irritability and negative affect.

Cognitive theories of aggression closely intersect with cognitive behavioral models of depression [39] in which negative, distorted thoughts about oneself, the future, and one's experiences are the predominant characteristics of the depressed individual [40]. Seligman's learned helplessness theory and Rehm's self-control model [40] also attribute aggression to deficits in self-evaluation to and in responses to life events that lead to cognitive distortions.

Individuals with extremely positive perceptions of themselves and their functioning are the most likely to become angry and violent [41]. For these individuals, experiences that threaten positive self-esteem and self-view can give rise to anger and hostility, which in turn may generate aggression. Because cognitive distortions in the shape of negative self-view and low self-esteem are also intrinsic to a state of depression, this theory provides another perspective on the relationships between mood and aggression.

Developmental perspectives

In normal development, aggressive behavior peaks by the ages of 2 to 3 years and declines thereafter [42]. A child's ability to use language to express negative emotions is an important factor in decreasing the use of physical aggression to express negative emotions [43]. Studies of children with language impairment indicate that such children have higher rates of depression and aggression [44,45].

From a developmental perspective, aggression is a common reaction to frustration in childhood. The child's interpretation of the frustrating situation may be more significant than the level of frustration in determining the child's reaction. The child's underlying mood state is also critical in determining whether an experience of frustration will lead to aggression. Strategies for behavioral and emotional regulation, such as self-comforting, seeking help, and distraction, help the child manage early temperament-driven frustration and fear responses when the control of negative emotions is necessary. Children who are unable to use such strategies may become aggressive. By the end of the second year of life, behavioral and emotional regulation patterns are established sufficiently to influence early personality and social-interaction skills and to contribute to problematic patterns of behavior, including mood disorders and aggressive behaviors [46]. Not surprisingly, toddlers who show persistent aggression in childhood tend to have particularly severe problems with aggression later in life [47].

The developmental relationship between mood and aggression is further clarified by examining the different stages of childhood. For example, in toddlers, the tendency to initiate aggression may be associated with a perception of hostile intent in others [47]. A study by Calkins [46] found an intriguing physiologic correlation between a decreased autonomic reactivity (cardiac respiratory sinus arrhythmia [RSA]) and aggressive or destructive symptomatology in young children. When coping and emotional regulation were needed, decreased RSA predicted increased emotional reactivity, decreased attentional abilities, more negative affect, and more dysregulated emotional behaviors.

Temperament may exert a stronger effect on early-emerging problem behaviors when internal or external sources of regulation are not functioning or are unavailable. As development progresses, the presentation of aggressive symptoms may change, but such symptoms remain problematic and reflect continuous underlying difficulties. Children who fail to develop impulse control at early stages are at the highest risk for lifelong difficulty in resisting temptations to demonstrate antisocial behavior [48].

Studies of aggressive behavior in school-aged children suggest that aggressive behavior tends to be sustained throughout the early elementary school years. Children with a combination of aggressive and withdrawn behaviors may have the most difficulty [49,50]. It has been speculated that these children withdraw as a means of reducing social anxiety or to limit interference from others; however, high levels of aggressive reactivity make them vulnerable to provocation and abuse [51]. The role of negative mood states and their relation to withdrawal in aggressive children deserves further study.

Violent behavior by boys during adolescence (ie, as seen in the social organization of gangs) has been viewed as a socialization pattern necessary for some boys to prove their manhood [15]. It is certainly true that aggressive behavior can be a healthy aspect of adolescence, as when the adolescent asserts his or her independence from parental authority. Misinterpretations of normal patterns of aggression have led to the minimizing the significance of even relatively extreme aggression or belligerence, however. Gender stereotyping may lead to minimizing aggressive behaviors in girls.

Depression becomes a significant health problem during adolescence, with current rates reported to be between 2.0% and 8.0% [52]. Epidemiologic and clinical studies have found that 40% to70% of depressed children and adolescents have comorbid psychiatric disorders. The frequency of comorbid disruptive behavior disorders varies widely and has been estimated to be between 10% and 80% [53,54]. Aggression also increases during adolescence. For instance, rates of violent crimes committed by youth also increase significantly in adolescence, further suggesting that aggression in this age group is a significant public health issue [55].

Depressive disorders and aggression in children and adolescents

Historically, comorbidity was probably addressed as masked depression or depressive equivalents, terms implying that aggressive and other acting-out behaviors are the means by which children express depressed mood [56]. The use of systematic interviews to ask children how they feel [57,58] has shown that the symptoms previously thought to mask depression are, in fact, definitive components of a depressive disorder or comorbid conditions. The major difference in depression in youths and adults is that in youths pure depression is unusual, and rates for any type of comorbidity range from 33% to 100% [59].

Aggression and depression co-occur phenomenologically for a variety of reasons. Irritability precedes episodes of aggression. It is also a basic symptom of depression and dysthymia, as well as of anxiety, and anxiety disorders are often antecedents to depression in children [60]. Irritability occurs frequently in adults as well as in children, and *The Diagnostic and Statistical Manual of Mental Disorders–III* (DSM–III) included irritability as one of the manifestations of dysphoric mood. Irritability was later eliminated as a proxy for depressed mood in adults to try to avoid misidentifying mania. Because of children's reduced ability to articulate feelings of disgruntlement, irritability is still allowed as a manifestation of dysphoria. Nevertheless, to keep from misdiagnosing a depressed, irritable child as having low level for frustration caused by attention deficit hyperactivity disorder (ADHD) or oppositional conduct disorder, recent editions of the DSM have a caveat that, for a diagnosis of depression, behaviors such as low tolerance of frustration and fighting should not occur exclusively during an episode of a mood disorder or be better accounted for by a mood disorder.

Behavior disorders (eg, conduct disorder and ADHD) are also frequently comorbid with child and adolescent depression [61]. Harrington [62] tried to clarify the relationship between aggression (in this case, conduct disorder) and depression in a follow-up study of children seen at the Maudsley Hospital with chart records of depressive symptoms. He found that for children the conduct disorder seemed to be the dominant problem. That is, children with conduct disorder and depression did not develop higher rates of depression as adults, but the behavior disorder persisted. His data and family studies suggest that, because rates of co-occurrence are so high, depression and conduct disorder in children may be distinct from pure depression in children and may merit a separate diagnostic category. The data are incompatible with the argument that the conduct disturbance is simply part of the depressive disorder [62]. As a result, International Classification of Disease (ICD-10) research diagnostic criteria [63] include a distinct diagnostic category for depressive conduct disorder.

The specific frequency of irritability and its consequences in dysthymic disorder are less well studied. A meta-analysis of relevant investigations in adults [64] found a direct relationship between a lifetime diagnosis of dysthymia with a history of criminal arrest or incarceration and physical altercations. The relationship of aggression to dysthymia in children and adolescents deserves further study [65–67].

Anxiety disorders, frequently comorbid with depression [68], are also frequently associated with aggressive behavior and intense anger. This association is particularly strong in posttraumatic stress disorder (PTSD) [69] and dissociative states. In one study [70] a self-reporting questionnaire administered to high school students found that exposure to violence, as victims or as witnesses, was correlated with emotional trauma, comorbid depression, anger, and dissociative symptoms. Dissociation has also been described as a frequent concomitant of acts of self-mutilation and of suicide attempts [7]. Finally, aggressive symptoms and severe conduct difficulties have been found to occur in 16.5% of teenagers with psychotic affective disorders [71,72].

Psychosis (eg, intermittent paranoid thinking and hallucinations) may also have a mood component and may be masked by aggression in children and adolescents [73]. As noted by Lewis and Yaeger [74] many aggressive adolescents would prefer to be thought of as "bad" rather than as "crazy." Although borderline personality traits are reported to be common in conduct-disordered youth, aggressive adolescents may be less likely to have borderline personality disorder than an underlying affective disorder [75]. The assessment of children and adolescents with conduct disorder is also complicated because many of them have experienced physical, psychologic, or sexual abuse. These traumatic experiences in early childhood are closely tied to the development of subsequent aggressive symptoms and mood disorders and confound the understanding of aggressive and mood symptoms for this group.

Bipolar disorder and aggression

Significant connections between aggressive behaviors in childhood and pediatric bipolar disorder have only recently been recognized [55,76–79]. Similar features of distractibility, impulsivity, hyperactivity, and emotional lability have led to diagnostic confusion between ADHD and bipolar disorder. Some cases of aggression attributed to ADHD may, in fact, have been caused by unrecognized bipolar disorder. Conversely, some have argued that mania is being too liberally diagnosed in the presence of symptoms of anger, irritability, or agitation alone. Clinical lore has handed down the untested concept that a positive response to mood stabilizers or a negative response to stimulants implies validation of a bipolar diagnosis. The question whether mania and comorbid ADHD with oppositional defiant conduct disorder represents a subtype of bipolar disorder [76], is continuous with adult mania with antisocial personality [80], or is a phenotypic red herring remains to be clarified.

As defined in manic children, the mood disturbance in bipolar disorder is usually irritability with affective storms, that is, prolonged and aggressive temper outbursts [79]. Patients become easily enraged and can engage in brutal physical altercations [55]. In one series [79] examples of aggression in manic states included assaultive behavior (using knives to threaten others, to stab furniture, or to cut off a cat's tail), throwing and breaking objects, kicking down doors, and otherwise destroying property. This severe irritability is the primary reason for the high rate of psychiatric hospitalization in manic children [79].

In a literature review, Carlson [81] found that children under 9 years of age with bipolar disorder presented with more irritability, crying, and psychomotor agitation than did older bipolar children who were more likely to exhibit the classic manic symptoms of euphoria and grandiosity. The prominence of irritability rather than euphoria as a manifestation of mania in younger age groups confounds the diagnosis, particularly because irritability is also a presenting complaint in childhood depression and other childhood psychiatric disorders. Irritability and its resultant aggressive symptoms may also be mis-diagnosed as exclusively caused by ADHD, oppositional defiant disorder, or conduct disorder, rather than as mania or comorbid mania with externalizing disorder. Because the irritability in manic children may be severe and persistent, it often leads to violence. In contrast to the predatory aggression seen in antisocial children with conduct disorder, aggressive symptoms in manic children tend to be associated with a pervasive irritable mood and are less organized and poorly goal-directed. The presence of episodes also helps distinguish bipolar disorder from other forms of psychopathology. The implications of mood disorder and severe aggression are illustrated in a recent study of juvenile offenders which emphasized the presence of mania in this group [82].

Depression, anger attacks and intermittent explosive disorder

In addition to the conditions just described, anger attacks are considered to be a component of other psychiatric diagnoses with mood components. The disorders in which intermittent outbursts of affective violence feature most prominently are classified as episodic dyscontrol syndromes. These outbursts are often related to a specific, stressful trigger. In some dyscontrol syndromes, violence is preceded by a sense of mounting tension, helplessness, and depression. Sometimes, violent behavior may occur without apparent warning, and the precipitating stress is evident only retrospectively. The attack may last minutes to hours and usually consists of biting, gouging, spitting, and verbal outbursts. The subject (child, adolescent, or adult) may subsequently be amnestic about the episode and demonstrate remorse when told what has occurred [35].

Fava and colleagues [83] suggest that anger attacks are actually atypical presentations of anxiety or depressive disorders. Patients presenting with brief, ego-dystonic episodes of anger that were grossly out of proportion to precipitating stressors describe autonomic features that resemble panic attacks but are unassociated with fear and anxiety. Treatment of these attacks with antidepressants produced marked behavioral improvements. General anxiety may be associated with intense anger in some patients [83].

Recent research suggests that intermittent explosive disorder is a bona fide impulse-control disorder related to mood disorders [84,85].

Intermittent explosive disorder is thought by some to be a form of pathologic affective aggression or a dysfunctional fight-versus-flight response to environmental danger, distinguished from other forms of aggression by its strong affective component. In one series of patients with intermittent explosive disorder [85], most patients described affective symptoms associated with their explosive episodes. These symptoms included maniclike symptoms (especially irritability or rage, increased energy, and racing thoughts) during the episode and rapid onset of depressed mood and fatigue after the act. These descriptions are reminiscent of brief but severe dysphoric mood swings of bipolar disorder. Patients who were actually diagnosed with bipolar disorder described mood and energy changes during aggressive episodes that were qualitatively similar but briefer than those associated with hypomanic or manic episodes. All patients demonstrated other axis-I psychopathology, including substance use, anxiety, and eating and other impulse-control disorders. Of 20 persons receiving monotherapy with a mood stabilizer, 12 (60%) reported reduction of aggressive impulses and acts. These findings strengthen a speculated association of intermittent explosive disorder with bipolar disorder.

Intermittent explosive disorder has been diagnosed in significant numbers of adult fire setters and alcoholic violent offenders who also had comorbid mood disorders. The decreased CSF concentrations of 5-HIAA in intermittent explosive disorder as well as in mood disorders suggest that both conditions are associated with dysfunctional central serotonergic neurotransmission. Favorable responses to antidepressant treatment in both disorders also argue for a commonality between these conditions. Because severe aggression shares many of the features of mood disorders, some investigators consider severe aggression, itself, as a type of mood disorder [15].

Although adult illness has been their predominant focus, studies of the childhood psychiatric histories of adult patients with intermittent explosive disorder are remarkable for hyperactivity, impaired attention, diagnosis of ADHD, treatment with stimulants, problematic temper tantrums, stealing, and fire setting [86]. First-degree relatives of these patients display high rates of substance use and of mood and other impulse-control disorders, including intermittent explosive disorder. Donovan et al reported a successful open trial of the anticonvulsant valproate in adolescents with explosive outbursts, substance abuse, and mood lability [87].

Epilepsy and head trauma are two conditions that have been associated with organic mood disorder, conduct disorder symptoms, and irritability. Behavioral disturbances in children with epilepsy have been described during the prodrome to a seizure, during the seizure, postictally, and even interictally. In adults, prodromal depressive symptoms have been noted in some individuals, whereas irritability has been described during the prodrome of seizures in children. Violence during the seizure has been invoked repeatedly as a legal defense for assorted crimes, but review by a panel of experts of ictal aggressive behavior documented by video–electroencephalogram (EEG) has shown that ictal violence is not purposeful, nor does it involve multistep, planned behaviors. Ictal aggressive behavior is usually associated with obvious confusion, alteration of consciousness, and amnesia for the event. Aggression may also occur during the resolving confusion experienced during the postictal phase. During both the ictal and postictal phases, attempts to restrain the patient may result in thrashing during which the health care provider can be injured [88,89]. A controversial syndrome termed interictal dysphoria characterized by dysthymia, irritability, and mood instability in adult epilepsy patients has not been described in children [90].

Head trauma, particularly when accompanied by objective findings of structural or functional brain abnormalities, is also notoriously associated with a predisposition toward poor impulse control and violent behavior. In some cases, this behavior may be caused by attenuation of the inhibitory role that the frontal lobe and its connections play in modulating behavior.

Suicidal and self-mutilating behaviors

In adolescents and adults, violent or aggressive behavior and depression are associated with a heightened risk of suicidal gestures [91], and adolescents who make multiple suicide attempts are more likely to be aggressive and to have experienced violence themselves. Depression is not always predictive of suicide attempts, however, nor is it always the presenting problem. Serotonin has been found to be reduced in men with violent, impulsive suicidal behaviors but not in those who engage in planned aggression or in suicide alone. Some speculate that there may be two types of suicidal behaviors, one associated with depression and another associated with violent behavior [92,93].

Impulsivity also increases the probability of aggressive or suicidal behavior. Among patients with borderline personality disorder, impulsivity is associated with suicidal behavior, independent of comorbid depression or substance abuse. Two predictors of the number of lifetime suicide attempts found in a study of adults were impulsive aggression in borderline personality disorder and hopelessness in major depressive disorder [94].

Depressed mood and higher levels of anxiety have been described as precursors to suicidal behavior and to self-mutilation [95]. A study by Guertin et al [96] examined the symptoms of adolescents attempting suicide with and without self-mutilating behavior. Carving on the skin and picking at a wound were the most commonly reported self-mutilating behaviors. The group engaged in suicidal and self-mutilating behaviors was significantly more likely than the group engaged in suicidal behaviors alone to be diagnosed with oppositional defiant disorder, major depressive disorder, and dysthymia and had higher scores on measures of hopelessness, loneliness, anger, risk taking, reckless behavior, and alcohol use. Loneliness increased the odds of self-mutilating behavior approximately sixfold. The authors concluded that adolescent suicide attempts with self-mutilating behavior are associated with greater cognitive/ affective and behavioral symptoms.

School shootings and the diagnosis of depression

The recent rash of school shootings may represent one of the most lethal and disturbing aspects of the relationships between mood disorder and violence in childhood and adolescence. In a recent review of characteristics of 34 adolescent mass murderers [97], depressive symptoms and a history of antisocial behaviors were pervasive. Unlike the persons with affective aggression previously described, however, the adolescent mass murderers manifested predatory aggression and did not show sudden or highly emotional warning signs [97]. Most of these adolescents were loners and substance abusers. Nearly half were bullied by others, were preoccupied with violent fantasy, and had a history of aggression. Most of them had made threatening statements to others regarding mass murder, and a number had also made suicidal gestures or later committed suicide.

Clinical assessment of mood and aggression

Disentangling aggressive symptoms from depressive symptoms can present a significant clinical challenge. Even without a concomitant mood disorder, the testy and oppositional nature of many aggressive youngsters makes them a difficult population to engage for evaluation or treatment. An overly formal interview style or excessive reliance on structured inventories may yield denial of symptoms or minimalist responses. In addition to a careful history obtained from parents and siblings, other relatives should be questioned, because immediate family members often minimize the severity of aggression reported. The history should probe for symptoms of depression and bipolar disorder, psychotic symptoms, anxiety in all of its iterations, prior exposure to violence and abuse, the antecedents of aggressive behavior, and triggers that exacerbate or terminate it.

Symptoms suggesting the presence of neurologic or medical conditions such as seizure disorders should be surveyed. Finally, given the developmental aspects of aggression, a baseline cognitive and psychoeducational battery, as well as assessment of executive functions, speech and language, visuospatial processes, and memory and learning, are invaluable in elucidating biologic contributors and concomitants of aggression.

Rating scales that assess children's' general behavior have some usefulness in providing information about symptoms and severity of violent behavior. Almost all standardized child behavior scales have an "aggression" factor, on which load items assessing oppositional behavior and physical aggression. Items on the Connor's scale [98] include "angry and resentful, argues with adults, loses temper, irritable." The Child Behavior Checklist [99] aggression factor includes, among other items, "argues a lot, cruelty/bullying, destroys own or other's property, gets in many fights, physically attacks people." Items such as "boasting, stubborn/sullen/irritable, sudden changes in mood or feelings, talks too much, temper tantrums/hot temper, showing off/clowning," however, also load on the aggression factor, complicating the distinction from mania. Other measures of the severity of aggression that have been used in research in adults include the Overt Aggression Scale [100], the Brown-Goodwin Assessment for Lifetime History of Aggression [31], and the Buss-Durkee Hostility Inventory [101]. Child and adolescent psychiatrists have either adapted adult measures for children [102,103] or have developed their own. The Measure of Aggression, Violence, and Rage in Children (MAVRIC) [104], a 19-item parent and adolescent self-reporting measure, has demonstrated good reliability and validity.

Personality measures such as the Minnesota Multiphasic Personality Inventory (MMPI) and the Millon Adolescent Clinical Inventory are also standardized, have a variety of factors that investigate mood and aggression, and may reveal previously masked emotional disturbances. Like behavior rating scales, they do not necessarily reflect long-term profiles but rather present a snapshot in time. The major problem with rating scales is that they do not easily allow for simple questions such as "How many times during the week does this event/rage/outburst occur?" "How long does it last?" "What starts it?" and "How does it end?"

All the structured and semistructured interviews for children and adolescents assess conduct disorder, oppositional defiant disorder, mania, depression, and anxiety [105]. There are, as well, interviews that examine personality changes caused by neurologic disorders [106]. Rating scales and structured interviews should be used to support rather than replace a thorough clinical interview. For the most part, a clinician is trying to understand the patient, and a diagnosis helps to that end. Standardized measures try to be comprehensive but certainly do not address everything that might be relevant to a specific child. Moreover, because the interviews are based on DSM criteria, and the goal of the criteria is to be as succinct as possible, considerable important detail is not included.

Issues in the psychopharmacologic treatment of mood disorders and aggression

The entangling of aggression and mood complicates treatment, as well as diagnosis, so that it is unclear whether reduced aggressiveness is a direct result of treatment or a byproduct of treating the underlying disorder such as depression. There are no evidence-based treatments for aggressive symptoms in the context of mood disorders. Malone [107] conducted a double-blind, placebo-controlled study of lithium in 86 hospitalized aggressive children and adolescents with conduct disorder. He concluded that lithium is a safe and effective short-term treatment for aggression in inpatients with conduct disorder. Pharmacologic studies of aggression are limited by the difficulty in measuring and differentiating reduction in irritability and mood lability from reduction in actual aggressive behaviors. This dilemma is also evidenced in the pharmacologic treatment of impulse control disorders in which treatment of the primary problem often leads to reduction of hostility and irritability. Aggressiveness with an explosive affective component was more responsive to pharmacologic therapies than aggression alone [108]. Fortunately, serotonergic agents are useful for treating both major depressive disorder and comorbid aggressive behavior problems. Similarly, mood stabilizers and antipsychotic medications decrease aggression, mania, and psychosis [109].

Finding the most effective agents to treat aggression is complicated by several factors. For reasons that vary from the political, to the definitional, to the methodologic, the Food and Drug Administration does not allow aggressive behavior to be directly targeted at this time.

Unlike panic symptoms that can be pharmacologically induced to study the psychotropic usefulness of agents for treating panic attacks, anger cannot be provoked by pharmacologic challenge. The effectiveness of psychotropic agents varies in different animal models of affective aggression [100]. Some agents such as, which can show antiaggressive effects in certain populations (eg, adolescents with ADHD), can precipitate aggressive responses in bipolar patients. The use of methylphenidate was also associated with nausea, vomiting, and urinary frequency in more than half of the subjects.

Currently, no specific antiaggressive drug is available. Instead, a variety of psychotropic agents, including antipsychotics, antidepressants (eg, selective serotonin-reuptake inhibitors [SSRIs]), anticonvulsants, mood stabilizers (eg, lithium), sedative-anxiolytics, and β-blockers are used for their secondary antiaggressive properties.

Because these therapies are directed against the psychiatric conditions that include aggression rather than against aggression itself, it is not surprising that aggressiveness associated with an explosive affective component is believed to respond more vigorously to pharmacotherapy than primary aggression [108]. Although SSRIs are used to treat depression and may reduce associated aggressiveness, SSRIs have not been well demonstrated to be effective in treating primary aggression in children and adolescents. The beneficial effects of SSRIs on aggressive symptoms associated with depression and other psychiatric disorders have not been the focus of most clinical trials of these agents and need further study. Although data to validate the claim that SSRIs can cause violent behavior are limited, this possibility continues to attract abundant media attention and has stirred much controversy [110]. If this reaction does occur, it may reflect vulnerability among a specific subset of depressed patients with severe serotonergic dysregulation leading to violence, murder, and suicide [15].

Lithium has been extensively studied for treatment of unprovoked aggressive outbursts in patients with diverse psychiatric diagnoses. At least six controlled studies have shown benefits of lithium in treating mania and disruptive behavior disorders in younger age groups [108,109,111]. Placebo-controlled studies have demonstrated the effectiveness of lithium in treating conduct disorder and severe aggression [111]. Lithium is most effective against affective or impulsive rather than predatory aggression. A subgroup of patients may be particularly vulnerable to developing cognitive impairment even at low lithium levels [112].

The efficacy of carbamazepine has not been as well demonstrated for these conditions, but potential benefits may have been obscured because trials were conducted in patients with heterogeneous conditions [113]. Concerns about agranulocytosis may also limit the clinical use of carbamazepine. Other drugs that may be useful in treating aggression or rage attacks include amitriptyline [114], clomipramine, desipramine, and clonazepam [115]. Valproic acid is also useful to treat irritability and aggression associated with adult bipolar disorder [116]. Controversies regarding side effects such as polycystic ovaries [117] raise potential concern about its use in adolescent girls.

There are numerous open-label reports of antiepileptic agent mood stabilizers, such as gabapentin [117–120] and lamotrigine [121–123], that have shown efficacy against aggression and agitation in adults, but there are far fewer investigations in children. Valproate, for example, has shown efficacy in treating explosive temper and mood lability in children and adolescents in several open-label trials [124]. The more recently introduced antiepileptic agents gabapentin, tiagabine, topiramate, levatiracetam, and zonisamide are currently being studied in adults and may prove to be helpful in younger populations as well [125,126].

Randomized trials of stimulants provide compelling evidence of significant efficacy in reducing aggression [127]. Because irritability is a concomitant of both mood disturbance and low frustration tolerance, it is relevant that measures of irritability also decline with adequate treatment of ADHD [128]. Given the common comorbidity of depressive symptoms in ADHD, the Texas Medication Algorithm Project [129], a consensus panel of experts, clinicians, administrators, and consumers, has provided a decision tree for managing these comorbidities. There is, however, no evidence base on which these guidelines have relied.

Antipsychotic medications such as risperidone have been studied for use in children with mood disorders and aggressive behavior. Schrier [130,131] conducted a retrospective chart review of 29 children with DSM–IV bipolar disorder and multiple comorbidities treated with risperidone. Significant improvements were seen in the severity of mania, psychosis, and aggression. This study again exemplifies the difficulty in distinguishing the direct effects on aggression from the favorable sequelae to treatment of the underlying disorder.

Anecdotal experience and limited studies suggest the efficacy of a number of agents. Clonidine has been shown to reduce aggression in several trials [132,133], and data from open-label studies of guanefacine are encouraging. The studies, however, are few in number and have some methodologic limitations. Although β-blockers have been exhaustively studied in the treatment of adults with neurologic impairments, these agents have not been adequately studied in the treatment of aggression in children. Anecdotal reports suggest that naltrexone may be helpful in treating self-mutilating adolescents. Benzodiazepines have been used to treat aggression in some adults with long-standing aggression by addressing symptoms of anxiety and irritability. This class of medications is also known to produce paradoxical agitation, however. Effect on mood was not examined. Table 1 summarizes medications that have been used to treat both aggression and mania.

Table 1
Treatments for mania and aggression

Treatment	Aggression	Bipolar disorder
Lithium	X	X
Valproate	X	X
Carbamazepine	X	X
Stimulants	X	A few case reports but not routinely
Neuroleptics	X	X
Atypical neuroleptics	X	X
Antidepressants	X	During the depressive phase
Anxiolytics	Buspirone	Benzodiazepines
β-Blockers	X	
Clonidine, Guanefacine	X	
Calcium channel blockers		X
Electroconvulsive therapy		X
New Antiepileptic	X	X
Drugs (ie, gabapentin, lamotrigine, topiramate, levatiracetam, tiagabine, zonisamide)	Case reports	Case reports and open-label studies in adults
Naltrexone	X	
Serenic compounds	X	
Eltoprazine	(New drug, under study)	

Adapted from G.A. Carlson, personal communication, 2002.

Finally, eltoprazine, a member of a new class of psychoactive agents known as serenic compounds, is currently being studied as a treatment for various forms of impulsive aggression, particularly in developmentally disabled patients [134,135].

Multidimensional treatment interventions

Psychosocial treatments are also essential and should include adaptive anger expression and the reduction of aggressive behavior and hostility. Treatment should facilitate understanding of the affective, physical, and cognitive precursors of aggressive behavior and the use of appropriate skills to de-escalate pending aggressive responses. Training in social skills and parenting skills programs are also believed to be helpful. There are a number of ongoing studies comparing the efficacy of medication, psychosocial treatment, and the combination of the two in young people with mood disorder. One hopes that these studies will also address comorbid conditions.

Violent behavior often requires an emergency room evaluation or a psychiatric hospitalization. Day-treatment programs or partial hospitalization programs can provide alternatives to hospitalization when available. If a parent has an untreated mood disorder, that condition also requires the clinician's attention. The prominence of comorbid conditions such as anxiety and conduct disorders requires that a treatment plan address several different disorders simultaneously for treatment to be successful.

References

[1] Max JE, Castillo CS, Kiele SL, et al. The Neuropsychiatric Rating Schedule: reliability and validity. J Am Acad Child Adolesc Psychiatry 1998;37:297–304.

[2] Knox M, King C, Hanna GL, et al. Aggressive behavior in clinically depressed adolescents. J Am Acad Child Adolesc Psychiatry 2000;39:611–8.

[3] Kashani J, Dahlmeier J, Bourduin C, et al. Characteristics of anger expression in depressed children. J Am Acad Child Adolesc Psychiatry 1995;34:322–6.

[4] Guertin T, Lloyd-Richardon E, Spirito A, et al. Self-mutilative behavior in adolescents who attempt suicide by overdose. J Am Acad Child Adolesc Psychiatry 2001;40:1062–9.

[5] Linnoila M, Virkkunen M, Scheinin M, et al. Low cerebrospinal fluid 5-hydroxyindoleacetic acid concentration differentiates impulsive from nonimpulsive violent behavior [abstract]. Life Sci 1983;33:2609–14.

[6] Cantwell DP, State MW, Voeller KKS. Speech and language disorders. In: Coffey CE, Brumback RA, editors. Textbook of pediatric neuropsychiatry. Washington, DC: American Psychiatric Association Press; 1998. p. 801–19.

[7] McElroy SL. Recognition and treatment of DSM-IV intermittent explosive disorder. J Clin Psychiatry 1999;60(Suppl 15):12–6.

[8] Blumer DP, Davies K. Psychiatric issues in epilepsy surgery. In: Ettinger AB, Kanner AM, editors. Psychiatric issues in epilepsy; a practical guide to diagnosis and management. New York (NY): Lippincott Williams & Wilkins; 2001. p. 231–49.

[9] Connors AK. Connor's Rating Scales-Revised. Toronto, Canada: Multi-Health Systems; 1977.

[10] Dodge KA, Coie JD. Social information processing factors in reactive and proactive aggression in children's peer groups. J Pers Soc Psychol 1987;53:389–409.

[11] Collins JJ, Bailey SL. Relationship of mood disorders to violence. J Nerv Ment Dis 1990;178: 44–7.

[12] Kashani JH, Beack NC, et al. Psychiatric disorders in a community sample of adolescents. Am J Psychiatry 1987;144:584–9.

[13] Lewis DO. The development of the symptom of violence. In: Lewis M, editor. Child and adolescent psychiatry a comprehensive textbook. Baltimore (MD): Williams & Wilkins; 1991. p. 331–40.

[14] Schwartz D, Proctor LJ. Community violence exposure and children's social adjustment in the school peer group: the mediating roles of emotion regulation and social cognition. J of Consult Clinical Psychology 2000;68:670–83.

[15] Cicchetti D, Rogosch R. Equifinality and multifinality in developmental psychopathology. Dev Psychopathol 1996;4:597–600.

[16] Weisbrot DM, Ettinger AB. Epilepsy and behavior: controversies and caveats. The Neurologist 1997;3:155–72.

[17] McCracken JT, Cantwell DP, Hanna GL. Conduct disorder and depression. In: Koplewicz HS, Klass E, editors. Depression in children and adolescents. Philadelphia (PA): Harwood Academic Publishers; 1993. p. 121–32.

[18] Singer M, Anglin RM, Song L, et al. Adolescents' exposure to violence and associated symptoms of psychological trauma. JAMA 1995;273:477–82.

[19] Donovan S, Stewart J, Nunes E, et al. Divalproex treatment for youth with explosive temper and mood lability: a double-blind, placebo-controlled crossover design. Am J Psychiatry 2000; 157:818–20.

[20] World Health Organization ICD-10. Mental and Behavioural Disorders. Geneva, Switzerland: World Health Organization; 1990.

[21] Rohde P, Lewisohn PM, Seley JR. Comorbidity of unipolar depression.II: comorbidity of other mental disorders in adolescents and adults. J Abnorm Psychol 1991;100:214–22.

[22] Dollard J, Doob L, Miller N, et al. Frustration and aggression. New Haven (CT): Yale University Press; 1939.

[23] Garcia-Sellers MJ, Church K. Avoidance, frustration, and hostility during toddlers' interaction with their mothers and fathers. Infant-Toddler Intervention 2000;10:259–74.

[24] Klein RG, Abikoff H, Klass E, et al. Clinical efficacy of methylphenidate in conduct disorder with and without attention deficit hyperactivity disorder. Arch Gen Psychiatry 1997;54: 1073–80.

[25] Knoll J, Stegman K, Suppes T. Clinical experience using gabapentin adjunctively in patients with a history of mania or hypomania. J Affect Disord 1998;49:229–33.

[26] Kashani JH, McNaul JP. Mood disorders in adolescents. In: Wiener JM, editor. Textbook of child and adolescent psychiatry. 2nd edition. Washington, DC: American Psychiatric Association Press; 1997. p. 343–82.

[27] Soloff PH, Lunch KG, Kelly TM, et al. Characteristics of suicide attempts of patients with major depressive episode and borderline personality disorder: a comparative study. Am J Psychiatry 2000;157:601–8.

[28] Bowden CL. Treatment of bipolar disorder. In: Schatzberg AF, Nemeroff CB, editors. Textbook of psychopharmacology. Washington, DC: American Psychiatric Association Press; 1998. p. 431–54.

[29] Arango V, Ernsberger P, Marzuk P, et al. Autoradiographic demonstration of increased serotonin 5–HT2 and beta-adrenergic receptor binding sites in the brain of suicide victims [abstract]. Arch Gen Psychiatry 1990;47:1038–47.

[30] Dunn DW. Attention-deficit hyperactivity disorder, oppositional defiant disorder, and conduct disorder. In: Ettinger AB, Kanner AM, editors. Psychiatric issues in epilepsy; a practical guide to diagnosis and management. New York (NY): Lippincott Williams & Wilkins; 2001. p. 111–26.

[31] Alessi N. Juvenile offenders and affective disorder. Am J Psychiatry 2001;158:146–7.

[32] Buitelaar JK. Open label treatment with resperidone of 26 psychiatrically hospitalized children and adolescents with mixed diagnoses and aggressive behavior. J Child Adolesc Psychopharm 2000;10:19–26.

[33] Kovacs M, Gatsonis C, Paulauskas SL, et al. Depressive disorders in childhood: IV. a longitudinal study of comorbidity with and risk for anxiety disorders. Arch Gen Psychiatry 1989;46:776–82.

[34] Carlson G, Cantwell D. Unmasking masked depression in children and adolescents. Am J Psychiatry 1980;137:445–9.

[35] Civic D, Holt VL. Maternal depressive symptoms and child behavior problems in a nationally-representative normal birthweight sample. Matern Child Health J 2000;4:215–21.

[36] Lion JR. Aggression. In: Kaplan HI, Sadock BJ, editors. Comprehensive textbook of psychiatry, vol 1. Baltimore (MD): Williams and Wilkins; 1995. p. 310–7.

[37] Fava M, Anderson K, Rosenbaum J. "Anger attacks": possible variants of panic and major depressive disorders. Am J Psychiatry 1990;147:867–70.

[38] Harrington R. Epidemiology. Depressive disorder in childhood and adolescence. West Sussex, UK: J Wiley and Sons; 1993. p. 65–83.

[39] Mattes JA. Comparative effectiveness of carbamazepine and propranolol for rage outbursts. J Neuropsychiatry Clin Neurosci 1990;2:159–64.

[40] Davidson RJ, Putnam KM, Larson CL. Dysfunction in the neural circuitry of emotion: a possible prelude to violence. Science 2000;289:591–4.

[41] Carlson GA. Clinical features and pathogenesis of child and adolescent mania. In: Shulman KI, Tohen M, Kutscher SP, editors. Mood disorders across the life span. New York (NY): Wiley-Liss; 1996. p. 127–47.

[42] Jensen PS, Hinshaw SP, Kraemer HC, et al. ADHD comorbity findings from the MTA study: comparing comorbid subgroups. J Am Acad Child Adolesc Psychiatry 2001;40:147–58.

[43] Achenbach TM, Edelbrock CS. Manual for the Child Behavior Checklist and Revised Child Behavior Profile. Burlington (VT): University of Vermont, Department of Psychiatry;1983.

[44] Beitchman JHJ, Brownlie EB, Inglis A, et al. Seven-year follow-up of speech/language impaired and control children: psychiatric outcome. J Child Psychol Psychiatry 1996;37:961–70.

[45] Coie JD, Dodge KA, Terry R, et al. The role of aggression in peer relations: an analysis of aggressive episodes in boys' play groups. Child Dev 1991;62:812–26.

[46] Thase ME. Mood disorders: biology. In: Sadock BJ, Sadock VA, editors. Comprehensive textbook of psychiatry, vol 2. Philadelphia (PA): Lippincott Williams & Wilkins; 2001. p. 1318–27.

[47] Lewis DO, Yeager CA. Diagnostic evaluation of the violent child and adolescent. Child Adolesc Psychiatr Clin North Am 2000;9:815–39.

[48] Lewis DO. From abuse to violence: psychophysiological consequences of maltreatment. J Am Acad Child Adolesc Psychiatry 1992;31:383–91.

[49] Cicchetti D, Ganiban J, Barnett D. Contributions from the study of high-risk populations to understanding the development of emotion regulation. In: Garber J, Dodge KA, editors. The development of emotion regulation and dysregulation. Cambridge (UK): Cambridge University Press; 1991. p. 15–48.

[50] Lewis DO. Neuropsychiatric vulnerabilities and violent juvenile delinquency. Psychiatr Clin North Am 1983;6:707–14.

[51] Kohen D. Eltoprazine for aggression in mental handicap. Lancet 1993;341:628–9.

[52] Rosack J. Called on carpet over violence claims. Psychiatric News 2001;XXVI(19):6–31.

[53] Ghaemi SN, Katzow JJ, Desai SP, et al. Gabapentin treatment of mood disorders: a preliminary study. J Clin Psychiatry 1997;59:426–9.

[54] Swann AC. Treatment of aggression in patients with bipolar disorder. J Clin Psychiatry 1999; 60(Suppl 15):25–8.

[55] Weisbrot DM, Ettinger AB. Psychiatric aspects of pediatric epilepsy. In: Ettinger AB, Kanner AM, editors. Psychiatric issues in epilepsy; a practical guide to diagnosis and management. New York (NY): Lippincott Williams & Wilkins; 2001. p. 127–45.

[56] Coccaro EF, Siever LJ, Klar HM, et al. Serotonergic studies in affective and personality

disorders: correlates with suicidal and impulsive aggressive behavior [abstract]. Arch Gen Psychiatry 1989;46:587–99.

[57] Buss AH, Durkee A. An inventory for assessing different kinds of hostility. J Consult Psychol 1957;21:343–9.

[58] Rutter M, Tizard J, Whitmore K. Education, health and behaviour. London (UK): Longman; 1970.

[59] Shields A, Cicchetti D. Reactive aggression among maltreated children: the contributions of attention and emotion dysregulation. J Clin Child Psychol 1998;27:381–95.

[60] Biederman J, Mick E, Faraone SV, et al. Pediatric mania: a developmental subtype of bipolar disorder? Biol Psychiatry 2000;48:458–66.

[61] Malone RP. A double-blind placebo-controlled study of lithium in hospitalized aggressive children and adolescents with conduct disorder. Arch Gen Psychiatry 2000;57:649–54.

[62] Charles LB, Calabrese JR, McElroy SL, et al. The efficacy of lamotrigine in rapid cycling and non-rapid cycling patients with bipolar disorder. Biol Psychiatry 1999;45:953–8.

[63] Gurvits IG, Koenigsberg HW, Siever LJ. Neurotransmitter dysfunction in patients with borderline personality disorder. Psychiatr Clin North Am 2000;23:27–40.

[64] Fava M. Psychopharmacologic treatment of pathologic aggression. Psychiatr Clin North Am 1997;20:427–51.

[65] Hughes CW, Emslie GJ, Crismon ML, et al. The Texas Children's Medication Algorithm Project: report of the Texas Consensus Conference Panel on Medication Treatment of Childhood Major Depressive Disorder. J Am Acad Child Adolesc Psychiatry 1999;38:1442–54.

[66] Donovan SJ, Susser ES, Nunes EV, et al. Divalproex treatment of disruptive adolescents: a report of 10 cases. J Clin Psychiatry 1997;58:12–5.

[67] Coccaro EF, Kavoussi RJ, Berman ME, et al. Intermittent explosive disorder-revised: development, reliability, and validity of research criteria. Compr Psychiatry 1998;39:368–76.

[68] Weinberg WA, Rutman J, Sullivan L, et al. Depression in children referred to an educational diagnostic center: diagnosis and treatment. J Pediatr 1971;3:1065–72.

[69] Winchel RM, Stanley M. Self-injurious behavior: a review of the behavior and biology of self-mutilation. Am J Psychiatry 1991;148:306–17.

[70] Isojarvi J, Laatikainen TJ, Pakarinen AJ, et al. Polycystic ovaries and hyperandrogenism in women taking valproate for epilepsy. N Engl J Med 1993;329:1383–8.

[71] Shaw SC. Aggression as an adverse drug reaction. Adverse Drug React Toxicol Rev 2000; 19:34–45.

[72] Wozniak J, Biederman J, Kiely K, et al. Mania-like symptoms suggestive of childhood-onset bipolar disorder in clinically referred children. J Am Acad Child Adolesc Psychiatry 1995;34: 867–76.

[73] Walrath CM, Mandell DS, Liao Q, et al. Suicide attempts in the "comprehensive community mental health services for children and their families" program. J Am Acad Child Adolesc Psychiatry 2001;40:1197–205.

[74] Bass JW, Geenens DL, Popper C, et al. Measure of aggression, violence, and rage in children [abstract]. In: Proceedings of the Annual Meeting of the American Academy of Child and Adolescent Psychiatry. San Francisco: American Academy of Child and Adolescent Psychiatry; 1993.

[75] Gabbard GO. Theories of personality and psychopathology: psychoanalysis. In: Kaplan HI, Sadock BJ, editors. Comprehensive textbook of psychiatry, vol 2. Baltimore (MD): Williams and Wilkins; 1995. p. 431–78.

[76] Fleming JE, Offord DR. Epidemiology of childhood depressive disorders: a critical review. J Am Acad Child Adolesc Psychiatry 1990;29:571–80.

[77] David CF, Kistner JA. Do positive self-perceptions have a "dark side"? Examination of the link between perceptual bas and aggression. J Abnorm Child Psychology 2000;28:327–37.

[78] Harrington R: Overlap with other disorders. Depressive disorder in childhood and adolescence. New York (NY): J Wiley and Sons; 1993. p. 84–96.

[79] Coccaro EF, Kavoussi RJ, Hauger RL, et al. Cerebrospinal fluid vasopressin levels correlate

with aggression and serotonin function in personality disordered subjects [abstract]. Arch Gen Psychiatry 1998;55:708–14.

[80] Vitiello B, Stoff DM. Subtypes of aggression and their relevance to child psychiatry. J Am Acad Child Adolesc Psychiatry 1997;36:307–15.

[81] Siassi I. Lithium treatment of impulsive behavior in children. J Clin Psychiatry 1982;43:482–4.

[82] McElroy SL, Soutullo CA, Beckman DA, et al. DSM-IV intermittent explosive disorder: a report of 27 cases. J Clin Psychiatry 1998;59:203–10.

[83] Yeager CA, Lewis DO. Mental illness, neuropsychologic deficits, child abuse, and violence. Child and Adolescent Psychiatry Clinics of North America 2000;9:793–813.

[84] Gjone H, Stevenson J. A longitudinal twin study of temperament and behavior problems: common genetic or environmental influences? J Am Acad Child Adolesc Psychiatry 1997;36:1456–1488.

[85] Eichelman B. Neurochemical and psychopharmacologic aspects of aggressive behavior. In: Meltzer HY, editor. Psychopharmacology: the third generation of progress. New York (NY): Raven Press; 1987. p. 697–704.

[86] Calabrese JR, Fatemi SH, Woyshville MJ. Antidepressant effects of lamotrigine in rapid cycling bipolar disorder [letter]. Am J Psychiatry 1996;153:1236.

[87] Kaplan ML, Erensaft M, Sanderson WC, et al. Dissociative symptomatology and aggressive behavior. Compr Psychiatry 1998;39:271–6.

[88] Calkins SD, Dedmon SE. Physiological and behavioral regulation in two-year-old children with aggressive/destructive behavior problems. J Abnorm Child Psychol 2000;28:103–18.

[89] Campbell M, Gonzalez NM, Silva RR. The pharmacologic treatment of conduct disorders and rage outbursts. Pediatric Psychopharmacology 1992;15:69–85.

[90] Angold A, Costello EJ, Erkanli A. Comorbidity. J Child Psychol Psychiatry 1999;40:57–87.

[91] Chess S, Thomas A. Temperament. In: Lewis M, editor. Child and adolescent psychiatry: a comprehensive textbook. Baltimore (MD): Williams & Wilkins; 1991. p. 145–59.

[92] Chu JA, Dill DL. Dissociative symptoms inrelation to childhood physical and sexual abuse. Am J Psychiatry 1990;147:887–92.

[93] Brown GL, Goodwin FK, Ballenger JC, et al. Aggression in humans: correlates with cerebrospinal fluid amine metabolites. Psych Res 1979;1:131–9.

[94] Berkowitz L. Frustration-aggression hypothesis: examination and reformation. Psychol Bull 1989;106:59–73.

[95] McElroy SL, Soutullo CA, Keck PE, et al. A pilot trial of adjunctive gabapentin in the treatment of bipolar disease. Ann Clin Psychiatry 1997;6:99–103.

[96] Mussen H, Conger JJ, Kagan J. Preschool personality development–hostility and aggression. Child development and personality. New York (NY): Harper and Row; 1974. p. 370–9.

[97] Apter A, Gothelf D, Orbach I, et al. Correlation of suicidal and violent behavior in different diagnostic categories in hospitalized adolescent patients. J Am Acad Child Adolesc Psychiatry 1995;34:912–8.

[98] Schubiner H, Scott R, Tzelepis A. Exposure to violence among intercity youth. J Adolesc Health 1993;14:214–9.

[99] Miller D. Affective disorders and violence in adolescence. Hosp Community Psychiatry 1986; 37:591–5.

[100] Meloy JR, Hempel AG, Mohandie K, et al. Offender and offense characteristics of a nonrandom sample of adolescent mass murderers. J Am Acad Child Adolesc Psychiatry 2001;40:719–28.

[101] Hay DF, Castle J, Davies L. Toddlers' use of force against familiar peers: a precursor of serious aggression? Child Dev 2000;71:457–67.

[102] Lewis DO, Pincus J, Shanok S, et al. Psychomotor epilepsy and violence in a group of incarcerated adolescent boys. Am J Psychiatry 1982;139:882–7.

[103] Silver JM, Yudofsky SC. Violence and the brain. In: Feinberg TE, Farash MJ, editors. Behavioral neurology and neuropsychology. New York: McGraw Hill; 1997, p. 711–17.

[104] Ladd GW, Burgess KB. Charting the relationship trajectories of aggressive, withdrawn and aggressive/withdrawn children during early grade school. Child Dev 1999;70:910–29.

[105] Mammen OK, Pilkonis PA, Kolko DJ. Anger and parent-child aggression in mood and anxiety disorders. Compr Psychiatry 2000;41:461–8.

[106] Coccaro EF, Lawrence T, Trestman RL, et al. Growth hormone responses to intravenous clonidine challenge correlate with behavioral irritability in psychiatric patients and in healthy volunteers [abstract]. Psychiatry Res 1991;39:129–39.

[107] Delga I, Heinssen RK, Fritsch RC, et al. Psychosis, aggression, and self-destructive behavior in hospitalized adolescents. Am J Psychiatry 1989;146:521–5.

[108] Harrington R, Fudge H, Rutter M, et al. Adult outcomes of childhood and adolescent depression: II. links with antisocial disorders. J Am Acad Child Adolesc Psychiatry 1991;30: 434–9.

[109] Pine DS, Cohen E. Therapeutics of aggression in children. Paediatr Drugs 1999;1:183–96.

[110] Geller B, Luby J. Child and adolescent bipolar disorder. a review of the past 10 years. J Am Acad Child Adolesc Psychiatry 1997;36:1168–76.

[111] Bates JE. Concepts and measures of temperament. In: Honstamm GA, Bates JE, Rothbart MK, editors. Temperament in childhood. Chichester (UK): Wiley; 1989. p. 3–26.

[112] Fogelson D, Sternbach H. Lamotrigine treatment of refractory bipolar disorder. J Clin Psychiatry 1997;58:271–3.

[113] Puig-Antich J. Major depression and conduct disorder in prepuberty. J Am Acad Child Adolesc Psychiatry 1982;21:118–28.

[114] Yudofsky SC, Kopecky HJ, Kutnik M, et al. The Overt Agitation Severity Scale for the objective rating of agitation. J Neuropsychiatry Clin Neurosci 1997;9:541–8.

[115] Hirschfeld RM, Shea MT. Mood disorders: psychosocial treatments. In: Kaplan HI, Sadock BJ, editors. Comprehensive textbook of psychiatry, vol 2. Baltimore (MD): Williams and Wilkins; 1995. p. 1178–89.

[116] Engel J. Seizures and Epilepsy, vol 31. 1st edition. Philadelphia (PA): F.A. Davis Co; 1989.

[117] Alessi NE, McManus M, Grapentine WL, et al. The characterization of depressive disorders in serious juvenile offenders. J Affect Disord 1984;6:9–17.

[118] Campbell M, Silva RR, Kafantaris V, et al. Predictors of side effects associated with lithium administration in children. Psychopharmacol Bull 1991;27:373–80.

[119] Quimby LG, Putnam FW. Dissociative symptoms and aggression in a state mental hospital. Dissociation 1994;4:21–4.

[120] Carlson GA, Bromet EJ, Jandorf L. Conduct disorder and mania–what does it mean in adults. J Affect Disorders 1998;148:199–205.

[121] Inamdar SC, Lewis DO, Siomopuoulos G, et al. Violent and suicidal behavior in psychotic adolescents. Am J Psychiatry 1982;139:932–5.

[122] Loeger R, Schmaling KB. Empirical evidence for overt and covert patterns of antisocial conduct problems: a meta-analysis. J Abnorm Child Psychol 1985;13:337–52.

[123] Kazdin AE, Esveldt-Dawson K, Unis A, et al. Child and parent evaluations of depression and aggression in psychiatric inpatient children. J Abnorm Child Psychol 1983;11:401–13.

[124] Carlson GA. Affective disorders in childhood and adolescence-An update. In: Cantwell CG, editor. Bipolar affective disorders in childhood and adolescence. New York (NY): Spectrum Publications; 1983. p. 61–84.

[125] Jaselskis CA, Cook EH, Fletcher KE, et al. Clonidine treatment of hyperactive and impulsive children with autistic disorder. J Clin Psychopharmacol 1992;12:322–7.

[126] Yehuda R. Managing anger and aggression in patients with posttraumatic stress disorder. J Clin Psychiatry 1999;60(Suppl 15):33–7.

[127] Beck AT, Ward CH, Mendelson M, et al. An inventory for measuring depression. Arch Gen Psychiatry 1961;4:561–71.

[128] Lindberg L, Asberg M, Sunquist-Stensman M, et al. 5-hydroxyindoleacetic acid levels in attempted suicides who have killed their children [letter]. Lancet 1984;2:928.

[129] Delini-Stula A, Vassout A. Differential effects of psychoactive drugs on aggressive responses in mice and rats. In: Sandler M, editor. Psychopharmacology of aggession. New York (NY): Raven Press; 1979. p. 41–60.

[130] Ulloa RE, Bermaher B, Axelson D, et al. Psychosis in a pediatric mood and anxiety disorders clinic: phenomenology and correlates. J Am Acad Child Adolesc Psychiatry 2000;39:337–45.
[131] Verhoeven WMA, Tuinier S, Sijben NAS. Eltoprazine in mentally retarded self-injuring patients. Lancet 1992;340:1037–8.
[132] Malone RP, Luebbbert J, Pena-Ariet M, et al. The Overt Aggression Scale in a study of lithium in aggressive conduct disorder. Psychopharmacol Bull 1994;30:215–8.
[133] King RA, Apter A. Psychoanalytic perspectives on adolescent suicide. Psychoanal Study Child 1996;51:491–511.
[134] Frazier JA, Meyer MC, Biederman J, et al. Risperidone treatment for juvenile bipolar disorder: a retrospective chart review. J Am Acad Child Adolesc Psychiatry 1999;38:960–5.
[135] Hunt RD, Ruud MB, Cohen DJ. The therapeutic effect of clonidine in attention deficit disorder with hyperactivity: a comparison with placebo and methylphenidate. Psychopharmacol Bull 1986;22:229–36.

Child Adolesc Psychiatric Clin N Am
11 (2002) 673–683

CHILD AND
ADOLESCENT
PSYCHIATRIC
CLINICS

Index

A

Adolescence
  bipolar disorder in, **461–475**. *See also Bipolar disorder, in adolescence and young adulthood.*
  depression in
    as indication for further episodes of depression, 626–630
    major depressive disorder in childhood and, 622–623

Adult(s)
  depression in
    major depressive disorder in childhood and, 623–625

Affective disorders
  prefrontal–subcortical limbic circuits in, 502–505

Age
  as factor in bipolar disorder, 534–535

Aggression
  bipolar disorder and, 659
  defined, 652
  depressive disorders and, 657–659
  in mood disorders, **651–673**. *See also Mood disorders, aggression and violence in.*
    biologic mechanisms of
      commonalities in, 654
    causes of, 653–657
    clinical assessment of, 662–664
    cognitive influences on, 655
    developmental perspectives on, 656–657
    psychodynamic perspectives on, 654–655
    psychopharmacologic treatment of
      issues in, 664–667
    subtypes of, 652–653

Amitryiptyline
  for depressive illnesses in children and adolescents, 557–558

Anger attacks
  in mood disorders, 660

Anticonvulsant(s)
  for bipolar disorder
    valproate, 604–605

D

Diagnostic Interview Schedule for Children-Version 4 (DISC-IV)
    in bipolar disorder evaluation, 464

E

Early-onset bipolar disorder
    imaging studies of, 507

Early-onset mood disorders
    causes of, **499–518**
    continuity of, 500–501
    familial, 500–501
        comorbidity as subtyping approach to, 501
    functional and structural changes in
        lateralization of, 508
    genetics of, **499–518**
        molecular, 501–502
    heritability of, 511–512
    imaging studies of, 505–507
    MRI imaging of
        cortical differences on
            neuropathology of, 508–509
    prevalence of
        assessment of, 511–512

ECT. *See Electroconvulsive therapy (ECT).*

Electroconvulsive therapy (ECT)
    for bipolar disorder, 610–611
    for depressive illnesses in children and adolescents, 572–573

Emotion(s)
    and mood, 520–522
    regulation of
        and normal development, 522–524
        normal and abnormal
            study of, **519–531**
                applications in childhood-onset bipolar disorder, 528–529
            physiological correlates of, 524–528

F

Fluoxetine
    for depressive illnesses in children and adolescents, 561, 566

Fluvoxamine
    for depressive illnesses in children and adolescents, 567

G

Gabapentin
    for bipolar disorder, 607–608